Third Edition

Gerontological Nursing

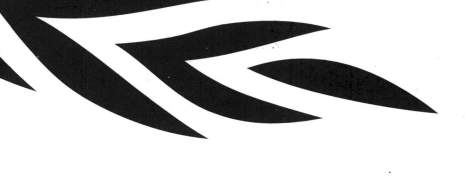

Review and Resource Manual

CONTINUING EDUCATION SOURCE
NURSING CERTIFICATION REVIEW MANUAL
CLINICAL PRACTICE RESOURCE

Patricia A. Tabloski, PhD, GNP-BC, FAAN, FGSA

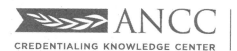

ANCC
CREDENTIALING KNOWLEDGE CENTER

Conferences.
Consultation.
Education.

8/13
MATT.
a 99.00

Library of Congress Cataloging-in-Publication Data

Tabloski, Patricia A.
 Gerontological nursing : review and resource manual. – 3rd ed. / by Patricia Tabloski.
    p. ; cm.
 Rev. ed. of: Gerontological nursing. 2nd ed. 2009.
 Includes bibliographical references and index.
 ISBN 9781935213291
 I. American Nurses Credentialing Center. Institute for Credentialing Innovation. II. Gerontological nursing. III. Title.
 [DNLM: 1. Geriatric Nursing–methods–Outlines. 2. Education, Nursing, Continuing–Outlines. WY 18.2]

 618.97′0231–dc23
                        2012044563

The American Nurses Credentialing Center (ANCC), a subsidiary of the American Nurses Association (ANA), provides individuals and organizations throughout the nursing profession with the resources they need to achieve practice excellence. ANCC's internationally renowned credentialing programs certify nurses in specialty practice areas; recognize healthcare organizations for promoting safe, positive work environments through the Magnet Recognition Program® and the Pathway to Excellence® Program; and accredit providers of continuing nursing education. In addition, ANCC's Institute for Credentialing Innovation provides leading-edge information and education services and products to support its core credentialing programs.

ISBN 13: 9781935213291

GERONTOLOGICAL NURSING REVIEW AND RESOURCE MANUAL, 3RD EDITION

DECEMBER 2012

Please direct your comments and/or queries to: revmanuals@ana.org

The healthcare services delivery system is a volatile marketplace demanding superior knowledge, clinical skills, and competencies from all registered nurses. Nursing autonomy of practice and nurse career marketability and mobility in the new century hinge on affirming the profession's formative philosophy, which places a priority on a lifelong commitment to the principles of education and professional development. The knowledge base of nursing theory and practice is expanding, and while care has been taken to ensure the accuracy and timeliness of the information presented in the **Gerontological Nursing Review and Resource Manual,** clinicians are advised to always verify the most current national guidelines and recommendations and to practice in accordance with professional standards of care used with regard to the unique circumstances that apply in each practice situation. In addition, every effort has been made in this text to ensure accuracy and, in particular, to confirm that drug selections and dosages are in accordance with current recommendations and practice, including the ongoing research, changes to government regulations, and the developments in product information provided by pharmaceutical manufacturers. However, it is the responsibility of each nurse practitioner to verify drug product information and to practice in accordance with professional standards of care. In addition, the editors wish to note that provision of information in this text does not imply an endorsement of any particular products, procedures or services.

Therefore, the authors, editors, American Nurses Association (ANA), American Nurses Association's Publishing (ANP), American Nurses Credentialing Center (ANCC), and the Institute for Credentialing Innovation cannot accept responsibility for errors or omissions, or for any consequences or liability, injury, and/or damages to persons or property from application of the information in this manual and make no warranty, express or implied, with respect to the contents of the **Gerontological Nursing Review and Resource Manual.** Completion of this manual does not guarantee that the reader will pass the certification exam. The practice examination questions are not a requirement to take a certification examination. The practice examination questions cannot be used as an indicator of results on the actual certification.

PUBLISHED BY

American Nurses Credentialing Center
The Institute for Credentialing Innovation
8515 Georgia Avenue, Suite 400
Silver Spring, MD 20910-3402
www.nursecredentialing.org

INTRODUCTION TO THE CONTINUING EDUCATION (CE) CONTACT HOUR APPLICATION PROCESS FOR *GERONTOLOGICAL NURSING REVIEW AND RESOURCE MANUAL, 3RD EDITION*

The Credentialing Knowledge Center now offers the continuing education contact hours for this manual online at www.NursingWorld.org, the American Nurses Association's Web site. This process involves answering approximately 25–30 questions that test knowledge of the information contained within this manual. The continuing education contact hours can be completed at any time and a certificate can be printed from the Web site immediately upon successful completion of the test.

After studying the manual and given an online multiple-choice test, the exam candidate will be able to:

1. Pass the posttest with at least 75% of the answers correct.

2. Select responses to test questions based on key principles, standards of practice, and theoretical basis of nursing practice.

3. Choose accepted therapeutic interventions in answering questions related to quality nursing practice.

4. Utilize direct and indirect professional role responsibilities and applications regarding nursing practice in answering test questions.

Upon completion of this manual *and* the online CE test, a nurse can receive a total of 26 continuing education contact hours at a price of $52, only $2 per CE. (ANA members receive a discount on CEs.) **The entire process—online test and evaluation form—must be completed by December 31, 2014 in order to receive credit.** To begin the process, please e-mail **revmanuals@ana.org**. Your patience with this process is greatly appreciated.

Inquiries or Comments

If you have any questions about the CE contact hours, please e-mail the Credentialing Knowledge Center at revmanuals@ana.org. You may also mail any comments to Editor/Project Manager, at the address listed below.

Duplicate CE Certificates

Once you have successfully passed the CE test, you may go back and re-print your certificate as often as you wish.

Conflicts of Interest

A conflict of interest occurs when an individual has an opportunity to affect educational content about health-care products or services of a commercial company with which she/he has a financial relationship.

The planners and presenters of this CNE activity have disclosed no relevant financial relationships with any commercial companies pertaining to this activity.

Credentialing Knowledge Center
American Nurses Credentialing Center
Attn: Editorial Project Manager
8515 Georgia Avenue, Suite 400
Silver Spring, MD 20910-3492
Fax: (301) 628-5342

A maximum of 26 contact hours may be earned by learners who successfully complete this continuing nursing education activity.

ANA's Center for Continuing Education and Professional Development is accredited as a provider of continuing nursing education by the American Nurses Credentialing Center's Commission on Accreditation.

ANCC Provider Number 0023.

ANA's Center for Continuing Education and Professional Development is approved by the California Board of Registered Nursing, Provider Number CEP6178 for 31.2 contact hours.

The ANA Center for Continuing Education and Professional Development includes ANCC's Credentialing Knowledge Center.

ACKNOWLEDGEMENTS

The author gratefully acknowledges the foundational work provided by Paula Gillman, MSN, RN, ANP-BC, GNP-BC, and Patti Parker, MSN, APRN, CNS, ANP-BC, GNP-BC, on the previous edition of this manual.

CONTENTS

TAKING THE CERTIFICATION EXAMINATION

When you sign up to take a national certification exam, you will be instructed to go online and review the testing and renewal handbook (www.nursecredentialing.org/documents/certification/application/generaltestingandrenewalhandbook.aspx). Review it carefully and be sure to bookmark the site so you can refer to it frequently. It contains information on test content and sample questions. This is critical information; it will give you insight into the nature of the test. The agency will send you information about the test site; keep this in a safe place until needed.

GENERAL SUGGESTIONS FOR PREPARING FOR THE EXAM

Step One: Control Your Anxiety

Everyone experiences anxiety when faced with taking the certification exam.

- ► Remember, your program was designed to prepare you to take this exam.
- ► Your instructors took a similar exam, and have probably talked to students who took exams more recently, so they know how to help you prepare.
- ► Taking a review course or setting up your own study plan will help you feel more confident about taking the exam.

Step Two: Do Not Listen to Gossip About the Exam

A large volume of information exists about the tests based on reports from people who have taken the exams in the past. Because information from the testing facilities is limited, it is hard to ignore this gossip.

► Remember that gossip about the exam that you hear from others is not verifiable.

► Because this gossip is based on the imperfect memory of people in a stressful situation, it may not be very accurate.

► People tend to remember those items testing content with which they are less comfortable; for instance, those with a limited background in women's health may say that the exam was "all women's health." In fact, the exam blueprint ensures that the exam covers multiple content areas without overemphasizing any one.

Step Three: Set Reasonable Expectations for Yourself

► Do not expect to know everything.

► Do not try to know everything in great detail.

► You do not need a perfect score to pass the exam.

► Learn the general rules, not the exceptions.

► The most likely diagnoses will be on the exam, not questions on rare diseases or atypical cases.

► Think about the most likely presentation and most common therapy.

Step Four: Prepare Mentally and Physically

► While you are getting ready to take the exam, take good physical care of yourself.

► Get plenty of sleep and exercise, and eat well while preparing for the exam.

► These things are especially important while you are studying and immediately before you take the exam.

Step Five: Access Current Knowledge

General Content
You will be given a list of general topics that will be on the exam when you register to take the exam. In addition, examine the table of contents of this book and the test content outline, available at www.nursecredentialing.org/cert/TCOs.html.

▶ What content do you need to know?

▶ How well do you know these subjects?

Take a Review Course

▶ Taking a review course is an excellent way to assess your knowledge of the content that will be included in the exam.

▶ If you plan to take a review course, take it well before the exam so you will have plenty of time to master any areas of weakness the course uncovers.

▶ If you are prepared for the exam, you will not hear anything new in the course. You will be familiar with everything that is taught.

▶ If some topics in the review course are new to you, concentrate on these in your studies.

▶ People have a tendency to study what they know; it is rewarding to study something and feel a mastery of it! Unfortunately, this will not help you master unfamiliar content. Be sure to use a review course to identify your areas of strength and weakness, then concentrate on the weaknesses.

Depth of Knowledge

▶ How much do you need to know about a subject?

▶ You cannot know everything about a topic.

▶ Study the information sent to you from the testing agency, what you were taught in school, what is covered in this text, and the general guidelines given in this chapter.

▶ Look at practice tests designed for the exam. Practice tests for other exams will not be helpful.

▶ Consult your class notes or clinical diagnosis and management textbook for the major points about a disease. Additional reference books can be found online at www.nursecredentialing.org/cert/refs.html.

▶ For example, with regard to medications, know the drug categories and the major medications in each. Assume all drugs in a category are generally alike, and then focus on the differences among common drugs. Know the most important indications, contraindications, and side effects. Emphasize safety. The questions usually do not require you to know the exact dosage of a drug.

Step Six: Institute a Systematic Study Plan

Develop Your Study Plan

▶ Write up a formal plan of study.

 » Include topics for study, timetable, resources, and methods of study that work for you.

 » Decide whether you want to organize a study group or work alone.

 » Schedule regular times to study.

 » Avoid cramming; it is counterproductive. Try to schedule your study periods in 1-hour increments.

▶ Identify resources to use for studying. To prepare for the examination, you should have the following materials on your shelf:

 » A good pathophysiology text.

 » This review book.

 » A physical assessment text.

 » Your class notes.

 » Other important sources, including: information from the testing facility, a clinical diagnosis textbook, favorite journal articles, notes from a review course, and practice tests.

 » Know the important national standards of care for major illnesses.

 » Consult the bibliography on the test blueprint. When studying less familiar material, it is helpful to study using the same references that the testing center uses.

▶ Study the body systems from head to toe.

▶ The exams emphasize health promotion, assessment, differential diagnosis, and plan of care for common problems.

▶ You will need to know facts and be able to interpret and analyze this information utilizing critical thinking.

Personalize Your Study Plan

▶ How do you learn best?

 » If you learn best by listening or talking, attend a review course or discuss topics with a colleague.

▶ Read everything the test facility sends you as soon as you receive it and several times during your preparation period. It will give you valuable information to help guide your study.

▶ Have a specific place with good lighting set aside for studying. Find a quiet place with no distractions. Assemble your study materials.

Implement Your Study Plan

You must have basic content knowledge. In addition, you must be able to use this information to think critically and make decisions based on facts.

- ▶ Refer to your study plan regularly.
- ▶ Stick to your schedule.
- ▶ Take breaks when you get tired.
- ▶ If you start procrastinating, get help from a friend or reorganize your study plan.
- ▶ It is not necessary to follow your plan rigidly. Adjust as you learn where you need to spend more time.
- ▶ Memorize the basics of the content areas you will be required to know.

Focus on General Material

- ▶ Most of what you need to know is basic material that does not require constant updating.
- ▶ You do not need to worry about the latest information being published as you are studying for the exam. Remember, it can take 6 to 12 months for new information to be incorporated into test questions.

Pace Your Studying

- ▶ Stop studying for the examination when you are starting to feel overwhelmed and look at what is bothering you. Then make changes.
- ▶ Break overwhelming tasks into smaller tasks that you know you can do.
- ▶ Stop and take breaks while studying.

Work With Others

- ▶ Talk with classmates about your preparation for the exam.
- ▶ Keep in touch with classmates, and help each other stick to your study plans.
- ▶ If your classmates become anxious, do not let their anxiety affect you. Walk away if you need to.
- ▶ Do not believe bad stories you hear about other people's experiences with previous exams.
- ▶ Remember, you know as much as anyone about what will be on the next exam!

Consider a Study Group

- ▶ Study groups can provide practice in analyzing cases, interpreting questions, and critical thinking.
  - » You can discuss a topic and take turns presenting cases for the group to analyze.
  - » Study groups can also provide moral support and help you continue studying.

Step Seven: Strategies Immediately Before the Exam

Final Preparation Suggestions

▶ Use practice exams when studying to get accustomed to the exam format and time restrictions.

  ▹ Many books that are labeled as review books are simply a collection of examination questions.

  ▹ If you have test anxiety, such practice tests may help alleviate the anxiety.

  ▹ Practice tests can help you learn to judge the time it should take you to complete the exam.

  ▹ Practice tests are useful for gaining experience in analyzing questions.

  ▹ Books of questions may not uncover the gaps in your knowledge that a more systematic content review text will reveal.

  ▹ If you feel that you don't know enough about a topic, refer to a text to learn more. After you feel that you have learned the topic, practice questions are a wonderful tool to help improve your test-taking skill.

▶ Know your test-taking style.

  ▹ Do you rush through the exam without reading the questions thoroughly?

  ▹ Do you get stuck and dwell on a question for a long time?

  ▹ You should spend about 45 to 60 seconds per question and finish with time to review the questions you were not sure about.

  ▹ Be sure to read the question completely, including all four answer choices. Choice "a" may be good, but "d" may be best.

The Night Before the Exam

▶ Be prepared to get to the exam on time.

  ▹ Know the test site location and how long it takes to get there.

  ▹ Take a "dry run" beforehand to make sure you know how to get to the testing site, if necessary.

  ▹ Get a good night's sleep.

  ▹ Eat sensibly.

  ▹ Avoid alcohol the night before.

  ▹ Assemble the required material—two forms of identification and watch. Both IDs must match the name on the application, and one photo ID is preferred.

  ▹ Know the exam room rules.

    ▹ You will be given scratch paper, which will be collected at the end of the exam.

    ▹ Nothing else is allowed in the exam room.

    ▹ You will be required to put papers, backpacks, etc., in a corner of the room or in a locker.

▷ No water or food will be allowed.

▷ You will be allowed to walk to a water fountain and go to the bathroom one at a time.

The Day of the Exam

▶ Get there early. You must arrive to the test center at least 15 minutes before your scheduled appointment time. If you are late, you may not be admitted.

▶ Think positively. You have studied hard and are well-prepared.

▶ Remember your anxiety reduction strategies.

Specific Tips for Dealing With Anxiety

Test anxiety is a specific type of anxiety. Symptoms include upset stomach, sweaty palms, tachycardia, trouble concentrating, and a feeling of dread. But there are ways to cope with test anxiety.

▶ There is no substitute for being well-prepared.

▶ Practice relaxation techniques.

▶ Avoid alcohol, excess coffee, caffeine, and any new medications that might sedate you, dull your senses, or make you feel agitated.

▶ Take a few deep breaths and concentrate on the task at hand.

Focus on Specific Test-Taking Skills

To do well on the exam, you need good test-taking skills in addition to knowledge of the content and ability to use critical thinking.

All Certification Exams Are Multiple Choice

▶ Multiple-choice tests have specific rules for test construction.

▶ A multiple-choice question consists of three parts: the information (or stem), the question, and the four possible answers (one correct and three distracters).

▶ Careful analysis of each part is necessary. Read the entire question before answering.

▶ Practice your test-taking skills by analyzing the practice questions in this book and on the ANCC Web site.

Analyze the Information Given

▶ Do not assume you have more information than is given.

▶ Do not overanalyze.

▶ Remember, the writer of the question assumes this is all of the information needed to answer the question.

▶ If information is not given, it is not relevant and will not affect the answer.

▶ Do not make the question more complicated than it is.

What Kind of Question Is Asked?

▶ Are you supposed to recall a fact, apply facts to a situation, or understand and differentiate between options?

  ▻ Read the question thinking about what the writer is asking.

  ▻ Look for key words or phrases that lead you (see Figure 1–1). These help determine what kind of answer the question requires.

FIGURE 1–1.
EXAMPLES OF KEY WORDS AND PHRASES

▶ avoid	▶ initial	▶ most
▶ best	▶ first	▶ significant
▶ except	▶ contributing to	▶ likely
▶ not	▶ appropriate	▶ of the following
		▶ most consistent with

Read All of the Answers

▶ If you are absolutely certain that answer "a" is correct as you read it, mark it, but read the rest of the question so you do not trick yourself into missing a better answer.

▶ If you are absolutely sure answer "a" is wrong, cross it off or make a note on your scratch paper and continue reading the question.

▶ After reading the entire question, go back, analyze the question, and select the best answer.

▶ Do not jump ahead.

▶ If the question asks you for an assessment, the best answer will be an assessment. Do not be distracted by an intervention that sounds appropriate.

▶ If the question asks you for an intervention, do not answer with an assessment.

▶ When two answer choices sound very good, the best one is usually the least expensive, least invasive way to achieve the goal. For example, if your answer choices include a physical exam maneuver or imaging, the physical exam maneuver is probably the better choice provided it will give the information needed.

▶ If the answers include two options that are the opposite of each other, one of the two is probably the correct answer.

▶ When numeric answers cover a wide range, a number in the middle is more likely to be correct.

▶ Watch out for distracters that are correct but do not answer the question, combine true and false information, or contain a word or phrase that is similar to the correct answer.

▶ Err on the side of caution.

Only One Answer Can Be Correct

▶ When more than one suggested answer is correct, you must identify the one that best answers the question asked.

▶ If you cannot choose between two answers, you have a 50% chance of getting it right if you guess.

Avoid Changing Answers

▶ Change an answer only if you have a compelling reason, such as you remembered something additional, or you understand the question better after rereading it.

▶ People change to a wrong answer more often than to a right answer.

Time Yourself to Complete the Whole Exam

▶ Do not spend a large amount of time on one question.

▶ If you cannot answer a question quickly, mark it and continue the exam.

▶ If time is left at the end, return to the difficult questions.

▶ Make educated guesses by eliminating the obviously wrong answers and choosing a likely answer even if you are not certain.

▶ Trust your instinct.

▶ Answer every question. There is no penalty for a wrong answer.

▶ Occasionally a question will remind you of something that helps you with a question earlier in the test. Look back at that question to see if what you are remembering affects how you would answer that question.

ABOUT THE CERTIFICATION EXAMS

The American Nurses Credentialing Center Computerized Exam

The ANCC examination is given only as a computer exam, and each exam is different.

The order of the questions is scrambled for every test, so even if two people are taking the same exam, the questions will be in a different order. The exam consists of 175 multiple-choice questions.

- ▶ 150 of the 175 questions are part of the test and how you answer will count toward your score; 25 are included to refine questions and will not be scored. You will not know which ones count, so treat all questions the same.

- ▶ You will need to know how to use a mouse, scroll by either clicking arrows on the scroll bar or using the up and down arrow keys, and perform other basic computer tasks.

- ▶ The exam does not require computer expertise.

- ▶ However, if you are not comfortable with using a computer, you should practice using a mouse and computer beforehand so you do not waste time on the mechanics of using the computer.

Know What to Expect During the Test

- ▶ Each ANCC test question is independent of the other questions.

  - ▹ For each case study, there is only one question. This means that a correct answer on any question does not depend on the correct answer to any other question.

  - ▹ Each question has four possible answers. There are no questions asking for combinations of correct answers (such as "a and c") or multiple-multiples.

- ▶ You can skip a question and go back to it at the end of the exam.

- ▶ You cannot mark key words in the question or right or wrong answers. If you want to do this, use the scratch paper.

- ▶ You will get your results immediately, and a grade report will be provided upon leaving the testing site.

Internet Resources

- ▶ ANCC Web site: www.nursecredentialing.org

- ▶ ANA Bookstore: www.nursesbooks.org. Catalog of ANA nursing scope and standards publications and other titles that may be listed on your test content outline

- ▶ National Guideline Clearinghouse: www.ngc.gov

THE OLDER ADULT

Older adults constitute a heterogeneous population with varying needs. Chronological age is a constant for older individuals; however, functional age varies. This chapter discusses the past and projected demographic trends of aging in the United States (see Figure 2–1).

GENERAL PROFILE OF OLDER ADULTS

According to the U.S. Administration on Aging (AoA, 2011), currently there are almost 40.4 million Americans age 65 years or older, an increase of almost 15% since 2000. Approximately 13% (about 1 in 8) of all Americans are older than 65. This number will grow to more than 71 million (20% of all Americans) by the year 2030, and to 80 million by 2050. Decreases in infant and young adult mortality contribute to longevity, but death rates for older adults have also decreased in the past two decades. From 2009 to 2010, the death rate for older people age 65 to 74 decreased by 0.8%, and by 0.7% for those age 75 to 84, while it increased by 1.9% in those over the age of 85. These numbers reinforce the prediction that people reaching the age of 65 have an increased life expectancy of an average additional 18 years (20.0 years for women and 17.3 years for men).

From 2009 to 2010, age-adjusted death rates decreased significantly for 7 of the 15 leading causes of death, including:

- ▶ Diseases of the heart
- ▶ Malignant neoplasms
- ▶ Chronic lower respiratory diseases
- ▶ Cerebrovascular diseases
- ▶ Accidents (unintentional injuries)
- ▶ Influenza and pneumonia
- ▶ Septicemia

Assault (homicide) fell from among the top 15 leading causes of death in 2010, replaced by pneumonia due to aspiration.

The age-adjusted death rate increased for five leading causes of death, including:

▶ Alzheimer's disease

▶ Nephritis, nephrotic syndrome, and nephrosis

▶ Chronic liver disease and cirrhosis

▶ Parkinson's disease

▶ Pneumonia due to aspiration

Other important trends and expectations include the following:

▶ The 85+ population is projected to increase from 5.5 million in 2010 to 6.6. million by 2020, making the oldest old the fastest-growing segment of the older adult population.

▶ A child born in 2011 can expect to live 78.7 years, or 31 years longer than a child born in 1900.

▶ People older than age 85—more than 4 million Americans, and the fastest-growing age group—are most likely to have chronic care needs. This number is expected to surpass 9 million by 2030 and be more than 20 million by 2050.

▶ Racial and ethnic minority populations have increased from 5.7 million in 2000 (16.3% of the older adult population) to 8.1 million in 2010 (20% of the older adult population) and are projected to increase to 13.1 million in 2020 (24% of the older adult population).

▶ Older women outnumber older men at 23.0 million to 17.5 million.

▶ Older men are much more likely to be married than older women; 72% of men are married, as opposed to 42% of women, while 40% of older women are widows.

▶ Older adults are often divided into groups: *young-old*, 65–75 years; *middle-old*, 75–84 years; *old-old*, 85 plus; and *elite-old*, or centenarians (see Figure 2–1).

▶ Almost 15.9% of older adults were below the poverty level as a result of out-of-pocket medical expenses in 2011.

▶ In 2011, the first of the baby boom generation reached what used to be known as retirement age. For the next 18 years, boomers will turn 65 at a rate of about 8,000 a day (AoA, 2011).

FIGURE 2-1.
OLDER AMERICAN POPULATION BY AGE: 1900-2050

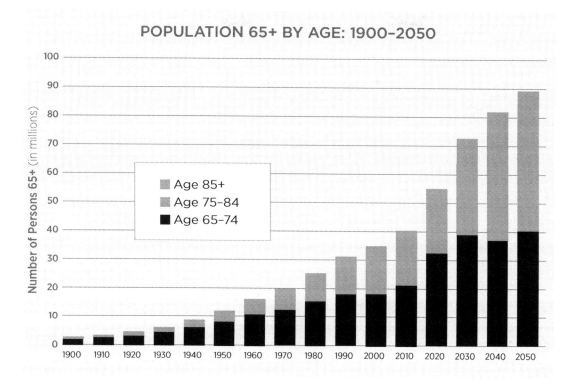

Adapted from "Projected Future Growth of the Older Population," U.S. Administration on Aging, 2011, http://www.aoa.gov/AoARoot/Aging_Statistics/future_growth/future_growth.aspx#age

OLDER ADULTS WHO ARE MEMBERS OF A MINORITY GROUP

Currently, minority older adults make up more than 20% of the older population in the United States. Between 2010 and 2050, it is projected that 77% of older Americans will be White, down from 87% in 2010. Within the same age group, 12% are projected to be Black (up from 9% in 2010), and 9% are projected to be Asian (up 3% from 2010 levels; AoA, 2011).

WHERE OLDER AMERICANS LIVE

According to AoA data (2011), of the 24 million households headed by older people in 2010, 77% were owners and 21% were renters. The median family income in 2010 was $25,704 for men and $15,072 for women. Households containing families headed by people over the age of 65 reported a median income of $45,763. Social Security constituted 90% or more of the income received by 35% of beneficiaries (22% of married couples and 45% of nonmarried beneficiaries). About 29% of older people residing in the community live alone (8.1 million women and 3.2 million men). The proportion of older people living alone increases with advancing age, especially for women, with 47% of women over the age of 75 living alone (AoA, 2011).

About 485,000 grandparents age 65 or over maintain households in which grandchildren are present (AoA, 2011). Relatively few adults age 65 or older live in nursing homes (about 1.25 million, or 3.1% of older Americans), occupying about 85% of the 1.7 million nursing home beds; the number of persons over the age of 85 living in nursing homes is 14% those in that age group. From 2002 to 2007, the numbers of persons over the age of 85 increased by 6.5%, while the number of nursing home beds increased by 1.7%, and nursing home occupancy rates increased only slightly, by 0.9% (AARP, 2009). The decreased rate of nursing home usage is reflective of the increase in healthcare options for older adults, including home care services, adult day care, assisted living, and other options to delay or prevent nursing home placement. Table 2–1 illustrates the rates of residence in skilled nursing facilities (SNFs) by age.

TABLE 2-1.
POPULATION 65 YEARS AND OLDER IN SKILLED NURSING FACILITIES

GENDER AND AGE	TOTAL POPULATION	IN SNFS - NUMBER	IN SNFS - PERCENT
Both genders, all ages	308,745,538	1,502,264	0.5%
Total, age 65 & older	40,267,984	1,252,635	3.1%
65–74 years	21,713,429	197,310	0.9%
75–84 years	13,061,122	420,790	3.2%
85–94 years	5,068,825	529,689	10.4%
95–99 years	371,244	87,621	23.6%
100 years & over	53,364	17,225	32.3%

Adapted from *The Older Population: 2010–2010 Census Briefs* (p. 18), by C. A. Werner, 2011, Washington, DC: U.S. Census Bureau. Available at http://www.census.gov/prod/cen2010/briefs/c2010br-09.pdf

Geographically, compared with other states, Florida had the greatest share of the population age 65 and older in both 2000 and 2010 (17.6% and 17.3%, respectively), followed by West Virginia (16.0%), Maine (15.9%), Pennsylvania (15.4%), and Iowa (14.9%). The state with the lowest share of the population age 65 and older was Alaska in both 2000 and 2010 (5.7% and 7.7%, respectively). Alaska also exhibited the largest growth rate for the 65-and-over population, which grew from 35,699 in 2000 to 54,938 in 2010, representing a 53.9% increase in the number of older persons (U.S. Census Bureau, 2011).

The state or area of residence greatly affects older adults' access to health care and social services. Metropolitan areas generally offer more options for medical treatment. Those states in which a greater proportion of the population is over 65 usually provide a larger variety of services for older adults. Proximity of neighbors and other caregivers is also affected by location of residence. Many older persons relocate to be nearer to family, especially after the death of a spouse.

MARITAL STATUS

In 2010, older men were much more likely to be married than older women—72% of men, compared to 42% of women. Widows accounted for 40% of all older women in 2010. There were more than four times as many widows (8.7 million) as widowers (2.1 million; AoA, 2011).

Divorced and separated (including married with spouse absent) older adults represented only 12.4% of all older persons in 2010. However, this percentage has increased since 1980, when approximately 5.3% of the older population were divorced, separated, or married with spouse absent (AoA, 2012; see Figure 2–2). Seniors living alone are at greater risk for adverse events, institutionalization, and poor health outcomes. Children and extended family or informal caregivers are needed to assist many older persons who lose the ability to care for themselves and do not have a spouse or significant other.

More than half (54.8%) of the older persons residing in the community lived with a spouse in 2009. Approximately 11.4 million, or 72.0%, of older men, and 8.7 million, or 40.7%, of older women lived with a spouse (Figure 2–2). The proportion living with a spouse decreased with age, especially for women. Only 28.2% of women 75+ years old lived with a spouse (AoA, 2011).

FIGURE 2–2.
MARITAL STATUS OF OLDER AMERICANS, 2009

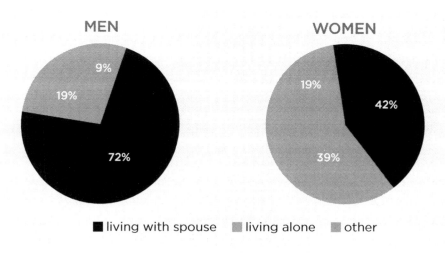

Based on data from U.S. Census Bureau, including the *2009 Current Population Survey, Annual Social and Economic Supplement* and the *2009 American Community Survey*, by U.S. Administration on Aging, 2011. See: *A Profile of Older Americans, 2010*, Administration on Aging, 2011. Available at http://www.aoa.gov/aoaroot/aging_statistics/Profile/2010/6.aspx

FINANCIAL STATUS

Adequate financial resources are essential to provide for housing, nutrition, and health care. Almost 3.5 million older adults (9.0%) were below the poverty level in 2010. This poverty rate is not statistically different from the poverty rate in 2009 (8.9%). Another 2.3 million, or 5.8% of older adults, were classified as "near-poor" (income between the poverty level and 125% of this level).

PHYSICAL CHANGES OF AGING

Each system of the body is affected by aging. Most of these changes are progressive and gradual, beginning sometimes as early as the 20s and 30s. There is a growing understanding of what constitutes normal aging changes and what is the result of disease. Normal aging consists of changes that occur in all older people.

Skin, Hair, and Nails

Many of the skin changes of aging result from loss of elasticity and subcutaneous tissue, coupled with sun damage. In general, skin appears thinner and more transparent (especially in light-skinned persons). Areas of increased or decreased pigmentation are common. The skin is drier, especially on the extremities, and can have a scaly appearance. Wrinkling is evident, and skin "tenting" over the extremities is common because of the loss of subcutaneous fat. As a result, skin turgor is not a reliable indicator of hydration status in older adults. If used at all, testing of turgor on the abdomen or chest wall, under the clavicles, or on the inner thigh is recommended, rather than on the forearm or sternum, as is done in younger adults (ConsultGeriRn.org, 2005).

Various types of skin lesions are common in older adults. Many are the result of sun damage accumulated through the years. Benign conditions include seborrheic keratoses, skin tags, senile lentigines, cutaneous horns, and cherry angiomas. The incidence of premalignant and malignant lesions is also higher, especially in light-skinned people. These lesions include actinic keratoses, basal cell carcinomas, squamous cell carcinomas, and malignant melanomas. Table 2–2 details characteristics of these lesions.

Skin changes, coupled with decreased circulation, increase the risk of pressure ulcer development in frail older adults who are immobile. Persons who are malnourished and diagnosed with multiple comorbidities are at even greater risk. Assessment of bony prominences and areas of pressure is critical, including the heels, sacrum, elbows, scapulae, back of the head, and ears.

Age-related changes in hair and nails also may be seen. Melanocytes stop functioning, which leads to graying of hair; hair also becomes thinner and drier. As they age, both men and women tend to develop more coarse hair on the face, ears, nose, and eyebrows. Symmetrical balding (male pattern baldness) is common in men. Fingernails and toenails generally thicken and become less transparent.

TABLE 2-2.
BENIGN AND MALIGNANT SKIN LESIONS COMMON IN OLDER PERSONS

BENIGN LESION	DESCRIPTION
Seborrheic keratosis	Raised, pigmented, warty lesions with a "stuck-on" appearance; often called "barnacles"
Acrochordon (skin tag)	Raised tag of skin occurring in areas of high friction, connected by a narrow stalk (pedunculated)
Senile lentigines (age spots)	Irregular pigmented lesions with a rough surface; occur in sun-exposed areas
Cutaneous horn	Small projection that is hard and arises from epidermis; common on face
Cherry angioma	Tiny cherry-red papule that is made up of blood vessels

MALIGNANT LESION	DESCRIPTION
Actinic keratosis	Small crusty or scaly area, same color as or different color than skin; often recognized by touch
Basal cell carcinoma	Raised pearly, pink papule; may have central umbilication or ulcerate; occurs in sun-exposed areas
Squamous cell carcinoma	Soft, elevated, scaly mass that ulcerates; occurs in sun-exposed areas
Malignant melanoma	Asymmetric lesion with irregular borders and color variation; occurs anywhere on body

Adapted from *Understanding Physiology*, by S. Huether & K. McCance, 2012, St. Louis, MO: Elsevier Mosby; *Geriatrics at Your Fingertips*, by D. Reuben, K. Herr, J. Pacala, B. Pollock, J. Potter, & T. Semla, 2011, New York: American Geriatrics Society; and *Promoting Sun Safety in Your Community: Senior Centers*, by the Skin Cancer Foundation, 2012, retrieved from http://www.skincancer.org/get-involved/your-community/senior-centers.

Functional Implication of Skin Changes

▶ Skin becomes more prone to injury and infection.

▶ Skin becomes dryer, sometimes resulting in itching and irritation.

▶ Onychomycosis, or fungal infection of toenails, can occur.

▶ A decrease in touch receptors may slow reflexes and reduce the sensation of pain.

▶ Vitamin D production becomes less efficient.

The Braden Scale can be used to assess pressure ulcer risk (Consultgeri.org, 2012; available at http://consultgerirn.org/uploads/File/trythis/try_this_5.pdf).

Cardiovascular

Age-related changes in the cardiovascular system affect both the heart and blood vessels. The left ventricle becomes thicker and less compliant. This change is exaggerated in those with longstanding hypertension. This thickening leads to a decrease in filling during diastole, which results in a lower stroke volume and, thus, a reduction in cardiac output. Tachycardia is poorly tolerated, because an increased heart rate further reduces diastolic filling time. In addition, the thickened myocardium is more prone to irritability, leading to arrhythmias and to ischemia. Fibrosis and sclerosis of the cardiac muscle can also affect the SA node, other conduction tissue, and the valves. These changes can lead to arrhythmias (such as sick sinus syndrome, heart block, premature beats) and stenotic or incompetent valves. In addition, decreased baroreceptor sensitivity can lead to postural hypotension (Huether & McCance, 2012).

Aging blood vessels become more calcified and tortuous as people age. The arteries lose elasticity and vasomotor tone and are less able to selectively regulate blood flow. Blood pressure increases because of increased peripheral resistance and can be worsened by atherosclerosis, which is a pathologic process, but occurs almost universally in "aging" arteries.

Functional Implications of Cardiovascular Changes

▶ Decreased cardiac reserve

▶ Increased risk of arrhythmias

▶ Increased risk of postural hypotension

▶ Increased risk of varicosities or dependency edema, or both, in lower extremities

Pulmonary

Lung expansion is diminished in the older population. This change results from several factors, including weakness of respiratory muscles, calcification of rib articulations leading to stiffness of the chest wall, and kyphosis. Pathologic conditions such as chronic obstructive lung disease (COPD) further reduce chest expansion because of air trapping at end-exhalation with emphysema, and excess mucous production and plugging with chronic bronchitis. COPD can lead to an increased anterior–posterior (AP) diameter of the chest, referred to as a "barrel chest."

Functional Implications of Pulmonary Changes

▶ Reduced pulmonary reserve

▶ Decreased cough reflex with increased risk of aspiration pneumonia

▶ Increased risk of infection and bronchospasm with airway obstruction

Sensory

Age-related sensory changes are common and can be a source of frustration for older adults and their caregivers. Decreased vision can greatly affect function and independence, and is feared by many older adults. Skin changes around the eye can lead to lid laxity and senile ptosis and can obstruct vision. Age-related vision changes (presbyopia) begin around age 40. Loss of lens elasticity and increased thickness cause a decrease in the ability to see contrast, need for higher light requirements, and increased susceptibility to glare.

"Dry eyes" are another common complaint of some older adults. The constant sensation of a foreign body in the eye and "dryness" is often accompanied by excessive tearing. In addition, many older persons may develop ringlike deposits around the iris of the eye, or arcus senilis. It is caused by lipid deposits deep in the edge of the cornea, but is not related to high cholesterol levels, does not affect vision, and does not require treatment (Behrenbeck, 2012).

"Normal" aging changes can be accompanied by pathologic changes in the eyes. Further thickening and yellowing of the lens can lead to the formation of cataracts, which affect about one-third of the population by the time they reach age 80. The increased intraocular pressure is associated with glaucoma and causes diminished peripheral vision. These and other conditions of the eye are discussed further in Chapter 20.

Hearing acuity diminishes with aging, which may be the reslut of presbycusis, a sensorineural hearing loss that probably has many causes. Presbycusis is caused by degeneration of the cochlea and changes in central auditory processing. These changes lead to loss of awareness of high-frequency tones and problems with word discrimination.

Conductive hearing loss due to cerumen in the ear canals is also common. Accumulation of cerumen is aggravated by dryness and flaking skin in the canal, as well as proliferation of aural hairs.

Alterations in taste can result from medication side effects, poor dentition or improperly fitting dentures, tobacco use, or other systemic problems. Dry mouth is a common complaint among older adults, and is considered by many to be a normal age-related change; however, it can also be exacerbated by cigarette smoking, medications, dehydration, and other lifestyle-related factors (Gonsalves, Wrightson, & Henry, 2008).

Functional Implications of Sensory Changes
- ► Increased risk of falls, burns, and motor vehicle accidents
- ► Increased risk of social isolation, boredom, and depression due to inability to participate with others in activities
- ► Increased risk of communication difficulties due to hearing loss

Musculoskeletal

The aging process has a profound effect on bone mineralization. Once women reach menopause, the process of bone resorption (osteoclast activity) outpaces the rate of bone building (osteoblast activity). By age 80, a woman may have lost up to 30% of her bone mass. This decrease in bone density and strength (osteoporosis) leads to an increased possibility of fracture, particularly in the weight-bearing bones and vertebrae. Loss of subcutaneous fat may make bony prominences more visible. Joint cartilage erodes and synovial fluid thickens, possibly leading to more painful joint movement. Muscle mass usually declines and tendons become less elastic, which leads to decreased tone and strength.

Like the cardiovascular system, the musculoskeletal system experiences the effects of a sedentary lifestyle. Maintaining a healthy lifestyle and proper nutrition, with calcium and vitamin D supplementation, can help prevent or reduce age-related musculoskeletal changes.

Functional Implications of Musculoskeletal Changes
- ▶ Increased risk of falls with injury
- ▶ Greater osteoarthritis pain and limited movement, leading to deconditioning
- ▶ Loss of muscle mass; general weakening may occur

Gastrointestinal

Functional Implications of Gastrointestinal Changes
- ▶ Becoming laxative-dependent, with negative effect on nutrient absorption
- ▶ Increased risk of drug toxicity due to decreased liver function
- ▶ Dysphagia and aspiration pneumonia more common
- ▶ Gastroesophageal reflux disease (GERD) more common with increased use of antacids, potentially affecting digestion and medication absorption

Female Genitourinary

Ovarian function decreases during the fourth decade of life, and the ovaries atrophy. About 1 or 2 years later, menstrual periods stop, usually between the ages of 40 and 55. This marks a decline in estrogen levels, followed by atrophy of the tissues. The labia and clitoris become smaller. The vaginal introitus constricts, and vaginal mucosa become pale, thin, and dry. These changes can lead to pain during sexual intercourse and also affect urinary continence. In addition, ligaments and connective tissues in the pelvis lose elasticity, causing a "shift" of the pelvic structures and occasionally bladder or vaginal prolapse. Pelvic laxity also has an adverse effect on urinary continence, especially during times of increased intra-abdominal pressure, such as with coughing or sneezing (stress incontinence). Bladder capacity decreases by about 50%, and sensory changes may delay the signal that the bladder is full, which can lead to overflow incontinence.

Functional Implications of Female Genitourinary Changes

▶ Pain and discomfort during vaginal intercourse (dyspareunia)

▶ Increased risk of vaginosis

▶ Increased risk of urinary incontinence

Male Genitourinary

Structural changes in the older man include thinning of pubic hair and sagging of the scrotum. Erections may develop more slowly. Ejaculatory volume can decrease, and the viability of sperm decreases with age. Hypertrophy of the prostate gland may close off the urethra and cause obstructive urinary symptoms, such as hesitancy, decrease in force of stream, increased urinary frequency, nocturia, or retention.

Functional Implications of Male Genitourinary Changes

▶ Increased risk of erectile dysfunction

▶ Increased risk of urinary retention, nocturia, and overflow incontinence

Renal

Renal function begins to decline in middle age, and that decline continues slowly through the remainder of life. Much of this decline may be attributed to undocumented pathology, such as hypertension or impaired glucose metabolism. Creatinine clearance remains the most reproducible clinical measure of golmerular filtration rate (GFR). It is important to remember that creatinine clearance is affected by the amount of creatinine (a byproduct of muscle metabolism) produced in an individual. Persons of advanced age with decreased muscle mass and cachexia may have a serum creatinine within "normal limits," despite a markedly reduced glomerular filtration rate. Diminished production of creatinine does not require much effort for the kidneys to clear, thus maintaining a normal serum level. The most common formula to calculate creatinine clearance is the Cockcroft-Gault formula: $\{(140 - Age) \times wt\ (kg) \times F\} / (Plasma\ Creatinine * 0.8136)$, where $F = 1$ if male and 0.85 if female.

Functional Implications of Changes in Renal Function

▶ Increased half-lives of medication, contributing to potential toxicity

▶ Increased risk of fluid overload or dehydration

Neurological

Age-related changes in the nervous system result from decreased velocity of nerve impulse conduction and diminished sensory perception. Responses to stimuli take longer. Cerebral neurons decrease slowly after age 50, but the excessive number of neurons present prevents this decrease from producing clinical signs or symptoms of cognitive impairment. Slowing of the autonomic nervous system may contribute to orthostatic hypotension.

Functional Implications of Neurological Changes

▶ Slowed speed of cognitive processing

▶ Increased risk of sleep disorders, neurologic diseases, and delirium

▶ Increased risk of sensory overload or deprivation

SUMMARY

This chapter has provided the necessary background information for the nurse to develop a perspective on the older person in America. Subsequent chapters will address the healthcare needs of this group.

The concept of *health* for older adults must be expanded beyond "disease-free." Felner and Williams (1979) crafted a definition of health that is most appropriate for older adults: "The ability to live and function effectively in society and to exercise self-reliance and autonomy to the maximum extent feasible, but not necessarily as total freedom from disease." This definition was incorporated into the Healthy People 2000+ documents (http://www.healthypeople.gov/2020).

Disease should not be the hallmark of old age; the definitioon of old age should include healthy independence. This goal can be achieved through careful follow-up and disease management, health promotion and screening, provisions for advance directives, healthy coping with physical and emotional loss, attention to housing and social services, and involving families and informal caregivers in aspects of care.

REFERENCES

AARP. (2009). *Across the states: Profiles of long-term care and independent living.* Retrieved from http://assets.aarp.org/rgcenter/il/d19105_2008_ats.pdf

Behrenbeck, T. (2012). *What's the relationship between arcus senilis and cholesterol?* Retrieved from http://www.mayoclinic.com/health/arcus-senilis/AN01493

ConsultGeriRN.org. (2005). *Consider this: Function.* Retrieved from http://consultgerirn.org/topics/function/need_help_stat/

Felner, B., & Williams, T. (1979). *Health promotion for the elderly: Reducing functional dependency.* In *Healthy People 2000* (pp. 365–387). Washington, DC: U.S. Government Printing Office.

Gonsalves, W., Wrightson, A., & Henry, R. (2008). Common oral conditions in older person's. *American Family Physician, 78(7),* 845–852.

Huether, S., & McCance, K. (2012). *Understanding physiology.* St. Louis, MO: Elsevier Mosby.

Koc, D., Dogan, A., & Bek, B. (2010). Bite force and influential factors on bite force. *European Journal of Dentistry, 4(2),* 223–232.

Lindeman, R. D. (2006). *Renal function and failure.* In T. Rosenthal, B. Naughton, & M. Williams. (Eds.), *Office Care Geriatrics* (pp. 414–431). Philadelphia: Lippincott.

Reuben, D., Herr, K., Pacala, J., Pollock, B., Potter, J., & Semla, T. (2011). *Geriatrics at your fingertips.* New York: American Geriatrics Society.

Seidel, H. M., Ball, J. W., Dains, J. E., & Benedict, G. W. (2006). *Mosby's guide to physical examination* (6th ed.). St. Louis, MO: Mosby.

Skin Cancer Foundation. (2012). *Promoting sun safety in your community: Senior centers.* Retrieved from http://www.skincancer.org/get-involved/your-community/senior-centers

U.S. Administration on Aging. (2011). *Profiles of older Americans.* Retrieved from http://www.aoa.gov/AoARoot/Index.aspx

U.S. Bureau of the Census. (2010). *Population 65 years and older in the United States.* Retrieved from http://factfinder2.census.gov/faces/tableservices/jsf/pages/productview.xhtml?pid=ACS_10_1YR_S0103&prodType=table

U.S. Bureau of the Census. (2011). *2010 Census shows 65 and older population growing faster than the total U.S. population.* Retrieved from http://2010.census.gov/news/releases/operations/cb11-cn192.html

U.S. Social Security Administration. (2012). *How work affects your benefits [electronic leaflet].* Retrieved from http://www.ssa.gov/pubs/10069.html#a0=0

Werner, C. A. (2011). *The older population: 2010–2010 Census briefs.* Washington, DC: U.S. Census Bureau. Retrieved from http://www.census.gov/prod/cen2010/briefs/c2010br-09.pdf

ADDITIONAL RESOURCES

Tabloski, P. (2010). *Gerontological nursing* (2nd ed.). Upper Saddle River, NJ: Pearson.

DEVELOPMENT OF GERONTOLOGICAL NURSING PRACTICE

This chapter discusses many issues related to the development of the specialty of gerontological nursing and is divided into the following sections:

- ► History of Gerontological Nursing Practice
- ► Regulatory Guidelines That Affect Gerontological Nursing Practice
- ► Trends Related to Patient Rights, Care, and Ethics
- ► Research in Gerontological Nursing

HISTORY OF GERONTOLOGICAL NURSING PRACTICE

In the 1920s, a few visionary nurses started to identify the challenges of caring for older adults and identified the need for specialization in this area of care. These nurses also recognized that specialized care of older adults could be delivered outside of acute care hospitals and described the need for rest homes and old-age homes to fill that gap. In 1925, the medical specialty of geriatrics began to emerge, and nursing quickly followed suit. Nurses and physicians recognized the need for specialized knowledge regarding health, disease, and aging because they realized that there were increasing numbers of older people and gains in life expectancy.

Today, the American Nurses Association (ANA) is responsible for defining the scope of practice and standards of nursing care, and it includes gerontological nursing in its ambit. Some of the significant events and policy changes that led to the specialty practice of gerontological nursing include:

▶ 1950: *Geriatric Nursing,* by Newton and Anderson, the first textbook on this topic, is published.

▶ 1961: ANA makes recommendations for specialty practice.

▶ 1962: The ANA Conference on Geriatric Nursing Practice meets for the first time, in Detroit, Michigan.

▶ 1966: ANA forms the Geriatric Nursing Division; Dr. Virginia Stone develops the first clinical specialty nursing program, at Duke University.

▶ 1969: ANA completes the first *Standards of Gerontological Nursing,* which was revised in 1976, 1981, 1987, 1995, 2004, and 2010.

▶ 1975: ANA offers the first Gerontological Nursing Certification Examination; the *Journal of Gerontological Nursing* publishes its first issue.

▶ 1976: The Division of Geriatric Nursing Practice changes to Gerontologic Nursing Practice to reflect the roles of nurses in providing care to healthy, ill, and frail older adults; Irene Mortenson Burnside writes the first gerontological nursing (not geriatric nursing) textbook, titled *Nursing and the Aged* (Burnside, 1988).

▶ 1979: The *Journal of Gerontological Nursing* sponsors the first National Conference on Gerontological Nursing.

▶ 1981: The first International Conference on Gerontological Nursing takes place.

▶ 1984: The National Gerontological Nursing Association (NGNA) is formed.

▶ 1993: A total of 12,000 nurses are certified in gerontological specialties.

▶ 1995: The John A. Hartford Foundation Institute for Geriatric Nursing is established at New York University to shape the quality of U.S. health care for older adults.

The *Scope and Standards of Practice for Gerontological Nursing* (2010) defines the goal of gerontological nursing practice as:

> . . . to provide the highest quality of care to the older adults within a healthcare system facing an unprecedented increase of their numbers. To do so, gerontological nurses employ a shared body of skills and knowledge to address the full range of needs related to the process of aging, the specialized care of older adults, and the uniqueness of older adults as a group and as individuals. These specialists lead interprofessional teams and collaborate with older adults and their significant others to promote autonomy, wellness, optimal functioning, comfort, and quality of life from healthy aging to the end of life. The Scope and Standards of Practice for Gerontological Nursing is the most succinct one-volume guide to the essentials of gerontological nursing: its practice environments and settings, its science and other evidence- and research basis, its education and professional development, and its ethical , societal, and cultural context. (ANA, 2010, p. 5)

Early in the 1980s, the National League for Nursing (NLN) and the American Association of Colleges of Nursing (AACN) supported the inclusion of gerontological nursing content in the basic nursing curriculum. Although the amount of gerontological content and experiences in nursing programs has increased in the last decade, it is still uneven, and a lack of faculty with expertise in gerontological nursing compounds the problem. Nursing leaders have called for more gerontological content and increased opportunities for students to care for older persons outside of the acute care hospital setting (Tanner, 2010).

The American Nurses Credentialing Center (ANCC) currently offers three certifications in this specialty, including the Gerontological Nurse, the Adult-Gerontological Nurse Practitioner, and the Adult-Gerontological Clinical Nurse Specialist. The American Academy of Nursing (AAN) has established a long-term-care (LTC) expert panel that includes nursing leaders to help set policy, testify to promote quality of life for older adults, publish texts and articles, and promote the science that will affect gerontological nursing for future decades.

REGULATORY GUIDELINES THAT AFFECT GERONTOLOGICAL NURSING PRACTICE

This section includes a brief description of the following regulatory guidelines that affect the older population and the nurses who care for them:

- ► Health Insurance Portability and Accountability Act (HIPAA)
- ► Informed consent and self-determination
- ► Healthcare reimbursement
- ► Nurse Practice Act
- ► Omnibus Budget Reconciliation Acts (OBRAs)
- ► Older Americans Act (OAA)
- ► Americans with Disabilities Act (ADA)
- ► Adult protective services (APS)

Health Insurance Portability and Accountability Act (HIPAA)

HIPAA (P.L. 104–191), signed into law in 1996, was the first federal law that protects patient health information. Initially enacted to assist people with insurance portability problems when they change jobs, this act now is more commonly known for its healthcare information components, which were brought into focus because of potentially stigmatizing diseases such as HIV/AIDS and the large amount of healthcare data being transmitted—and potentially intercepted—electronically.

Most large healthcare organizations have their own HIPAA training programs, which usually are updated annually, for employees. Privacy and confidentiality in healthcare information are integral to the delivery of health care and are the responsibility of healthcare providers. Patients must be informed of HIPAA privacy measures at any initial visit to a healthcare provider or facility. HIPAA classifies the following healthcare information as confidential:

► Patient-identifying data

► Data related to past or present medical, psychosocial, or functional issues

► Healthcare provider information

► Past or present reimbursement data

If HIPAA standards are not followed, civil or criminal penalties can occur.

Informed Consent and Self-Determination

Informed consent is granted by a patient in a legal document that discloses information about a proposed treatment before the treatment is performed. Professional standards limit the duty to disclose information to what a reasonable medical practitioner would disclose under the same or similar circumstances. "Reasonable" patient standards require that the healthcare provider give information that the patient needs to decide whether or not to have a particular treatment.

Consent is required before touching a patient or performing a medical or surgical procedure, and is required before helping a patient with bathing, taking vital signs, or administering medications. Patients can revoke consent at any time during patient care by refusing care or simply stating that they have changed their mind. If a healthcare provider proceeds with treatment after consent has been revoked, it may be considered assault and battery.

Gerontological nurses are obligated to give patients information about activities before those activities take place, including administration of medications. Any invasive treatment requires written informed consent. If in doubt about whether written informed consent is needed, assume that it *is* needed.

Exceptions to the requirement for informed consent include emergency situations; situations in which a patient waives his or her right to informed consent; and *therapeutic privilege,* whereby medical judgment concludes that revealing such information would be extremely harmful to the patient and may lead to suicide or violent behavior. Healthcare providers should invoke therapeutic privilege with great caution (U.S. Department of Health and Human Services, 2012).

The responsibility for obtaining informed consent rests with the person performing the procedure or treatment that requires the consent. For medical or surgical procedures, it is the physician; for nursing procedures, it is the nurse. If the responsibility for obtaining consent for a medical or surgical procedure is delegated to the nurse, then the nurse is legally accountable for the information that he or she gives the patient.

The most fundamental patient right is the right to decide, and it is possessed by all competent adults. Older adults have the right to give or deny informed consent for all healthcare treatment decisions unless a court of law has deemed them to be incompetent for decision-making. The statute that protects the competent patient's right to choose is the Patient Self-Determination Act of 1991 (PSDA; P.L. 101-508), which is discussed in more detail below.

Healthcare Reimbursement

The current healthcare reimbursement system includes social insurance, private insurance, and means-tested insurance. *Social insurance* includes Medicare, *private insurance* covers most working adults aged 20 to 65, and *means-tested insurance* includes Medicaid and disability insurance (Supplemental Security Income; SSI). The latter insurances are for those who are poor or have a disability (no age limitation), and eligibility depends on the person's meeting certain requirements, most of which are financial. These programs change according to federal or state guidelines and budgetary allocations.

Gerontological nurses should have some knowledge of the development of Medicare, the major health insurance coverage for older adults in the United States. The following timeline lists some important events in the evolution of Medicare:

- ► 1935: Congress passes the Social Security Act.
- ► 1945: Disability insurance is added to Social Security.
- ► 1965: Medicare Part A is enacted as national health insurance for older adults; it covers hospital care and, now, hospice care.
- ► 1966: Medicare Part B is enacted; it covers outpatient care such as physician visits and outpatient diagnostics; the patient pays a monthly premium; Medicare pays 80% of the charges, and the patient is responsible for the remaining 20%.
- ► 1972: Medicaid is enacted; it covers those who are poor, regardless of age.
- ► 1984: Medicare establishes diagnosis-related groups (DRGs) as the basis for payment for hospital care in the Medicare system; hospitals are reimbursed a set amount per admitting diagnosis, regardless of patient length of stay (LOS); this payment system begins the cycle of earlier hospital discharge and increased use of home health care to decrease costs.
- ► 1984: Medicare Part B begins reimbursing outpatient care under a relative value unit (RVU)–based system; in this system, Medicare decides on "approved charges" for all outpatient care. For instance, a doctor's office charges $30 for a urine analysis; Medicare approves $20 as the reasonable charge; therefore, Medicare pays 80% of $20, and the patient pays the remaining $4. If the physician "takes assignment," that $10 difference between the original charge ($30) and what Medicare approves ($20) is written off or ignored; if the physician does not take assignment, the patient is billed the $10 difference.

▶ 1989: The Omnibus Budget Reconciliation Act (OBRA) is enacted with two goals: (1) to develop tools to collect data on patients that would determine how Medicare is reimbursed, essentially saving money and making Medicare more of a capitated reimbursement; and (2) to develop training and standards for LTC and home health agencies to improve patient care.

▶ 1995: The Health Care Financing Administration (HCFA) mandates use of standardized assessment tools for LTC facilities, including the Resident Assessment Instrument (RAI), which includes the Minimum Data Set (MDS) and Resident Assessment Protocols (RAP); facilities are required to become computerized to use clinical data for federal reimbursement (U.S. Government Accounting Office, 1999).

▶ 1996: The Balanced Budget Act restructures Medicare Part A reimbursement, allowing Medicare to offer managed care options, and changing reimbursement in ambulatory care centers, LTC facilities, home health agencies, and rehabilitation hospitals to a prospective payment system (PPS). Under this system, these facilities receive a certain daily rate to care for the patient, and all care must be paid for out of that rate; this arrangement put the facilities in charge of how they used their daily allotment (in terms of ancillary departments and outside providers). Physician reimbursement continues to be covered under Medicare Part B and is not part of this PPS system. Advanced practice nurses covered under the Medicare fee structure are reimbursed at only 85% of the physician rate.

▶ 1998: HCFA mandates that the PPS system be phased into all skilled nursing facilities (SNFs) that are, at that time, hospital-based.

▶ 2007: Medicare Part D is added, which helps cover prescription drugs for older adults.

▶ 2010: The Affordable Healthcare Act is passed by Congress and signed by the president on March 23, 2010. Provisions of the law allow parents to insure their dependent children until age 26, prohibit insurance companies from denying insurance to dependent children under the age of 19 because of preexisting conditions, and strengthen Medicare by eliminating copays for preventive health services to encourage their use. Visit Healthcare.gov for further information on the Affordable Healthcare Act at http://www.healthcare.gov/law/features/rights/index.html.

Sources of reimbursement include Medicare Parts A, B, and D; Medigap; Medicare Managed Care; Medicaid; and out-of-pocket fee-for-service:

▶ *Medicare Part A:* Covers hospital and skilled nursing care (whether in a hospital, rehabilitation center, or LTC facility). The patient has an inpatient deductible for hospital care with each hospital admission; skilled nursing care is paid at 100% for the first 20 days, then a copayment is required for days 21 to 100. The patient is 100% responsible if the LOS is greater than 100 days, and a hospital stay of 3 days must take place before a skilled nursing facility admission. Home health, durable medical equipment, hospice, blood transfusions, and inpatient psychiatric services are all covered under this part of Medicare.

▶ *Medicare Part B:* Patients pay a monthly premium for this part, which covers medically necessary physician and advanced practice nurse services; outpatient hospital care; outpatient physical, occupational, and speech therapy; diagnostic tests; durable medical equipment (for patients who have not been hospitalized); prosthetics and orthotics; dialysis; emergency room care; organ transplant outpatient services; and some medical supplies, such as ostomy equipment and casts. Preventive services also are covered, such as annual physical examinations, mammograms, colonoscopies, or sigmoidoscopies; Pap/pelvic exams for women; diabetes-monitoring supplies; bone mineral density testing for osteoporosis; and certain vaccines, such as an annual flu shot and pneumococcal and hepatitis B shots in high-risk individuals.

▶ *Medicare Part D:* This plan helps cover prescription drugs. Currently, in 2012, patients pay a monthly premium and, after an annual deductible, prescription medications are covered until $2,930 worth of medications have been purchased. At that point, patients fall into the "donut hole" and pay 100% out of pocket for prescriptions until expenses reach $4,700. While in the donut hole, the enrollee pays 50% of the cost of brand-name drugs and 86% of the cost of generic drugs. After $4,700, the remaining prescription medications are covered at 90%. These plans, which vary by state, have many options and many formulas; each year, patients must assess what is offered in their states and evaluate which medications are covered before selecting a plan. (See www.medicare.gov for further information on Medicare.)

▶ *Medigap or Medicare supplemental insurance:* Private insurance companies offer plans that cover the 20% of uncovered (or patient copayment) charges that Medicare does not pay. These policies often cover annual Medicare deductibles and any Medicare Part A deductibles; the government mandates that these Medigap policies be one of 10 standard types that are labeled A–J (A is the least expensive and covers the least services, and J is the most costly and most comprehensive). Patients pay a monthly premium for a Medigap policy on the basis of their financial status and healthcare needs. Most recently, Medicare SELECT Medigap policies have come into vogue; these plans are the least expensive of all Medigap policies but require that patients receive services from certain providers at certain facilities to receive full benefits.

▶ *Medicare PLUS CHOICE:* These options, which were part of the Balanced Budget Act of 1996, have extended from traditional Medicare to Medicare managed care (which includes health maintenance organizations [HMOs], point of service options [POSs], or preferred provider organizations [PPOs]). All Medicare managed care options require that patients use certain providers and certain facilities, and are required to cover all the traditional services covered by Medicare.

▶ *Medicaid*: Eligibility criteria for this joint federal and state program for poor Americans are set each year at the federal level. Medicaid and the Children's Health Insurance Program (CHIP) provide health coverage to nearly 60 million Americans, including children, pregnant women, parents, older adults, and persons with disabilities. To participate in Medicaid, federal law requires states to cover certain population groups (mandatory eligibility groups) and gives them the flexibility to cover other population groups (optional eligibility groups). States set individual eligibility criteria within federal minimum standards. A state can apply for a waiver of federal law to expand health coverage beyond these groups (Medicaid.gov, 2012). Medicaid is funded by the state, with matching contributions from the federal government. To qualify for Medicaid, participants must meet federal poverty levels as specified by the federal government. Many residents of long-term-care facilities are subsidized by Medicaid as they "spend down" their financial resources and become indigent. For further information, visit http://www.medicaid.gov/Medicaid-CHIP-Program-Information/By-Topics/Eligibility/Eligibility.html.

▶ *Out-of-pocket fee-for-service*: This term refers to the amount that patients have to pay for healthcare services not covered by any insurance plan, such as copayment for drugs and physician office visits.

Because healthcare reimbursement has changed over the years, some methods may be confusing to gerontological nurses who have always worked in acute care. Table 3–1 lists common types of healthcare reimbursement mechanisms used today.

TABLE 3–1.
TYPES OF HEALTHCARE REIMBURSEMENT

TYPE	DESCRIPTION
Retrospective payment	Payment based on cost of services received
Prospective payment	Payment at predetermined, fixed rate for a specific set of healthcare services
Third-party reimbursement	Reimbursement from someone or some agency other than the person receiving care; usually a form of public or private insurance
Fee-for-service	Payment given for certain services; patient pays healthcare provider
Per diem payment	Specific cost or payment per day for specific services
Diagnosis-related groups (DRGs)	Hospitalization payment method used by Medicare; based on patient diagnosis at admission
Capitation	Payment based on number of people enrolled in the plan, regardless of amount of use or nonuse of services; usually this amount is per day or per month per "covered life"
Managed care organizations (health maintenance organizations [HMOs])	Patient pays a monthly amount for the service and then a small copayment each time the service is used; the idea is to provide preventive and curative care to individuals, thus decreasing the long-term expense of undiagnosed medical issues
Resource utilization groups (RUGs)	Predetermined reimbursement based on patient acuity and staff needed to care for the patient; Medicare and Medicaid use this type of reimbursement in skilled nursing and rehabilitation settings

Adapted from *Acute Inpatient PPS* by CMS.gov, 2012, retrieved from http://www.cms.hhs.gov/Medicare/Medicare-Fee-for-Service-Payment/AcuteInpatientPPS/index.html?redirect=/AcuteInpatientPPS/.

In addition to those in Table 3–1, the following terms appear in healthcare financing literature:

▶ *Coinsurance:* An insurance policy that covers the 20% not covered by Medicare Part B. A patient usually purchases a Medigap policy to cover this amount or may opt to pay out of pocket (rather than paying a monthly policy premium).

▶ *Entitlements:* Federal programs enacted through legislation, with eligibility requirements, such as Medicaid. *Medically indigent* refers to those who cannot afford healthcare services and do not have health insurance.

▶ *Fiscal intermediary:* The company that manages the financial aspects of health care for another agency. Medicare uses fiscal intermediaries in each state to supervise and distribute payments according to the claims received.

▶ *Peer review organizations (PROs):* Healthcare professionals paid by the federal government to review care given to Medicare patients.

▶ *Preferred provider organizations (PPOs):* Healthcare providers selected by a third party to deliver care to a selected group at a reduced or preset rate.

▶ *Primary payor:* The company or person responsible for the majority of the healthcare payments for an individual. For the majority of Americans aged 60 or older, Medicare is the primary payor.

▶ *Supplemental insurance:* A second policy that covers the deductible and the 20% not paid by the primary payor.

▶ *Spending down:* A term applied to older adults reducing their assets to become eligible for Medicaid; usually done to pay for nursing home care.

▶ *Universal coverage:* Accessible health care for all U.S. citizens. This topic is part of an ongoing debate among American policymakers.

Nurse Practice Act

Nurses have a professional responsibility to perform up to accepted or customary standards of care and are responsible for providing care that reflects those established standards. The standards are measured according to the expected performance of a reasonable and prudent nurse possessing the same or similar skills or knowledge under the same or similar circumstances.

A *standard of care* is a guideline for nursing practice that sets an expectation for the nurse to give safe, high-quality care. These standards are used to determine whether a nurse has provided the expected level of care for his or her level of skill, education, and experience.

Standards come from state and federal laws, the Joint Commission (previously the Joint Commission for Accreditation of Health Care Organizations [JCAHO]), internal organizational rules or bylaws, and published standards from professional organizations. In 2004, ANA combined the scope of practice into one book for all practice areas, and they updated it in 2010. Gerontological nurses should be familiar with these standards (available for purchase at http://www.nursesbooks.org/Main-Menu/Foundation/Nursing-Scope-and-Standards-of-Practice.aspx).

In 2007, the Robert Wood Johnson Foundation (RWJF) funded the Quality and Safety Education for Nurses (QSEN) project. The goal of QSEN is to address the challenge of preparing future nurses with the knowledge, skills, and attitudes (KSA) necessary to continuously improve the quality and safety of the healthcare systems in which they work.

To accomplish this goal, six competencies were defined in the project, including patient-centered care, teamwork and collaboration, evidence-based practice, quality improvement, and informatics, as well as safety. In addition to these definitions, sets of knowledge, skills, and attitudes for each of the six competencies were created for use in nursing prelicensure programs (Cronenwett et al., 2007). This project is ongoing and continues to promote innovation in education. Please see http://www.qsen.org/overview.php#overview for further details.

As health care changes dramatically, nurses are encountering better informed patients. It is not uncommon for patients, including older adults, to have researched possible treatments on the Internet and come to their primary care provider to discuss such treatments for themselves. As health care shifts from hospitals to community-based sites, older adults are becoming more interested in health promotion and disease prevention programs. Gerontological nurses must understand and be an integral part of this change in method of healthcare delivery.

Omnibus Budget Reconciliation Acts

The United States Census Bureau reports that in 2010, 3.1% of older adults in the United States were living in LTC facilities. The Federal Nursing Home Reform Act, or the Omnibus Budget Reconciliation Act (OBRA, 1987), creates a set of national minimum standards of care and rights for people living in certified nursing facilities. OBRA applies to all Medicare- and Medicaid-certified LTC facilities, including beds in acute care hospitals certified as separate units and *swing beds*—those in a hospital that can be used for either acute care or LTC. The goal of OBRA is to improve care for nursing home residents.

The changes OBRA brought to nursing home care are enormous. Some of the most important provisions include:

▶ Emphasis on a resident's quality of life, as well as the quality of care

▶ New expectations that each resident's ability to walk, bathe, and perform other activities of daily living will be maintained or improved, unless there are medical reasons otherwise

▶ A resident assessment process with data collected leading to development of an individualized care plan

▶ 75 hours of training and testing for paraprofessional staff

▶ Rights to remain in the nursing home as long as there are no non-payment matters, dangerous resident behaviors, or significant changes in a resident's medical condition

▶ New opportunities for potential and current residents with mental retardation or mental illnesses for services in and outside of a nursing home

▶ A right to safely maintain or bank personal funds with the nursing home; rights to return to the nursing home after a hospital stay or an overnight visit with family and friends; the right to choose a personal physician and have access to medical records

▶ The right to organize and participate in a resident or family council

▶ The right to be free of unnecessary and inappropriate physical and chemical restraints

▶ Uniform certification standards for Medicare and Medicaid homes

▶ Prohibitions on turning to family members to pay for Medicare and Medicaid services

Under the provisions of OBRA, a facility must have an ombudsman who is available to investigate any potential or actual violations of these standards and seek remediation if necessary. OBRA has improved the quality of life for nursing home residents through its provision for comprehensive care planning and limiting the use of chemical and physical restraints.

The *enforcement mechanisms and sanctions* section addresses corrective action plans and their use to ensure that a substandard facility comes into compliance. Sanctions can include monetary penalties and the appointment of independent managers to run a facility until the problems can be corrected or the facility is closed. See http://oig.hhs.gov/oei/reports/oei-01-01-00090.pdf for further information on this important legislation.

Older Americans Act

Enacted in 1973, the Older Americans Act (OAA; P.L. 89-73) set up nutrition programs, transportation options, and social services focused on older adults. The OAA also includes a statute for training and research. Over the years, this act has ensured congregate low-cost meals at senior centers and nutrition sites. OAA is responsible for the home-delivered meals programs, most commonly known as Meals on Wheels.

The OAA provides funds for local bus and van services for older adults to go to grocery stores or medical appointments. The availability of these services varies from city to city, depending on the amount of matching state funds. The act also addresses social needs such as physical and mental health, housing, LTC ombudsmen programs, and information and referral services for low-income older adults. In addition, the act includes the expansion and dissemination of information about aging, aging services, and programs available for older adults in the United States.

Americans with Disabilities Act

The Americans with Disabilities Act (ADA; P.L. 101-336), an expansion of the Rehabilitation Act of 1973 (P.L. 93-112), became law in 1990. It prohibits discrimination against persons with disabilities by organizations that receive federal monies or federal assistance; promotes the rights of persons with disabilities; and allows them to use local, state, or federal regulations to fight discrimination. Some important parts of the ADA are Titles II, III, and IV (see Table 3–2).

TABLE 3-2.
IMPORTANT TITLES OF THE AMERICANS WITH DISABILITIES ACT

TITLE	SERVICES COVERED	IMPACT
II	Public services and transportation	▶ Prohibits discrimination in public transportation systems ▶ Paratransit must be provided for people with disabilities who cannot use public ground transportation ▶ All must be in full compliance by 2010
III	Public accommodations	▶ Requires private enterprises to provide public accommodations for people with disabilities (private clubs and religious organizations are exempt, based on the Civil Rights Act of 1964)
IV	Telecommunications	▶ Federal Communication Commission must provide interstate and intrastate telecommunication services to people with speech and hearing impairments; covers ▶ Telecommunication devices for the deaf (i.e., TDD) to allow people with speech and hearing impairments to communicate on a level equal to that of those without impairments

Adapted from Americans with Disabilities Act of 1990. Pub. L. 101–336, 42 U.S.C. § 12101. Retrieved from http://www.ada.gov/pubs/adastatute08.htm.

Adult Protective Services

Adult Protective Services (APS) refers to a group of laws and regulations that have been enacted to deal with abuse and mistreatment of older adults. Usually, APS is administered by a state's department of social services. Most states designate certain professionals or other caregivers as *mandatory reporters*—those required by law to report elder abuse or mistreatment whenever they have a high degree of suspicion. Failure to report can result in civil or criminal penalty.

In most states, nurses are mandated reporters. More detailed information on abuse and mistreatment of older adults is included in Chapter 10 and online at The National Adult Protective Services Organization (http://www.apsnetwork.org/).

TRENDS RELATED TO PATIENT RIGHTS, CARE, AND ETHICS

This section covers several trends important to the care of older adults: patient rights across the continuum of care, life expectancy and retirement, culture, and ethical issues and decision-making.

Patient Rights

Bills of rights are guides that institutions use to help them deal with patients who enter the institution. They do not have the force of law, but are required by the Joint Commission for facilities to be accredited. Hospitals and LTC facilities have patient bills of rights and are held to the standards stated in those rights.

The Joint Commission requires that two patient rights be respected: privacy and confidentiality. Privacy is guaranteed to all in the United States under the 14th Amendment's concept of personal liberty. Confidentiality is based on statutes that give legal status to relationships between certain individuals. Confidentiality is controlled by the person who receives the private information (U.S. Department of Health and Human Services, 2012). The ANA Code of Ethics for Nurses addresses the rights of privacy and confidentiality in relation to patient information.

Disclosure of confidential information may be required for public protection and is governed by federal and state laws. Healthcare providers are permitted to report such information, usually a patient's medical record, in good faith as allowed by law or ordered by a court. The healthcare facility that creates the record owns it; however, use and disposition of the record are subject to many laws and regulations (e.g., HIPAA). Patients have the right to access to their own medical records.

The most fundamental patient right is the right to decide. This right is possessed by all competent adults and is not lost when a person becomes incompetent; the right can be maintained by using advance directives and surrogate decision-makers.

Healthcare facilities must develop policies that address advance directives, which come in many forms and are not in effect until a patient is incapable of making a decision for him- or herself. These directives include living will, durable power of attorney (DPOA), appointment of a healthcare representative, do not resuscitate (DNR) orders, and other forms of declaration of preference regarding life extension measures and care.

A *living will* states a patient's preferences for end-of-life issues. A *DPOA* is a legal document that designates an alternative decision maker in the event that a patient becomes incapacitated. The DPOA has an advantage over the living will in that the designated agent can assess a current situation and ask questions. If a person does not have either of these (or a DNR order), the law requires that all efforts to sustain life be taken by healthcare providers.

Appointment of a healthcare representative is appropriate for a patient who is declared incompetent by a court of law or who lacks the clinical capacity to provide informed consent, which often occurs with older patients. The legal standards are:

▶ *Substituted judgment*: Attempting to reach the same decision that the patient would make if he or she could do so.

▶ *Best interests*: Attempting to make a decision that benefits the patient by promoting his or her current welfare, with no consideration given to previously stated preferences.

DNR orders are specific orders from healthcare providers that direct that cardiopulmonary resuscitation not be provided in the event of sudden death. A *life-prolonging procedures declaration* involves a patient's statement that he or she does not want specific interventions to prolong life, such as placement of a feeding tube or use of a ventilator. This scenario is particularly applicable to older adults. Many of these aggressive medical interventions are not appropriate for use in the frail older adult, those with advanced dementia, and those with multiple comorbidities. The use of aggressive interventions may prolong life, but the underlying disease process cannot be reversed, and overall quality of life may suffer. It is recommended that everyone (not just older persons) discuss their preferences for health care and establish advance directives so that there is no confusion or family conflict when and if an older person cannot speak for him- or herself.

Five Wishes is a movement that encourages people to give specific instructions (more than those included in a living will) that address five categories (Masters-Farrell, 2006):

1. The person chosen to make decisions when the patient no longer can speak for himself or herself (DPOA)

2. The kind of treatment the patient wants or does not want

3. How comfortable the patient wants to be

4. How the patient wants to be treated by others

5. What information the patient wants loved ones to be told

Five Wishes is legal in 42 states and can be used in all 50 states. More information on this movement can be found at http://www.agingwithdignity.org/five-wishes-states.php.

The role of gerontological nurses in patient rights and self-determination is delineated by the ANA (1997), which states that nurses should know their own state laws, be familiar with all types of advanced directives, and be responsible for facilitating informed decision-making. Although the Patient Self-Determination Act (PSDA) has been in effect for almost two decades, and most adults are aware of advanced directives, the vast majority have not completed them. Gerontological nurses are charged with helping patients understand the importance of these documents and helping patients complete an advance directive while healthy, not at the end of life.

Life Expectancy and Retirement

Life expectancy for both men and women has increased dramatically, from 46 years in 1900 to 75.7 for men and 80.8 for women today (U.S. Census Bureau, 2012). This increase in longevity is largely due to improved medical technology throughout life, as well as changes in public health; the advent of vaccines, antibiotics, and insulin; and caregiver support. With longevity comes the need to address social policy and support legislation to meet the needs of older workers planning to retire.

Retirement from work necessitates a pension or other income, such as Social Security. Availability of medical care, goods and services, and other protections is an important feature of retirement. According to current census data, the average American retiree has 18–25 years to spend in retirement.

Certain organizations and groups that focus on the older population or issues related to aging should be noted, because patients and those caring for them may find these organizations useful as resources for aging research and policy questions. Table 3–3 provides a brief, partial listing of some of the more prominent organizations focused on older adults.

TABLE 3–3.
ORGANIZATIONS FOCUSED ON OLDER ADULTS

ORGANIZATION	PURPOSE	MEMBERSHIP
AARP (formerly American Association of Retired Persons)	Advocates for improvement in all aspects of living for older adults; analyzes legislative policy and makes recommendations	People age 55 and older
American Society on Aging (ASA)	Provides networking, education, training, and advocacy	Older adults, academic community, policy makers, business community
Association for Gerontology in Higher Education (AGHE)	Supports development of academic programs in gerontology and aging via education, research, and public service	Academic institutions and organizations committed to gerontology education
Gray Panthers	Activist group working to combat ageism and promote human rights	Older and younger adults
National Council on Aging	Information and consultation center that addresses concerns of older adults; conducts research, demonstration programs, conferences, and workshops	Older and younger adults
Hartford Institute for Geriatric Nursing	Sets national agenda and shapes quality of health care for older adults by promoting competency in nurses who care for older patients	Nurses and other healthcare professionals

Culture

According to the U.S. Census Bureau (2010), certain groups who were once considered minorities will be part of an emerging majority by 2050. The largest growth areas of the older population are occurring in the Hispanic and Black cultures.

Each ethnic group includes much diversity, and gerontological nurses must be aware of these cultural trends and educate themselves appropriately. To deliver culturally competent care, nurses must approach each older adult as a unique individual. No assumptions should be made about the background, education, values, and preferences of each older adult. Each person's values and preferences must be considered along with cultural identity, and can influence the delivery of nursing care.

Ethical Issues and Decision-Making

Gerontological nurses often are faced with difficult choices that affect patients, and may be called on to use ethical principles to guide the decision-making process. *Ethics* involves standards of moral conduct; the ANA Code of Ethics guides the practice of all nurses (ANA, 2001). This document was developed as a guide for carrying out nursing responsibilities in a manner consistent with high quality of nursing care and the ethical obligations of the profession. The Code of Ethics delineates nine key provisions, including:

1. The nurse practices with compassion and respect for the inherent dignity, worth, and uniqueness of every individual, unrestricted by consideration of social or economic status, personal attributes, or the nature of health problems.

2. The nurse's primary commitment is to the patient, whether an individual, group, family, or community.

3. The nurse promotes, advocates for, and strives to protect the health, safety, and rights of the patient.

4. The nurse is responsible and accountable for individual nursing practice and determines the appropriate delegation of tasks consistent with the nurse's obligation to provide optimum patient care.

5. The nurse owes the same duties to self as to others, including the responsibility to improve integrity and safety, to maintain competence, and to continue personal and professional growth.

6. The nurse participates in establishing, maintaining, and improving health care environments, and conditions of employment conducive to the provision of quality healthcare and consistent with the values of the profession through individual and collective action.

7. The nurse participates in the advancement of the profession through practice, education, administration, and knowledge development.

8. The nurse collaborates with other health professions and the public in promoting community, national, and international efforts to meet healthcare needs.

9. The profession of nursing, as represented by associations and their members, is responsible for articulating nursing values, maintaining the integrity of the profession and its practice, and shaping social policy. (ANA, 2001, p. 7)

In addition, gerontological nurses should be familiar with the following ethical principles:

▶ *Advocacy:* Championing the needs of others. This principle involves ensuring that patients are fully informed and able to access all benefits to which they are entitled.

▶ *Autonomy:* The concept that each person has the right to make independent decisions. This belief is the foundation of patient self-determination and is considered the most important ethical principle.

▶ *Beneficence:* Doing good. For nurses, this includes finding alternative ways to provide the greatest good, and doing no harm to patients.

▶ *Nonmaleficence:* Doing no harm. All nurses should avoid harming patients.

▶ *Confidentiality:* The right to privacy. This concept is the basis of HIPAA.

▶ *Fidelity:* Keeping promises and being faithful to one's commitments and responsibilities. Nurses should keep commitments and honor their word to patients.

▶ *Justice:* Fairness of an act or situation. Nurses should treat patients fairly and ensure that they receive services that they deserve.

▶ *Quality and sanctity of life:* Quality of life is a perception based on personal values, which vary widely and may change depending on the situation. Sanctity of life is the belief that all life is valuable, regardless of someone's level of functioning.

▶ *Veracity:* Truthfulness. Nurses should be truthful with patients.

Ethics committees in institutions can assist families and healthcare professionals, including nurses, when they are making difficult healthcare decisions.

These ethical principles may seem reasonable, appropriate, and fairly straightforward; however, in actual practice, it may be difficult to discern with clarity the application of these principles. For example:

▶ An older patient may be fearful of and refuse a procedure that could be lifesaving; coercing the patient into consenting to the procedure could help keep him or her alive, but would violate the right to autonomy.

▶ A patient may have a history of falling and could avoid a fall-related injury by being confined to a Geri-chair or being otherwise restrained; harm may be avoided by using the restraint, but doing this could violate the patient's right to be free from restraints.

According to Tabloski (2010), some ethical issues that gerontological nurses commonly encounter include:

▶ Determining appropriateness of emergency treatment

▶ Obtaining, clarifying, and enacting advance directives

▶ Providing palliative care

▶ Eliminating or using chemical and physical restraints

▶ Accessing complementary and alternative treatments

▶ Handling disclosure, especially of patient prognosis

▶ Making economic decisions

▶ Distributing resources fairly

In addition, both federal and not-for-profit agencies establish criteria to guide individuals and agencies in the care and treatment of older adults. The following agencies have avenues for addressing ethical issues related to older adults:

▶ *Centers for Medicare and Medicaid Services:* Created specific oversight for these two programs and their respective components that is ethics-based

▶ *National Center for Elder Abuse:* Sets the standards for states' APS agencies (http://www.ncea.aoa.gov/ncearoot/Main_Site/index.aspx)

▶ *Resident Bill of Rights:* Part of the OBRA reform provisions; enforced as part of LTC facility survey and must be visible in all facilities (see above for more information; http://www.gao.gov/assets/230/228383.pdf)

▶ *Patient Self-Determination Act of 1990:* Ensures that clients are given information about the extent to which their rights already exist under state law (see above for more information; www.healthcare.gov)

RESEARCH IN GERONTOLOGICAL NURSING

Nursing research is important for many reasons, including the need to improve nursing practice, maintain professional credibility, and create an avenue to provide evidence to influence the development of health policy. In addition, research can help nurses learn new information, describe certain phenomena, explore phenomena that are not commonly known, explore how two phenomena are related (or not related) and why, and predict and control factors that can affect care.

The importance of research in developing evidence-based interventions cannot be overstated. In an era of scarce financial resources, with the need to treat patients effectively and the great risk inherent in many aggressive medical and nursing interventions, gerontological nurses must be aware of "best practices" to deliver the highest-quality care to their patients.

Gerontological nurses can participate in research by identifying clinical problems to study, or they may be involved in gathering data and interpreting findings related to patient care. Nurses often are part of research teams at hospitals and universities, and may be members of healthcare institutional review boards (IRBs), which work to protect the rights of human subjects in clinical trials (Tabloski, 2010). Currently, nurses are studying the following gerontology issues:

▶ Positioning to prevent skin breakdown

▶ Bathing patients who have Alzheimer's disease

▶ Urinary incontinence

▶ Constipation (NINR, 2012)

Nursing research often focuses on nonpharmaceutical ways to improve patient care. Doctoral programs in nursing have helped develop the role of nurse–researchers. Gerontological nurses have participated on and chaired IRBs in many healthcare organizations, such as the National Institutes of Health. Nurse–researchers can present their findings at local and national meetings and publish their work in healthcare-related journals (Tabloski, 2010).

Whenever nurses are involved in research, it is imperative that the rights of people always be protected. A facility's IRB can help ensure this protection through informed consent, anonymity and confidentiality in data collection, and explanation of the risks and benefits of the research (ANCC, 2007).

Research Process

The research process, regardless of the discipline, begins with identification of a problem. Gerontological nurses might identify a problem that occurs in their practice, or they might use research to guide their continuous quality improvement (CQI) efforts. In addition, nursing theory, geriatric literature, conferences, and organizational priorities might serve as sources for research questions. It is during this process that variables are identified that could affect the research. These include:

▶ *Patient-related variables:* Age, gender, procedure

▶ *Nurse-related variables:* Age, gender, education

▶ *System-related variables:* Length of hospital stay, referral to home care

Then the problem is assessed: Does it occur frequently? Can it be solved by collecting data? Will studying it lead to better patient care? These are just a few of the thoughts that must take place before a research study begins.

Next is establishing the research question, which can include the following:

▶ *Descriptive questions:* How is one concept related to another, such as anxiety in older adults and early hospital discharge?

▶ *Exploratory or relational questions:* Describing a relationship between two concepts, such as determining the relationship between predischarge anxiety and postdischarge behavior.

▶ *Predictive questions:* Does one concept predict the occurrence of another concept? For example, does predischarge anxiety or family structure best predict postdischarge behavior?

▶ *Experimental or quasi-experimental questions:* If one outcome can be predicted, then what happens if one modifies the input leading to that outcome? If one knows that intense patient teaching predicts posthospital discharge behavior, could one arrange to change or enhances the patient teaching component to assess whether postdischarge behavior change? (ANCC, 2007)

After the statement of the research problem comes deciding what type of research to do: qualitative or quantitative. *Qualitative methods* are thought to be inductive, while *quantitative methods* involve deductive reasoning.

Qualitative Research

Qualitative methods are used when little is known about the subject, to reach a deeper understanding of phenomena, for instrument development, or to generate a hypothesis about a relationship so that further testing can be done (ANCC, 2007). The data obtained are often expressed in words, not numbers, and data analysis occurs while the data collection is being carried out. Table 3–4 categorizes the five types of qualitative research.

TABLE 3-4.
TYPES OF QUALITATIVE RESEARCH

TYPE	PURPOSE
Phenomenological	Describe experiences as they are lived from the perspective of study participants
Grounded theory	Understand basic social processes; roots are in sociology
Ethnography	Understand a culture or subculture from its own perspective; roots are in anthropology
Historiography	Understand past events
Content analysis	Classify words in text by their theoretical importance

Adapted from *Medical-Surgical Nursing Review and Resource Manual* (2nd ed.), by ANCC, 2007, Silver Spring, MD: Author.

Quantitative Research

Quantitative research, which is more common in nursing, is used to explain and predict phenomena, generate cause and effect, test theory or instruments, or evaluate effectiveness of a nursing intervention (ANCC, 2007). This type of research is more common in all health-related disciplines.

Variables can be divided into four types: *independent, dependent, extraneous,* and *demographic* (see Table 3–5).

TABLE 3-5.
VARIABLES USED IN QUANTITATIVE RESEARCH

TYPE OF VARIABLE	DESCRIPTION
Independent	Stimulus or activity that is being manipulated by the researcher to create an effect on the dependent variable
Dependent	Response, behavior, or outcome that the researcher wants to predict or explain
Extraneous	Other factors that can change and may influence the dependent variable
Demographic	Characteristics of the participants that are collected for descriptive purposes

Causality is support for cause-and-effect relationships or evidence that a change in outcomes is the result of an intervention or action carried out by the researchers. *Validity* is the measure of truth or accuracy of the study. Many different issues in validity are important:

► *Statistical conclusion validity:* Whether the conclusions made through the analyses reflect the real world; this type of validity includes potential Type I and Type II errors.

  » *Type I error:* When the researcher concludes that a difference between two groups exists but, in reality, there is none (seen when multiple statistical analyses are used or when chance is the cause of the difference, rather than a true relationship).

  » *Type II error:* When the researcher concludes that no difference between two samples exists, even though there actually is a true difference (seen with low statistical power).

► *Internal validity:* Extent to which the effect detected in a study results from the relationship between the independent and dependent variable, not from an extraneous factor.

► *Construct validity:* Quality of the fit between the definition of a concept and its method of measurement.

► *External validity:* Extent to which research findings can be generalized beyond the sample used in the study (ANCC, 2007).

The design of a quantitative research study can be *descriptive, correlational, experimental,* or *quasi-experimental* (see Table 3–6).

TABLE 3-6.
DESIGNS OF QUANTITATIVE RESEARCH

TYPE OF STUDY	DESCRIPTION	OTHER PERTINENT INFORMATION
Descriptive	Used to delineate characteristics of a sample or setting	Purpose is to avoid generalizing to a larger population
Correlational	Used to study a population by systematically examining a representative sample; findings generalized to the population represented by the sample	▶ Cross-sectional: collect data at one point in time ▶ Longitudinal: collect data at more than one point in time ▶ Designs used to describe relationships between or among factors with the intent of not making inferences about the larger population
Experimental	Used to test hypotheses about causal relationships	▶ Control a basic characteristic: ability of the researcher to manipulate the independent variable and to eliminate, hold constant, or measure the effect of extraneous variables ▶ Elements include at least 2 groups, random assignment, and pretests and posttests of the independent variable
Quasi-experimental	Used to test hypotheses about causal relationships	▶ Control a basic characteristic: ability of the researcher to manipulate the independent variable and to eliminate, hold constant, or measure the effect of extraneous variables ▶ Elements include at least 2 groups, random assignment, and pretests and posttests of the independent variable—but all 4 of these elements cannot be met

Adapted from *Medical-Surgical Nursing Review and Resource Manual* (2nd ed.), by ANCC, 2007, Silver Spring, MD: Author.

After the study design is decided on, *sampling* occurs—a group of people or elements is selected to participate in the research study. *Population* refers to the entire set of people or elements that meet the *sampling criteria*—the characteristics essential for inclusion in the target population. Usually, researchers designate specific inclusion and exclusion criteria for the sample population. Also critical is obtaining a sample large enough to generate reliable results (ANCC, 2007). Three items depend on an adequate sample size:

1. *Effect size:* Amount of an impact or strength of the relationship between the independent and dependent variables.

2. *Power:* Capacity of a statistic to detect significant differences or relationships between groups in the sample. The minimal acceptable power for a study is 0.80, meaning an 80% probability of correctly teasing out a difference between groups.

3. *Significance level:* Set by the researcher to determine the probability of making a Type I error. Most often, probability level is .05 or less; at this level, the researcher can conclude to a 95% probability that the two groups are different.

Three other issues related to samples are important in research: *sampling error, random sampling,* and *nonprobability sampling* (see Table 3–7).

TABLE 3–7.
OTHER IMPORTANT ISSUES RELATED TO SAMPLES

ISSUE	DESCRIPTION	COMMENTS
Sampling error	Difference between a sample statistic and a population parameter	▸ If the sample does not reflect the population, the sampling error will be large ▸ Random variation: the expected difference when measuring a variable in different subjects from the same sample ▸ Systematic variation: when subjects vary in some specific way from the population as a whole
Random sampling	Way to ensure that every person in the population has an equal chance to be selected into the sample	▸ Ensure that the sample represents the population and decreases systematic variation ▸ Include simple random samples, stratified random samples, and cluster samples
Nonprobability sampling	Every person in the population does not have an equal chance of being selected into the sample	▸ Includes convenience and quota samples ▸ Random assignment to a group controls systematic bias within convenience samples

Adapted from *Medical-Surgical Nursing Review and Resource Manual* (2nd ed.), by ANCC, 2007, Silver Spring, MD: Author.

After ensuring the appropriate sample size and method of sampling, the researcher must assess how to measure the variable in the study. *Measurement* is the assigning of numbers to objects, events, or situations in the study and includes nominal, ordinal, interval, and ratio.

- ▸ *Nominal:* Lowest level of measurement. Numbers function as labels or categories (e.g., 1 is used for female, 2 is used for male).
  - » Categories are mutually exclusive.
  - » All data fit into one of the categories.
- ▸ *Ordinal:* Represents a sequence or order (e.g., the graduating registered nurse may be 1st or 10th in the class). The number is significant in terms of relative position.
  - » Categories are mutually exclusive.
  - » Categories can be placed in order, but intervals are not equal.
- ▸ *Interval:* Represents order and equal distance between intervals (e.g., temperature is measured on an interval scale; the difference between 10 and 20 degrees is the same as that between 40 and 50 degrees; 0 does not mean the absence of temperature).
  - » Categories are mutually exclusive.
  - » Categories can be placed in order.
  - » Intervals are equal, but the scale does not contain an absolute 0.

▶ *Ratio:* Highest form of measurement; exists on a continuum (e.g., weight, length, or volume; 0 represents no weight, length, or volume; scale does contain an absolute 0; therefore, 6 inches is twice as long as 3 inches).

　▸ Categories are mutually exclusive.

　▸ Categories are placed in order.

　▸ Intervals are equal, and the scale contains an absolute 0.

It is impossible to measure a concept perfectly. *Measurement error* is the difference between the concept in the real world and the way it is measured by an instrument. Whenever one attempts to measure something, there is always a *true score,* an *observed score*, and an *error score.* The observed score is the true score plus the error score (ANCC, 2007).

The error score has two parts: random error and systematic error. *Random error* is the score observed to vary around the true score; it cannot be eliminated. Random error will increase the amount of unexplained variance around the true mean score.

Systematic error causes the observed score to vary from the true score in a consistent (systematic) way. Systematic error will affect mean scores (ANCC, 2007). Researchers attempt to reduce this type of error as much as possible.

Other important measurement issues include *reliability, validity,* and *sensitivity* (see Table 3–8 for definitions). These terms are critical in assessing the rigor of any research study, and all nurses should be familiar with them.

TABLE 3-8.
TERMS USED TO ASSESS RIGOR OF A RESEARCH STUDY

MEASUREMENT ISSUE	DEFINITION	IMPORTANT POINTS	COMMENTS
Reliability	Reflects consistency or reproducibility of scores obtained within the measure	► Provides an indication of the amount of random error in the measurement of the concept in the study ► Expressed as a correlation coefficient, with 1.00 being perfectly reliable and 0.00 being unreliable	► Estimates are specific to the sample being used. ► Reliability coefficient of 0.80 is the minimal acceptable level for established instruments.
Validity	Reflects the extent to which an instrument represents the concept being measured within a specific situation	► Systematic error reduces validity. ► Validity of an instrument develops through repeated use over time.	► Validity of an instrument often is rated based on how it has been assessed by experts and as it has been compared to other instruments. ► Labels given for validity include content-related evidence, criterion-related evidence, or evidence that the instrument has been accurate in predicting future or concurrent events.
Sensitivity	Ability to measure or detect relevant change in the concept		

Adapted from *Medical-Surgical Nursing Review and Resource Manual* (2nd ed.), by ANCC, 2007, Silver Spring, MD: Author.

The next phase of the research process involves data collection. There are four ways to gather information for a study: observation, self-report, existing data, or physiological measurement.

► *Observation:* Allows the concept to be studied in its natural environment. It can answer questions about human behavior (e.g., facial expression, body language).

► *Self-report:* Is done through questionnaires, surveys, or interviews. It answers questions about facts, beliefs, feelings, and attitudes.

► *Existing data:* Include public records, medical records, and national databases. These data can be used to answer a new question.

► *Physiological measures:* Include blood pressure, heart rate, pulse, and so forth.

The final stage in the research process is data analysis, during which the researcher assesses the data using statistical methods. Statistics can be categorized in one of two ways: descriptive or inferential.

▶ *Descriptive statistics:* Give precise, standard ways to summarize and communicate complex information about a sample.

▶ *Inferential statistics:* Allow for probability inferences about a sample.

Descriptive statistics give information about central tendency (mean, median, and mode), distribution of the sample (symmetry, modality, and kurtosis), dispersion (range, standard deviation, and variance) and association (contingency tables, cross-tabulations, and correlation coefficients). For definitions, see Tables 3–9, 3–10, 3–11, and 3–12.

TABLE 3-9.
DESCRIPTIVE STATISTICS: CENTRAL TENDENCY MEASURES

MEAN	MEDIAN	MODE
Sum of scores divided by the number of scores in the sum	Score at the exact center of the distribution	Score that occurs with the highest frequency

TABLE 3-10.
DESCRIPTIVE STATISTICS: DISTRIBUTION MEASURES

SYMMETRY	MODALITY	KURTOSIS
▶ Left side of the curve is exactly the same as the right side of the curve ▶ If a distribution curve is symmetrical, all 3 measures of central tendency are equal; if a curve is not symmetrical, it is skewed ▶ Positive skew—largest portion of data falls below the mean; curve has a tail extending to the right ▶ Negative skew—largest portion of the data falls above the mean; curve has an initiating tail	▶ Curve may be unimodal, bimodal, or multimodal ▶ Symmetric curves are unimodal	Peakedness of the curve, related to the spread or variability of the scores

Adapted from *Medical-Surgical Nursing Review and Resource Manual* (2nd ed.), by ANCC, 2007, Silver Spring, MD: Author.

TABLE 3-11.
DESCRIPTIVE STATISTICS: DISPERSION MEASURES

RANGE	STANDARD DEVIATION	VARIATION
Difference between highest and lowest scores	Average amount by which scores vary around the mean	Average of the squared standard deviation

Adapted from *Medical-Surgical Nursing Review and Resource Manual* (2nd ed.), by ANCC, 2007, Silver Spring, MD: Author.

TABLE 3–12.
DESCRIPTIVE STATISTICS: ASSOCIATION MEASURES

CONTINGENCY TABLES AND CROSS-TABULATIONS	CORRELATION COEFFICIENTS
▸ Allows visual comparison of summary data related to two variables within the sample ▸ Contingency tables used for nominal and ordinal data ▸ Chi-square test used for differences between cells in a contingency table	▸ Provides information about the direction, strength, and shape of relationships ▸ Values range from –1.00 (perfect and inverse correlation) to 1.00 (perfect and positive correlation)

Adapted from *Medical-Surgical Nursing Review and Resource Manual* (2nd ed.), by ANCC, 2007, Silver Spring, MD: Author.

Inferential statistics are classified as parametric, nonparametric, and hypothesis testing of differences and association between variables. *Parametric statistics* require assumptions about the distribution of the data—normal and homogeneity of variance—while *nonparametric statistics* make no assumptions about the shape of the distribution (ANCC, 2007). Nonparametric statistics are relevant when the distribution is not normal or the sample size is small. They are used with nominal or ordinal type data.

When assessing differences and associations between the study variables, researchers can use the following statistical methods (ANCC, 2007):

▸ *Tests of difference*

    ▹ *Parametric:* *t*-test, analysis of variance

    ▹ *Nonparametric:* Mann-Whitney U test, sign test

▸ *Tests of association*

    ▹ *Parametric:* Pearson correlation coefficient

    ▹ *Nonparametric:* Spearman and Kendall correlation coefficients

Evidence-Based Practice

The term *evidence-based practice (EBP)* is used to describe activities or treatments that are based on the results of clinical research, not on hunches or suspicions. It is important for nurses to use research findings that affect patient care. Consumers and governing bodies expect professional nurses to provide care that is substantiated by research studies. Doing so will improve the quality of gerontological care. This type of information can come from a variety of sources, including national guidelines, professional organizations, and local organizational data (e.g., CQI data).

National guidelines can be based on research or opinions of experts. The Agency for Healthcare Research and Quality publishes practice guidelines on a variety of nursing and medical topics (see www.ahrq.gov and www.guideline.gov).

EBP guidelines contain comprehensive and summary information of existing research studies and rate the quality of the evidence. An example of one rating system follows:

▶ Level I: Evidence from at least one well-designed randomized controlled trial.

▶ Level II-1: Evidence from well-designed controlled trials without randomization.

▶ Level II-2: Evidence obtained from well-designed cohort or case-control analytic studies, preferably from more than one center or research group.

▶ Level II-3: Evidence from multiple cohort studies without intervention.

▶ Level III: Opinions of respected authorities based on clinical experience, descriptive studies, or reports of expert committees. (U.S. Preventive Services Task Force [USPSTF], 2012)

Professional organizations can publish research-based protocols, such as Nurses Improving Care to Healthsystem Elders (NICHE), which is sponsored by the Institute of Geriatric Nursing at New York University. Local organizations can disseminate their CQI data to help revise systems and processes within the organization.

Another component of EBP is *research utilization,* which involves analyzing and critiquing clinical nursing research before initiating it in clinical practice. Nurses must critically assess whether a published research study is sound and transferable to their own nursing practice.

Also important is the evaluation of outcomes: Are nurses maximizing the benefits associated with the resources being used to care for patients? An *outcome* is the way patient health status changes over time and can be positive, negative, or neutral. Outcomes depend on many factors, such as treatments and baseline condition. Some commonly used outcome measures are patient satisfaction, functional health status, and morbidity and mortality rates.

SUMMARY

As you can see, research involves thoughtful and well-planned design. The national standard is that healthcare providers of all types be well versed in research findings and use these as they care for patients. Doing so makes it likely that care of patients will improve.

REFERENCES

American Nurses Association. (2010). *Nursing: Scope and standards of practice*: *Gerontological nursing* Washington, DC: Author.

American Nurses Credentialing Center. (2007). *Medical–surgical nursing review and resource manual* (2nd ed.). Silver Spring, MD: Author.

Americans with Disabilities Act of 1990. Pub. L. 101–336, 42 U.S.C. § 12101.

Burnside, I. M. (1988). *Nursing for the aged: A self-care approach* (3rd ed.). New York: McGraw-Hill.

Center for Medicare and Medicaid Services. (2012). *Acute inpatient PPS*. Retrieved from http://www.cms.hhs.gov/Medicare/Medicare-Fee-for-Service-Payment/AcuteInpatientPPS/index.html?redirect=/AcuteInpatientPPS/

Cronenwett, L., Sherwood, G., Barnsteiner, J., Disch, J., Johnson, J., Mitchell, P., Sullivan, D., & Warren, J. (2007). Quality and safety education for nurses. *Nursing Outlook, 55*(3), 122–131.

Masters-Farrell, P. A. (2006). Ethical/logical principles and issues. In K. L. Mauk (Ed.), *Gerontological nursing: Competencies for care* (pp. 596–605). Sudbury, MA: Jones & Bartlett.

National Institute of Nursing Research. (2012). *Strategic plan*. Retrieved at http://www.ninr.nih.gov/

Newton, K., & Anderson, H.C. (1950). *Geriatric nursing*. St. Louis, MO: Mosby.

Tabloski, P. A. (2010). *Gerontological nursing*. Upper Saddle River, NJ: Pearson Education.

Tanner, C. (2010). Transforming pre-licensure nursing education: Preparing the new nurse to meet emerging healthcare needs. *Nursing Education Perspective, 31*(6), 347–353.

U.S. Census Bureau. (2010). *Census summary file*. Retrieved from http://www.census.gov/prod/cen2010/briefs/c2010br-09.pdf

U.S. Census Bureau. (2012). *Expectancy of life at birth*. Retrieved from http://www.census.gov/compendia/statab/2012/tables/12s0104.pdf

U.S. Department of Health and Human Services. (2012). *Summary of HIPAA privacy rule*. Retrieved from http://www.hhs.gov/ocr/privacy/hipaa/understanding/summary/index.html

U.S. Government Accounting Office. (1999). *Nursing home care*. Retrieved from http://www.gao.gov/assets/230/228383.pdf

U.S. Preventive Services Task Force. (2012). *Evidence report development*. Retrieved from http://www.uspreventiveservicestaskforce.org/uspstf08/methods/procmanual4.htm

THEORIES OF AGING

Aging adults interact with their physical and psychological environments in an attempt to define an order for themselves. Many theories attempt to explain the varied aspects of human development and conceptualize a framework to address the various stages of aging—physical, cognitive, and emotional. These theories provide a perspective from which to view developmental facts about aging; however, they are not a comprehensive explanation of the process of aging. No single theory encompasses the complexity of the aging process, because it is influenced by a composite of biological, psychological, social, functional, and spiritual factors that intervene along a continuum from birth to death.

BIOLOGICAL THEORIES

Aging is an individual process that differs from species to species and from one human being to another, with no two individuals aging identically. There are varying degrees of physiological changes, capacities, and limitations within given age groups. Biological theories are concerned with basic questions about physiological processes that occur in an organism over time. Some prominent biological theories include:

► Error

► Free-Radical

► Cross-Link

► Wear-and-Tear

► Programmed-Aging/Hayflick Limit

► Immunity

► Emerging Biological theories

It is important to note that biological theories are divided into two classes: stochastic and nonstochastic. *Stochastic theories* discuss aging as a random event that occurs and accumulates over time, while *nonstochastic theories* suggest that aging is a predetermined or timed process of events.

The stochastic theories include error, free-radical, cross-link, and wear-and-tear theories. The nonstochastic theories encompass the programmed-aging/Hayflick limit and immunity theories.

Various biological theories of aging have been more persuasive than others at various times, but no one unifying theory explains the mechanics and causes underlying the biological phenomenon of aging. Aging and disease are not synonymous, because all individuals age differently. Biological theories provide ideas about the physical aspects of aging. To be holistic, it is important to look at other theories, such as sociological and psychological ones that are also concerned with factors that affect aging.

Error Theory

This theory is based on the idea that errors can occur in the process of DNA transcription, and eventually lead to aging or death of the cell. These errors, if left unchecked, could result in a product that does not even represent the original cell (Sonneborn, 1979). As these cells continue to divide, eventually organ function can be lost when dysfunctional cells reach a large enough number.

Free-Radical Theory

Free radicals are the molecular byproducts of metabolic and environmental activities within the body that contain unpaired ions/electrons that exist momentarily and are highly reactive. In health, enzymatic activity neutralizes these radicals. When this process does not occur, molecular reactions within the cell membranes can interfere with RNA/DNA transcription. Parts of the molecules break off the loose electrons and attach to other molecules, causing alterations in cellular structures. This theory emphasizes the importance of the mechanism of oxygen use by the cell, because the greatest source of free radicals is the metabolism of oxygen (Jin, 2010).

Environmental pollutants are believed to promote free-radical activity. Certain foods (antioxidants) are thought to reduce free-radical activity (e.g., those containing Vitamins A, C, and E).

Cross-Link Theory

This theory proposes that, with advancing age, some proteins become increasingly cross-linked or entwined and impede metabolic processes. These cross-linkages obstruct the passage of nutrients and wastes between intracellular and extracellular compartments. These cross-linked proteins engage in a chemical process that impedes mitosis on the cellular level. As these cross-linked agents increase, they form aggregates that interfere with intracellular transport, which can then cause failure of the organs and, eventually, of body systems (Jin, 2010).

Cross-link theory proposes that the immune system declines with age, and the body's defense mechanism cannot remove the cross-linked agents. Although proposed as a probable cause of arteriosclerosis, this theory has little support in empirical evidence.

Wear-and-Tear Theory

This theory suggests that tissues and cells have vital parts that wear out with repeated use, resulting in many of the changes of aging. Over time, these aging effects accumulate, resulting in loss of organ function and, eventually, death. This theory is sometimes used to explain death from frailty and multisystem organ failure in old age (Jin, 2010).

Programmed-Aging Theory/Hayflick Limit Theory

While studying fetal fibroblastic cells and their reproductive capabilities, Dr. Leonard Hayflick (1961) found that cells were limited in the ability to replicate, and the life expectancy–aging phenomenon was a preprogrammed, species-specific biological clock. According to this theory, unlimited cell division does not occur; therefore, immortality of the human being would be an abnormal (as opposed to normal) occurrence.

Immunity Theory

Immune function diminishes with age. T and B cells implicated in cell-mediated immunity respond differently to invading organisms. In addition, there are changes in the humoral immune response that predispose older adults to cancer. This increased occurrence of cancer is a result of a decreased resistance to tumor cells and a heightened production of autoantigens, which can cause an increase in autoimmune disease (Huether & McCance, 2012).

Emerging Biological Theories

These theories, which currently are under investigation, include the neuroendocrine control theory (or pacemaker theory), metabolic theory of aging (or calorie restriction theory), and DNA-related research theory.

The *neuroendocrine control theory* addresses the interrelated role of the neural and endocrine systems. Over time, complex interactions that govern hormone production decline. Cornerstones of this theory are the roles of hypothalamus, DHEA, and melatonin in longevity, immune function, and the aging process (Jin, 2010).

The metabolic/caloric restriction theory originated in 1996, when Hayflick departed from studying fibroblastic cells to look at caloric restriction in rodents and then saw increases in life span. Thus, he proposed that each organism has a finite amount of metabolic lifetime, and those with higher metabolic rates have shorter life spans (Jin, 2010).

DNA mapping, or the discovery of the human genome, has led to the belief that there may be as many as 200 genes responsible for controlling aging in human beings. The discovery of *telomeres*—the regions at the ends of chromosomes—and their subsequent decrease in cell division with age explains the fact that cells have a limited capacity to divide (Carrascosa, Ros, Andres, Fernandez-Agullo, & Arribas, 2009).

SOCIOLOGICAL THEORIES

These theories deal with the roles and relationships assumed by individuals as they age. Historically, dating back to the 1960s, a focus on loss and its relevance to adjustment permeated the literature. With increased longevity, more active older adults, and the migration of families, other theories have emerged that deal with broadening the context of environment and the interrelationships between older adults and society. The most prominent sociological theories include:

▶ Disengagement

▶ Activity

▶ Continuity

▶ Age Stratification

▶ Person–Environment–Fit

Disengagement Theory

This theory was introduced in 1961 by sociologists Elaine Cumming and William E. Henry. They viewed the process of aging as a developmental task. They hypothesized that, as a person ages, he or she disengages and becomes self-centered, preferring to withdraw from society and becoming internally focused. The U.S. retirement system and aging retirement complexes sparked this theory, which has since been refuted. As a theory, disengagement met with immense controversy and had a relatively short life. However, it quickly led to the framework for other developmental theories.

Activity Theory

This theory, which is in direct contrast to the disengagement theory, was proposed by sociologists Robert James Havighurst and Ruth Albrecht in 1953, with the major premise being that people need to be active to promote life satisfaction and a positive self-concept. Essentially, this theory suggests that the person is in a constant process of trying to remain "middle-aged." It is based on three assumptions: (1) It is better to be active than to be nonactive, (2) it is better to be happy than to be unhappy, and (3) older people are the best judges of their own happiness (Havighurst, 1972).

Continuity Theory

This theory, which refutes the disengagement and activity theories, proposes that how a person has been throughout life is how that person will continue through the remainder of life. Because it says that life is continuous in its development, this theory is sometimes viewed as a developmental one. As we age, we continue previous habits, preferences, values, beliefs, and all that has previously contributed to our personalities (Havighurst, Neugarten, & Tobin, 1963).

Age Stratification Theory

This theory addresses societal values—interdependence between the aging person and society. Society determines which cohort groups individuals belong to, their roles in society, and how they collectively age. There is a dynamic interaction between the aging person and society.

According to sociologist Matilda White Riley (1985), the five major parts of this theory are: (1) each person is a process in society based on his or her cohort, and these cohorts age socially, biologically, and psychologically; (2) new cohorts will experience society differently from other cohorts; (3) society can be divided according to ages and roles; (4) people, roles, and society as a whole are continually changing; and (5) interactions between the older person and society are ever-changing.

Person–Environment–Fit Theory

This theory, as proposed by Dr. M. P. Lawton in 1982, posits that a person's competencies mold and shape him or her throughout life, and play a major role in helping a person deal with a changing environment.

Lawton identified these competencies as (1) ego strength, (2) motor skills, (3) individual biological health, (4) cognitive capacities, and (5) sensory-perceptual capacities. As competencies change in older age, so does an individual's ability to interrelate with the environment.

PSYCHOLOGICAL THEORIES

The assumption in these theories is that aging continues as a dynamic developmental process. These theories incorporate many of the concepts of the biological and sociological theories, and weave adaptive-coping mechanisms into the explanation of how the person behaves. Memory, learning, emotions, and motivation are all part of the psychological coping mechanisms that are challenged as one ages. Prominent approaches in this category include:

▶ Maslow's Hierarchy of Human Needs Theory

▶ Jung's Theory of Individualism

▶ Erikson's Eight Stages of Life

▶ Peck's Expansion of Erikson's Theory

▶ Selective Optimization With Compensation

Maslow's Hierarchy of Human Needs Theory

This theory, which was proposed by psychologist Abraham Maslow (1943), posits that each individual has an innate internal hierarchy of needs that motivate all human behaviors. This theory includes a stair-step hierarchy that begins with physiological needs, such as biological integrity; moves through safety, security, belonging, and self-esteem; and ends with self-actualization. A baby has to maintain his or her biological and physiological integrity, and then moves along the steps to the need for protection and attachment (safety) while acquiring self-esteem. It is at this final stage of self-actualization that the adult strives to achieve self-direction, have satisfying relationships with others, and maintain a sense of values.

Jung's Theory of Individualism

In this theory by Carl Jung (1960), a person's personality is visualized as oriented toward either the external or internal world. People are viewed as either extroverted or introverted. Jung posits that, in middle life, an individual begins questioning his or her life and unattained goals. The popular term *mid-life crisis* came into vogue with this theory.

Jung's theory suggests that this "crisis" is actually just a rite of passage along the continuum of successful aging. Jung suggests that, as human beings age, we become more inwardly focused, and can value the self despite physical limitations or losses. People should be able to accept themselves as they are, accentuating past accomplishments, not limitations.

Erikson's Eight Stages of Life

This developmental theory, developed by Erik Erikson (1950), focuses on a life span approach from birth to death. The seventh and eighth stages of generativity versus self-absorption, and stagnation and ego-integrity versus despair, pertain to the older adult.

Generativity is referred to as the process of being productive in life, and it begins around 45–65 years of age, or middle adulthood. This time is when one looks toward contributing to the next generation as opposed to being absorbed in and preoccupied with one's own personal well-being. Adults older than age 65 have integrated egos if they can look back with a sense of satisfaction and acceptance of life. Those who despair are individuals with unresolved conflicts who view their lives as a series of misfortunes, disappointments, and failures.

Peck's Expansion of Erikson's Theory

In 1968, M. Scott Peck expanded upon Erikson's eighth stage of older adulthood. Peck believed that, because people were living longer, this eighth stage of life should be further subdivided. He believed that this ego-integrity-versus-despair stage should be assessed in three parts: (1) ego differentiation versus work role preoccupation, (2) body transcendence versus body preoccupation, and (3) ego transcendence versus ego preoccupation.

In the first stage, the older person's task is to achieve feelings of worth and self-significance from areas other than work. During the second stage, the older person's task is to adjust to the declines in physical self that can occur with age; this stage can be achieved if the person has satisfying interpersonal and social activities.

The final stage involves the older adult accepting that death is inevitable, but not dwelling on it. Believing that there is a future beyond one's mortality helps one achieve this task of aging.

Selective Optimization With Compensation

P. B. Baltes (1987) credited with developing this theory, which focuses on the individual developing certain strategies to manage and adapt to the losses—both physical and emotional— that accompany older age. There are three elements in this adaptive framework: (1) selection, (2) optimization, and (3) compensation.

A person self-selects the domain of function that he or she knows best, optimizes that function, and compensates using these components. Baltes theorizes that older individuals can age successfully with declining function.

NURSING THEORIES

Since Florence Nightingale, many nurses have developed theoretical frameworks to guide nursing practice. Some prominent nursing theories that can be related to the aging process include:

- ▶ Orem's Self-Care
- ▶ Rogers's Force Field
- ▶ Roy's Adaptation Model

Orem's Self-Care Theory

Dorothea Orem's theory of nursing (1991) describes patients as self-care participants. Orem suggests that the role of the nurse is to help patients achieve the self-care skills needed to promote health, enhance recovery from disease, and facilitate a peaceful death.

This theory is helpful in planning care for older people because it focuses on maintaining independence while adapting to the changes of aging. This theory allows the older person to retain control and physical functioning, which would be lost if the nurse did not include the person in the caregiving process.

Rogers's Force Field Theory

Martha Rogers's force field theory (1970) defines a patient as a force field that interacts with other energy sources in the environment. The nurse is responsible for promoting synergistic actions that promote the patient's health. Older adults are forces to be dealt with in the healthcare environment. The nurse establishes the synergy among the many resources and programs that maintain the health and well-being of the older adult.

Roy's Adaptation Theory

Sister Callista Roy (1984) posited that patients are in constant contact with a dynamic environment. The adaptation theory states that the goal of nursing is to promote patients' innate and acquired mechanisms for adaptation to health and illness.

All of these theories have implications for nursing in developing appropriate interventions, planning activities, and promoting acceptance of chronic illness.

OTHER THEORETICAL CONSIDERATIONS

Gerontological nurses often advocate for their clients who transfer into and out of many facilities. Often they must advocate for them not only within their practice setting, but also in the community. Several theoretical models may assist them in the care of their older patients. Gerontological nurses should be familiar with these prominent models:

▶ Change Theory

▶ Conflict Resolution

▶ Adult Education Theory

Change Theory

Classic change theory was first introduced by sociologist Kurt Lewin in 1951. He sees behavior as a force that is dynamic, working in balance yet in opposite directions within an organization. Lewin discusses unfreezing, which moves people toward change; the actual process of change; and refreezing, which involves integrating the desired change.

Lewin describes force field analysis, which is identifying the need for a change, deciding what actions are needed to bring about the change, and then identifying moving and restraining forces within the organization or system. His research also elaborates on the many reasons that people and organizations are resistant to change, such as maintaining the status quo, lack of information, and perceived cost of the change. Recognizing that change in organizations and in people's behaviors is often a difficult task will enable gerontological nurses to use Lewin's ideas to provide better care for elderly patients.

Conflict Resolution

Gerontological nurses should recognize that conflict is a natural occurrence that can be beneficial. There are many reasons for a conflict to occur: attitudes, perception of scarce rewards, task interdependence, and power variances between two people.

Avoidance, compromise, forcing, collaboration, confrontation, and smoothing are ways to resolve conflict. Avoidance and smoothing are passive, while confrontation (used most widely) is active. Once the problem is assessed and identified, it must be addressed in an organized manner. Then, direct confrontation can be operationalized through collaboration and agreement on key issues (Epstein, Borrell, & Catarina, 2000). In gerontological nursing, decisions often are made by multiple professionals with caregivers or family of older adults. Resolving divergent opinions and conflicts is essential to arriving at a reasonable and ethical caring intervention.

Adult Learning Theory

According to Anderson (2001), this theory is based on the belief that adults learn differently from children. Adults are self-directed and are interested in information that will benefit them. Depending on the information being shared, the nurse may use a wide variety of teaching methods.

Behavioral therapy is appropriate for enhancing psychomotor skills and changing or stopping habits, such as smoking cessation. Cognitive therapy is useful for skills or lifestyle changes. Humanistic therapy helps with self-reflection and study to make major life changes.

Learning styles are the ways people absorb new information; they vary from person to person. Principles related to learning styles include:

▶ The learning styles of teacher and learner should be identified.

▶ Teachers should be cautioned against using their preferred style.

▶ A teacher is most effective when using the learner's style.

▶ Different learning styles should be encouraged in all learners.

▶ Learning styles can be learned and developed with practice and some direction by both the teacher and learner.

Some key points that the gerontological nurse should remember when teaching the older client are:

▶ New learning should relate to what the client already knows.

▶ Environmental factors affect the learning process (e.g., lighting, background noise, too much stimuli).

▶ The teacher must consider the motivation and desire of the learner to obtain the new information.

▶ The learner should be in control of what and how much is learned in each session.

▶ Ability to learn should always be considered (e.g., literacy in terms of reading, comprehension, problem-solving and application abilities).

▶ Congruence of language is important for successful adult learning (i.e., for the older person's understanding of the information that the teacher is trying to communicate should there be a language barrier).

▶ Physical wellness or illness can affect what the learner can learn.

▶ The physical environment should be comfortable.

Older adults, like younger people, want new and pertinent information. Nurses with special expertise in geriatrics have an obligation to keep abreast of the most pertinent and appropriate ways to teach older clients. An abundance of senior-focused education programs exist, and nurses should share these resources with patients as applicable (see Table 4–1).

TABLE 4–1.
SENIOR-FOCUSED EDUCATION WEB SITES

PROGRAM	WEB SITE	DESCRIPTION
RoadScholar (formerly Elderhostel)	http://www.roadscholar.org/	Nonprofit learning organization and travel adventure for people age 55 and older
Administration on Aging	http://www.aoa.gov	Overview of topics, programs, and services related to aging
USA.gov – government made easy for seniors	http://www.usa.gov/Topics/Seniors.shtml	Official U.S. site for all government information specific to seniors
OASIS	http://www.oasisnet.org/	Health information site for older adults; programs in the arts, humanities, wellness, and community service
Senior Net	http://www.seniornet.org	Nonprofit organization of computer resources for older adults; the purpose is to educate older adults about computer technologies

To teach older adults effectively, it is important to keep some basics in mind. Begin by assessing the sensory function and psychological state of the older adult. Areas to consider include:

▶ *Decreased vision:* These older adults will have difficulty reading educational materials.

▶ *Decreased hearing:* These older patients will have difficulty hearing instructions and may not ask questions.

▶ *Impaired cognitive ability:* These older patients may not understand or remember verbal instructions.

▶ *Depression:* These older patients may lack the motivation to participate actively in their health care.

▶ *Stress:* These older patients may not be able to process information and focus their attention in order to learn effectively.

▶ *Chronic illness:* These older patients may be uncomfortable or in physical distress, or lack the physical stamina to concentrate and process information.

To achieve a successful outcome, teachers should attempt to compensate for such issues.

COMMUNICATION

Whenever interacting with older clients, it is important to respect the communication issues that are relevant to this population:

▶ Confidentiality

▶ Therapeutic techniques

▶ Interviewing techniques

▶ Written communication

▶ Communication barriers

Confidentiality

Respecting confidentiality is critical with any type of patient interaction, regardless of the patient's age. Nurses must ensure privacy when discussing sensitive issues and should ask the patient if he or she prefers to discuss healthcare concerns alone or in the presence of family or significant others.

In addition, it is imperative to follow Health Insurance Portability and Accountability Act (HIPAA) guidelines in every patient encounter. In the field of gerontology, it is not uncommon to interface with family members and other care providers. The patient's wishes for exchange of information must be respected at all times.

Therapeutic Techniques

Good communication should be based on sound adult learning theory principles, as described above. However, therapeutic communication is more that just the spoken word; it also includes nonverbal communication, such as eye contact, tone of voice, rate of speech, facial gestures, and body posture.

Therapeutic communication between nurses and older patients is goal-oriented and designed to promote growth in the older patient. The basic components of therapeutic communication include trust, respect, rapport, genuineness, and empathy. The gerontological nurse should engage in the therapeutic use of self, which involves the use of one's personality consciously and in full awareness, in an attempt to establish relatedness and to structure nursing interventions (Epstein, Borrell, & Caterina, 2000). The gerontological nurse must be confident in his or her abilities and be willing to engage in conversations with older adults regarding life, death, pain, suffering, illness, and health as components of the human condition (Epstein, Borrell, & Caterina, 2000). The rushed or distracted nurse will send a signal that he or she is not really interested in what the older patient is saying.

It is also extremely important for the nurse to be an active and effective listener. Several nonverbal behaviors have been designed to facilitate attentive listening:

- ▶ **S**—Sit squarely facing the older adult
- ▶ **O**—Observe an open posture
- ▶ **L**—Lean forward toward the older adult
- ▶ **E**—Establish eye contact
- ▶ **R**—Relax (Epstein, Borrell, & Caterina, 2000)

Interviewing Techniques

Communication and interviewing older people can be facilitated by paying attention to basic principles of conversation. Virginia Satir (1976) believed that the following are critical to facilitating communication with another person:

- ▶ Invite
- ▶ Arrange environment
- ▶ Maximize communication
- ▶ Maximize understanding
- ▶ Follow through

An invitation suggests that we are interested in having another person present and with us. Using the invitation approach can be demonstrated by greeting the patient and asking him or her an informal and nonthreatening question, such as, "What brought you into the clinic today?"

The second technique, which is critical with gerontological clients, centers on making the environment conducive to the interaction. The environment should be comfortable, private, and have minimal distractions (see the information on adult learning theory).

The third technique is to use communication techniques that ensure the patient can understand the message. Use age-appropriate language; avoid using medical jargon that the patient cannot relate to; show respect for the client by calling him or her by his or her surname; and avoid using patronizing terms, such as "honey" or "sweetie." The nurse should ask the patient to clarify what he or she is hearing to ensure that the patient understands what is being asked or shared.

The next technique involves maximizing the patient's understanding by being open-minded and a good listener. The patient must be allowed to share his or her thoughts and feelings during the interview.

The final stage of therapeutic interviewing involves follow-through. Giving the patient actions to take that support what the nurse has said during the interview adds credibility to the nurse–patient relationship, which is important for positive health outcomes.

Written Communication

Most of those who work exclusively with geriatric clients recognize the value of writing down information and instructions. Written communication between patient and nurse becomes increasingly vital if the patient has memory impairment, aphasia, dysarthria, and hearing or vision impairments.

Patients with mild cognitive deficits may be able to compensate for memory loss with written reminders and instructions, especially in the early stages of deficits and with good family and social support. Patients with speech impairments, such as aphasia or dysarthria, may come to rely on written communication to meet their needs or get answers to questions.

Patients with a hearing impairment often pose some communication difficulty. It may not be possible to correct the hearing deficit, so written communication becomes vital. Patients with a vision impairment may or may not be able to use written communication to facilitate positive health outcomes because the patient may be, more often than not, legally blind (as opposed to totally blind). Glaucoma, cataracts, and age-related macular degeneration will impair a part of vision, but a person may retain certain parts of the vision field. For these patients, written communication, done in large dark block letters, can augment communication.

In addition, be aware of basic literacy principles and be certain that the patient can read the language used in written communication.

Communication Barriers

This category can apply to all types of communication. The adult learning theory section presents some physical barriers that might interfere with communication involving the older adult. Other areas to consider include:

▶ Poor listening habits

▶ Distractions

▶ Inconsistent verbal and nonverbal cues

▶ Credibility issues

▶ Lack of time

▶ Work pace that does not allow for proper therapeutic communication

▶ Harsh or indifferent tone of voice

▶ Biases from the nurse or patient

This is only a partial list, but it suggests items that can interfere with successful communication with older clients.

REFERENCES

Anderson, M. M. (2001). Communication process. In A. S. Luggen & S. E. Meiner (Eds.), *NGNA: Core curriculum for gerontological nursing* (pp. 36–38). St. Louis, MO: Mosby.

Baltes, P. B. (1987). *Life-span development and behavior.* New York: Lawrence Erlbaum.

Carrascosa, J., Ros, M., Andres, A., Fernandez-Agullo, T., & Arribas, T. (2009). Changes in the neuroendocrine control of homeostasis by adiposity signals during aging. *Experimental Gerontology, 44*(1), 20–26.

Epstein, F., Borrell, F., & Caterina, M. (2000). *Therapeutic communication in psychiatric nursing. Open access articles on mental health.* Retrieved from http://nursingplanet.com/pn/therapeutic_communication.html

Erikson, E. (1950). *Childhood and society.* New York: W.W. Norton.

Havighurst, R. J. (1972). *Developmental tasks and education.* New York: David McKay.

Havighurst, R. J., Neugarten, B. L., & Tobin, S. S. (1963). Disengagement, personality, and life satisfaction in later years. In P. Hanson (Ed.), *Age with a future* (pp. 201–209). Copenhagen, Denmark: Munksgaard.

Hayflick, L. (1996). *How and why we age.* New York: Ballantine Books.

Huether, S., & McCance, K. (2012). *Understanding pathophysiology.* St. Louis, MO: Elsevier Mosby.

Jin, K. (2010). Modern biological theories. *Aging Diseases, 1*(2), 72–74.

Jung, C. (1960). *The state of life in collected works: Vol. 8. The structure and dynamics of the psyche.* New York: Pantheon Books.

Lawton, M. P. (1982). Competence, environmental pressure, and the adaptation of older people. In M. P. Lawton, P. G. Windley, & T. O. Byers (Eds.), *Aging and the environment: Theoretical approaches* (pp. 65–76). New York: Springer.

Lewin, K. (1951). *Field theory in social science.* New York: Harper & Row.

Maslow, A. (1943). A theory of human motivation. *Psychological Review, 50,* 370–396.

Orem, D. (1991). *Nursing: Concepts of practice.* St. Louis, MO: Mosby-Year Book, Inc.

Peck, P. (1968). Psychological development in the second half of life. In B. Neugarten (Ed.), *Middle age and aging* (pp. 37–49). Chicago: University of Chicago Press.

Rogers, M. (1970). *Theoretical basis of nursing.* New York: F. A. Davis, Co.

Roy, C. (1984). *Introduction to nursing: Adaptation model.* Upper Saddle River, NJ: Prentice Hall.

Riley, M. W. (1985). Age strata in social systems. In R. H. Binstock & E. Shanas (Eds.), *Handbook of aging and the social sciences* (pp. 55–70). New York: Van Nostrand Reinhold.

Satir, V. (1976). *Making contact.* Berkeley, CA: Celestial Arts.

Sonneborn, T. (1979). The origin, evolution, nature, and causes of aging. In J. Behnke, C. E. Finch, & C. Moment (Eds.), *The biology of aging* (pp. 7–27). New York: Plenum Books.

ADDITIONAL RESOURCES

American Association of Retired Persons: www.aarp.org

American Society on Aging: www.asaging.org

Association for Gerontology in Higher Education: www.aghe.org

National Assessments of Adult Literacy: www.nces.ed.gov

National Institute on Aging: www.nia.nih.gov/health

Osher Lifelong Learning Institute at George Mason University: www.olli.gmu.edu

GERONTOLOGICAL NURSING ISSUES

The Standards of Professional Nursing Practice (American Nurses Association [ANA], 2010b) constitutes the authoritative set of the duties that all registered nurses, regardless of role, population, or specialty, are expected to perform competently. The standards may be used as evidence that care is provided as required, with the understanding that application of the standards depends on the context in which the care is being delivered. The standards are subject to change with the dynamics of the nursing profession, as new patterns of professional practice are developed and accepted by the nursing profession and the public. The standards are subject to formal, periodic review and revision.

STANDARDS OF GERONTOLOGICAL NURSING

The *Standards of Clinical Gerontological Nursing Care* (ANA, 2010a) describes the necessary competencies of care for each step of the nursing process, including assessment, diagnosis, outcome identification, planning, implementation, and evaluation. These competencies are the essential foundation of the actions taken by gerontological nurses when caring for their patients.

These standards enable the nursing profession to identify and meet the professional responsibility to deliver high-quality patient care to older people. Performance standards are defined, and each includes measurement criteria.

▶ **Standard I: Assessment. The gerontological nurse collects patient health data.**

> » **Rationale:** Interviewing, functional assessment, environmental assessment, physical assessment, and review of health records enhance the nurse's ability to make sound clinical judgments. Assessment is culturally and ethnically appropriate.

▶ **Standard II: Diagnosis. The gerontological nurse analyzes the assessment data in determining diagnosis.**

> » **Rationale:** The gerontological nurse, either independently or in collaboration with interdisciplinary care providers, evaluates health assessment data to develop comprehensive diagnoses that form the basis for care interventions.

▶ **Standard III: Outcome identification. The gerontological nurse identifies expected outcomes individualized to the older adult.**

> » **Rationale:** The ultimate goals of providing gerontological nursing care are to influence health outcomes and improve or maintain the aging person's health status. Outcomes often focus on maximizing the aging person's state of well-being, functional status, and quality of life.

▶ **Standard IV: Planning. The gerontological nurse develops a plan of care that prescribes interventions to attain expected outcomes.**

> » **Rationale:** A plan of care structures and guides therapeutic interventions and achieves expected outcomes. It is developed in conjunction with the older adult, his or her significant others, and interdisciplinary team members.

▶ **Standard V: Implementation. The gerontological nurse implements the interventions identified in the plan of care.**

> » **Rationale:** The gerontological nurse uses a wide range of culturally competent direct and indirect interventions designed for health promotion, health maintenance, prevention of illness, health restoration, rehabilitation, and palliation. The gerontological nurse implements the plan of care in collaboration with the older adult and others. The gerontological nurse selects evidence-based interventions according to his or her level of education and practice when available.

▶ **Standard VI: Evaluation. The gerontological nurse evaluates the older adult's progress toward attainment of expected outcomes.**

> » **Rationale:** Nursing practice is a dynamic and evolving process. The gerontological nurse continually evaluates the older adult's responses to treatment and interventions. Collecting new data, revising the database, changing nursing diagnoses, and modifying the plan of care are often essential. The effectiveness of nursing care depends on ongoing evaluation.

As health care continues to evolve, new roles have emerged for gerontological nurses. In addition to the traditional role of clinical practitioner, gerontological nurses also may serve in the roles of patient advocate, nurse educator, nurse manager, nurse consultant, and nurse researcher (ANA, 2010a).

▶ *Advocate:* Advances the rights of older persons and educates others about negative stereotypes of aging.

▶ *Educator:* Organizes and provides instructions about healthy aging, disease detection, treatment of disease, and rehabilitation to older patients and their families. Also participates in inservice education, continuing education, and training ancillary personnel as appropriate.

▶ *Manager:* Maintains current relevant information about federal and state regulations, and provides nursing leadership in a variety of healthcare settings.

▶ *Consultant:* Consults with and advises others who are providing nursing care to older patients with complex healthcare problems. Participates in developing clinical pathways and quality assurance standards and implementing evidence-based practices.

▶ *Researcher:* Collaborates with established researchers in developing clinically based studies, assists with data collection and identifying appropriate research sites, communicates relevant research findings to others, and participates in presenting findings at gerontological conferences and in publications.

Because they view patients holistically, nurses are in an ideal position to serve in these roles. Helping patients achieve their optimal levels of physical, mental, and psychosocial well-being is the primary goal of gerontological nurses.

Components of Comprehensive Geriatric Assessment

Despite variations in instruments, structure of the interdisciplinary team, and methods used, several strategies have been proven to make the evaluation process more effective. These include the development of a close-knit interdisciplinary team with minimal redundancy in the assessments performed, the use of carefully designed questionnaires that reliable older patients or their caregivers can complete beforehand, and the effective use of assessment forms that are incorporated into computer databases (Reuben et al., 2011).

Three underlying principles of comprehensive geriatric assessment are that (Reuben et al., 2011):

1. Physical, psychological, and socioeconomic factors interact in complex ways to influence the health and functional status of the older person.

2. Comprehensive evaluation of an older adult's health status requires an assessment in each of the following domains:

   ▹ Physical status: Medical diagnoses, medications, nutrition, dentition, hearing, vision, pain, continence, functional ability, balance and gait, falls

   ▹ Cognitive status: Mood, mental, and spiritual status

    » Environmental status: Social and financial status, environmental hazards

    ▶ Care preferences for life-sustaining treatments and establishment of advance directives

3. Functional abilities should be a central focus of the comprehensive evaluation. Other more traditional measures of health, such as medical diagnosis, nursing diagnosis, physical examination results, and laboratory findings, form the basic foundation of the assessment to determine overall health, well-being, and the need for social services.

The interrelationships among the physical, social, and psychological aspects of aging and, perhaps, illness present a challenge to gerontological nurses when beginning geriatric evaluations. Gerontological nurses often are charged with the responsibility of obtaining a history of a patient's past health and present illness. Contextual variables that should be considered in obtaining those histories include evaluation of the environment, accuracy of the health history, communication difficulties, underreporting of symptoms, vague or nonspecific complaints, multiple complaints, lack of time, social history, psychological history, home environment, and culture and education.

Evaluation Environment. To make the older patient and family comfortable, modifications may be made to the evaluation environment. These include adequate lighting, decreased background noise, comfortable seating, easily accessible restrooms, examination tables that can be raised or lowered as needed, and availability of water or juice. Patient comfort will ease communication and improve the data-gathering process.

Accuracy of the Health History. Before the healthcare visit, clear instructions should be given to the older patient and family about parking arrangements and the registration process. Many assessment clinics mail information packets in advance, so the patient can come prepared. This packet might include:

▶ A past medical history form, which can be completed at home and is helpful for older patients with complicated medical histories. The dates of hospitalizations, operations, serious injuries or accidents, procedures, and so on can be ascertained beforehand to save time during the assessment appointment. The form also would include history of adverse drug effects or allergies.

▶ Instructions to bring in all prescription and over-the-counter medications for review by the gerontological nurse.

▶ Instructions to bring any medical records, laboratory or X-ray reports, electrocardiograms, reports of vaccinations, and other pertinent health records.

▶ Instructions to write down and bring the names of all healthcare providers involved with the patient's health care, including primary care providers, specialists, and alternative medicine practitioners (e.g., acupuncturists, massage therapists, chiropractors).

The more information that older patients and their family can organize ahead of time, the better and more efficient the assessment will be. Patience is necessary when obtaining a history, because the thought and verbal processes are often slower in older adults. Older patients should be allowed adequate time to answer questions and report information (Kane et al., 2004).

The history should include emphasis on the following:

► Review of acute and chronic medical problems

► List of medications

► Disease prevention and health maintenance review (e.g., vaccinations, PPD [tuberculosis], cancer screenings)

► Functional status (e.g., activities of daily living [ADLs])

► Social supports (e.g., family, caregiver stress, safety of living environment)

► Finances

► Driving status and safety record

► Geriatric review of symptoms (e.g., patient/family perception of memory, dentition, taste, smell, nutrition, hearing, vision, falls, fractures, bowel and bladder function)

► Care preferences and advance directives (Kane et al., 2004)

Often, a standardized form is used to guide and direct the obtaining of health history. Gerontological nurses should be aware of potential difficulties in obtaining health histories from older adults (Reuben et al., 2011):

► *Communication difficulties:* Decreased hearing or vision, slow speech, and use of English as a second language can affect communication.

► *Underreporting of symptoms:* Fear of being labeled as a complainer, fear of institutionalization, and fear of serious illness can influence symptom reporting.

► *Vague or nonspecific complaints:* These may be associated with cognitive impairment, drug or alcohol use or abuse, or atypical presentation of disease.

► *Multiple complaints:* Associated "masked" depression, presence of multiple chronic illnesses, and social isolation often are an older adult's cry for help.

► *Lack of time:* Short appointments will result in a hurried interview with missed information. New patients scheduled for geriatric assessment should have a minimum of a 1-hour appointment with the gerontological nurse.

► *Social history:* Holistic evaluation is not complete without an assessment of the social support system. Many frail older adults receive support and supervision from family members and significant others to compensate for functional disabilities.

Key elements of the social history include the following:

- ► Past occupation and retirement status
- ► Family history (helpful to construct a family genogram)
- ► Present and former marital status, including quality of the relationship(s)
- ► Identification of family members, with designation of level of involvement and place of residence
- ► Living arrangements
- ► Family dynamics
- ► Family and caregiver expectations
- ► Economic status, adequacy of health insurance
- ► Social activities and hobbies
- ► Mode of transportation
- ► Community involvement and support
- ► Religious involvement and spirituality

Older adults who exhibit symptoms of sadness, social isolation, questioning of their existence, feeling they are being punished by God, or asking about availability of religious or spiritual counseling should be asked if they would like help with their spiritual concerns. Religion and spirituality can be a great source of hope and strength in times of need and crisis. Many healthcare facilities and community agencies have access to religious and spiritual counselors who can meet with older adults and their families if there is need and the older adult does not have an ongoing relationship with a priest, minister, rabbi, or spiritual counselor.

Psychological History. A significant proportion of older adults with mental illness remain unrecognized and untreated; when treated, their use of healthcare services decreases (Health Resources and Services Administration, 2008). The reported range of adults ages 65 or older with mental disorders, both in institutions and in the community, is estimated to be between 20% and 30%.

Mental and emotional problems are not a normal part of aging. Mental health problems that manifest themselves in older adults should be evaluated, diagnosed, and treated. By forming a trusting therapeutic relationship, gerontological nurses can demonstrate caring, warmth, respect, and support for an older adult who may be hesitant to verbalize feelings of low self-esteem, depression, bizarre thought patterns, or phobias and anxieties.

Key elements of the psychological history include

▶ Any history of past mental illness

▶ Any hospitalizations or outpatient treatments for psychological problems

▶ Current and past stress levels and coping mechanisms

▶ Current and past levels of alcohol or recreational drug use

▶ Medications taken for anxiety, insomnia, or depression

▶ Identification of any problems with memory, judgment, or thought processing

▶ Any changes in personality, values, personal habits, or life satisfaction

▶ Identification of feelings regarding self-worth and hopes for the future

▶ Feelings of appropriate emotions related to present life and health situation (e.g., feelings of sadness about losses)

▶ Presence of someone to love, support, and encourage the older patient

▶ Feelings of hopelessness or suicidal ideation (Health Resources and Services Administration, 2008)

The accuracy of the health history and identification of problems depend on adequate mental and affective functioning. The higher the level of cognitive impairment, the more likely the older patient is to report inaccurate information. Problems with short-term memory can cause older adults to forget to report adverse events such as falls, safety issues in the home, or other relevant problems that could influence the plan of care. Further, depressed older patients may score poorly on instruments used to assess psychological function because they do not have the energy or motivation to concentrate or answer questions. These older adults continuously appear sad and say "I don't know" or "I couldn't tell you" when responding to questions.

There are benefits to interviewing older adults with and without the family or significant others present. Some older patients will confide difficulties to the gerontological nurse in private that they may be hesitant to report in the presence of family. These issues may encompass family dynamics, sexuality, bowel and bladder function, or other personal concerns. Many older patients are hesitant to complain when their family is present because they are afraid to be seen as critical or to be labeled as a complainer or incompetent.

On the other hand, family can assist in obtaining an accurate health history for older patients with memory impairments. A good strategy is to seek permission from an older patient to include the family to verify or gather additional information. Older patients with depression may feel demoralized and be unable to take part in rehabilitation or health promotion activities because of lack of energy and motivation (Health Resources and Services Administration, 2008). Family members and involved caregivers often can report subtle changes in personality and function that may go undetected by others.

Instruments commonly used in clinical practice to assess psychological function include the following:

▶ *Geriatric Depression Scale:* The short form includes 15 questions and measures depression in the older adult. A score of > 5 for the responses in bold is suggestive of depression and indicates the need for further screening (Kurlowicz & Greenberg, 2007; Yesavage & Brink, 1983).

▶ *The Mini-Cog:* The Mini-Cog tests cognition, using three-item recall and a clock-drawing test. It takes about 3 minutes to administer and is not affected by language, education, or culture. The tool can differentiate older people with dementia from those without dementia (Borson, Scanlan, Chen, & Ganguli, 2003; Doerflinger, 2007).

▶ *Home Environment:* Some geriatric assessment teams have the time and resources to visit older patients' homes and conduct assessments of the environment. While this direct observation is the best way to gather accurate and reliable data, it is time-consuming and can be expensive. Therefore, many geriatric assessment teams question the older adult and the family regarding the adequacy of the home environment and the resources available to maintain adequate levels of function.

Factors to be considered when assessing the home environment include:

▶ *Stairs:* Narrow stairs with poor lighting, inadequate railings, and uneven steps are fall risks. Does the older adult have the strength and balance to climb stairs? If a wheelchair or walker is used, are there ramps, or space for them to be added?

▶ *Bathing and toileting:* Can the older adult safely move on and off the toilet? Is a raised toilet seat needed? Are grab bars present? Is there an adequate bathmat in the tub? Is a shower seat needed? Is lighting adequate?

▶ *Medications:* Where are medications stored? Are there grandchildren in the home who are at risk because of open storage or nonreplacement of caps? Are old and outdated medications disposed of to prevent accidents? Are medications refilled on time to prevent on-off dosing patterns? Is a list of medications available for emergencies?

▶ *Advance directives:* Has the older adult named a healthcare proxy or established a living will? If so, does the family and primary care provider have a copy? Is the proxy knowledgeable about the patient's preferences? Is the proxy's contact information posted in an easily visible position (e.g., on the refrigerator)? Does it specify the value or quality of life or length of life?

▶ *Nutrition and cooking:* Is there adequate food in the home? Is there a working stove or microwave oven? Are any safety problems associated with the stove or microwave? If a gas stove is used, is it safe? Is the pilot light functioning properly? Are there gas leak detectors? Is food storage adequate? Is spoiled food present? Is the food preparation environment clean? Who does the grocery shopping? How are trash and garbage disposed of?

▶ *Falls:* Are the floors free of cords, debris, and scatter rugs? Is there adequate lighting? Are there nightlights? Are there pets that dart around quickly? If there is a history of falls, would the older adult consider wearing an emergency alert system around his or her neck?

▶ *Smoke detectors:* Are there functioning smoke detectors? Are batteries changed yearly?

▶ *Emergency numbers:* Are emergency telephone numbers posted or preprogrammed into the phone?

▶ *Temperature of home:* Is there adequate heat in the winter and cooling in the summer?

▶ *Temperature of water:* Is the hot water set below 120° F?

▶ *Safety of the neighborhood:* Can the older person venture outside without fear of becoming a crime victim? Are there adequate door locks and latches? How close is the nearest neighbor? Is there nearby help if it is needed?

▶ *Financial:* Are there stacks of unpaid bills? Are services such as phone and electricity in good working order? Are there large amounts of cash hidden or stored around the house? Is there adequate money to purchase nutritious food?

The increasing need for healthcare providers to care for older adults from diverse backgrounds means that gerontological nurses must consider how assessment and development of a treatment plan may need to be modified to avoid misunderstandings or ineffective care. Be cautious about drawing conclusions from test scores that are derived from patients of different cultures and various educational backgrounds (Spector, 2008).

Some instruments, such as the Mini-Mental State Exam (Folstein, Folstein, & McHugh, 1975), have developed and validated scoring norms based on level of education. This examination has a component dependent on reading a sentence and following instructions, writing a sentence, performing complex mathematical calculations, and spelling a word backward. Older patients may be reticent to tell a healthcare provider that they are unable to read or write and may score poorly as a result—low scores could be attributed falsely to cognitive impairment, rather than low reading literacy. Gerontological nurses should always consider and assess educational level, language barriers, reading levels, and cultural background before using standardized instruments.

To provide culturally appropriate care, it is important to understand and elicit the beliefs, attitudes, values, and goals of older adults relating to their lives, illness, and health states. Cultural competence in healthcare consists of several components (Spector, 2008):

▶ Knowing the prevalence, incidence, and risk factors (epidemiology) for diseases in different ethnic groups

▶ Understanding how response to medications and other treatments varies with ethnicity

▶ Eliciting the culturally held beliefs and attitudes toward illness, treatment, and the healthcare system

▶ Keeping an open mind and approaching each older adult as a unique individual

To avoid stereotypical thinking, it is important to recognize that heterogeneity exists within various ethnic groups, and providing culturally sensitive care dictates that each person be approached as a unique individual. A patient's age, place of birth, where his or her childhood was spent, and how he or she was socialized to American culture all can affect performance on standardized assessment instruments. Many of the instruments used by clinicians to assess older patients have not been validated for use with cultural minorities (Spector, 2008). The members of some ethnic groups are less willing to report difficulty in taking care of themselves and may fear admitting their dependence on others.

After completing an assessment and reaching appropriate nursing diagnoses, the gerontological nurse formulates a plan of care, with the goal being to individualize the plan to reflect the older adult's values. The overall goals of nursing care are to influence health outcomes, improve or maintain the older patient's health status, or provide comfort care at the end of life. Gerontological nurses often will focus on improving a patient's quality of life, improving functional status, and promoting well-being.

The clarity and achievability of the goals of nursing care are critical to the development of an effective plan of care. These goals should:

▶ Be linked to the nursing diagnoses

▶ Be mutually formulated with the older adult, family, and interdisciplinary team whenever possible

▶ Be culturally appropriate

▶ Be attainable given available resources and the care setting

▶ Include a time frame for attainment

▶ Adequately reflect associated benefits and costs

▶ Provide direction for continuity of care

▶ Be measurable (ANA, 2010b)

A first step is to assign priority to the problems diagnosed. Problems with high priority include those that have a potential for immediately negatively affecting health status, those of concern to the older patient and the family, and those that negatively affect function and quality of life. Other problems can be deferred and addressed at a later time—patients can become overwhelmed when well-meaning healthcare providers attempt to do too much for them at one time. Some problems that need immediate attention can be resolved by nursing interventions, and some require referral to other people, including family members, nursing colleagues, or members of the interdisciplinary healthcare team. A well-functioning team demands that the participants take into account the contributions of other team members and communicate effectively in all phases of the care-planning process (Health Resources and Services Administration, 2008).

Another critical issue in goal formulation is the ability of gerontological nurses to set realistic and achievable goals. When nurses set goals that are unattainable, it sets up patients for failure. Once older patients feel they have failed to meet the goals established by their healthcare providers, they may not keep follow-up appointments, may become depressed and blame themselves for being weak or lazy, or may manufacture excuses to protect themselves from criticism.

After the goals of care have been carefully selected, gerontological nurses will choose appropriate direct and indirect interventions in collaboration with older adults, family (if appropriate), and the interdisciplinary care team. The nursing profession must identify its unique focus and demonstrate accountability in terms of that focus. The nursing interventions identified in the nursing care plan demonstrate that accountability and communicate to the nursing staff the particular problems of older patients and the prescribed interventions for directing and evaluating the care being given (Carpenito, 2009). The interventions are selected on the basis of the needs, desires, and resources of older adults and accepted nursing practice (ANA, 2010a).

Appropriate nursing interventions may include the following:

- Assisting older patients to a higher level of function or self-care
- Identifying health promotion activities
- Identifying disease-prevention and screening activities
- Teaching health practices and habits
- Counseling
- Seeking consultation
- Collecting data on an ongoing basis; refining the initial nursing assessment
- Exploring treatment choices, including pharmacological and nonpharmacological options
- Implementing palliative care and holistic care of patients who are dying or seriously ill
- Referring patients to community resources
- Managing patients' cases
- Evaluating and educating ancillary caregivers and family (ANA, 2010a)

Nursing interventions will be selected based on the following:

- Linkage to the desired outcome
- Characteristics of the nursing diagnosis
- Strength of the research associated with the intervention
- Probability of successfully implementing the intervention
- Acceptability of the intervention to the older patient and others involved in the plan of care
- Assurance that the intervention is safe, ethical, culturally competent, and appropriate
- Documentation of the intervention
- Knowledge, skills, experience, and creativity of the nurse (ANA, 2010b; Carpenito, 2009)

Gerontological nurses choose appropriate nursing interventions on the basis of their knowledge of practice and the supports available in the practice environment. In the dependent role, nurses will implement physician's orders according to safe and acceptable standards of practice. Administration of treatments, medications, therapeutic diets, and preparation for diagnostic testing usually will be specified in writing for implementation by the nursing staff. In the independent role, nurses will establish and implement nursing actions to carry out the nursing care plan. The goal of the nursing action is to direct individualized care to older patients and prescribe care to prevent, reduce, or eliminate the actual or potential problem identified in the nursing diagnosis.

During implementation of the nursing intervention, gerontological nurses will carefully monitor patient response, the responses of others involved in the care delivery, achievement of the outcome, alternative interventions that may supplement or replace the specified interventions, the accuracy and safety of the intervention, the competency of others in delivering the care, and validation of the appropriateness of the intervention (Carpenito, 2009). Nursing interventions can be added, deleted, or modified as part of the ongoing process of providing individualized care.

Evaluation is the final component of the nursing process, and gerontological nurses will undertake a systematic and ongoing process to compare patient response to the activities identified in the nursing care plan to the established outcome criteria. Nurses will seek input from the patient, family, and others involved in the care.

It is important to consider information from the physical, social, and psychological assessment of the patient; information from diagnostic testing; level of satisfaction with care; and documentation of the costs and benefits associated with the treatment. The initial assessment and nursing diagnosis may be revised with new goals and nursing interventions specified if appropriate: the problem has been resolved and the plan should be continued as specified, the problem has been resolved and the nursing interventions can be revised or discontinued, or the problem still exists.

A problem that still exists despite implementation of the nursing care plan may indicate that the interventions were not carried out as specified, the interventions were not effective in alleviating the problem, or an error or omission exists in the initial nursing assessment and diagnosis. At this point, nurses have the opportunity to modify and revise the nursing care plan.

Some healthcare institutions routinely gather evaluation data as part of an ongoing quality assurance project. By gathering outcomes data on large numbers of older patients, nurse managers and clinicians can identify opportunities for improvement. Quality assurance data often will focus on negative outcomes, such as falls with injuries, medication errors, unintentional weight loss, development of decubitus ulcers, and incidence of urinary tract infections. Should problems in these areas be identified, gerontological nurses may become involved in the development of policies, procedures, and practice guidelines to improve quality of care and quality of life for older adults (ANA, 2010a).

Gerontological nurses interpret, apply, and evaluate research findings to inform and improve gerontological nursing practice (Standard VII; ANA, 2010a). Gerontological nurse generalists participate by identifying clinical problems appropriate for study, gathering data, and interpreting findings to improve the nursing care provided to older adults. Additionally, gerontological nurses use research findings to provide evidence-based nursing interventions to their patients. Evidence-based practice is considered the best method for delivery of skilled and compassionate care to older adults.

Many gerontological nurses work as part of research teams and collaborate with nursing colleagues with advanced education and research training. Further, gerontological nurses may serve on institutional review boards to give input on the protection of rights for research participants involved in clinical research activities.

Nurses have long been recognized as direct healthcare providers, but the role of nurses as scientists is less recognized. In the United States, federal funding for nursing research began in the 1950s, but it was not until 1986 that the National Center for Nursing Research, later to become the National Institute of Nursing Research (NINR), was established within the National Institutes of Health (NIH; NINR, 2012). NINR's mission is to advance the science of health and will invest in research to:

▶ Enhance health promotion and disease prevention

▶ Improve quality of life by managing symptoms of acute and chronic illness

▶ Improve palliative and end-of-life care

▶ Enhance innovation in science and practice

▶ Develop the next generation of nurse scientists (NINR, 2012)

According to the NINR Strategic Plan released in 2012, there are four current areas of research emphasis at NINR: promoting health and preventing disease, advancing the quality of life with focus on symptom management, palliative and end-of-life care, and investment in innovation and development of nurse scientists. Often, nursing research focuses on the development of noninvasive, cost-efficient behavioral techniques as alternatives or supplements to the usual care provided to older patients.

Nursing research can lead to broad policy and practice changes. For instance, studies by nurse researchers identified the problems that can result from the use of physical restraints in the clinical setting. Increases in agitation, falls, decubitus ulcers, and urinary and fecal incontinence were documented as harm that can result from physical restraints (Strumpf & Evans, 2008). As a result, the standard of practice and federal law now mandate that physical restraints be used only in emergencies when all other methods have been tried without success. This change has improved the quality of life for many older patients.

The development of PhD programs in nursing has played a major role in the production of gerontological research. Nursing research can address basic science and clinical questions. Gerontological nurse researchers have participated in and chaired review panels across various institutes at NIH. PhD-prepared nurse researchers now are urged to seek postdoctoral positions and funding.

Many nurse researchers present their findings at specialized nursing meetings and interdisciplinary conferences, and also publish in nursing and interdisciplinary journals. The relationship between gerontological nursing practice issues and nursing research should be a dynamic one, with each informing the other. However, sometimes there is a lag between the dissemination of a research finding and the use of that finding in clinical practice. This may be the result of four factors:

1. Some nurses may have a natural reluctance to change the way things are done.

2. Some nurses lack training or education in the use and interpretation of research and are hesitant to endorse the findings of research studies.

3. Many practicing nurses do not read research-based journals and, therefore, are unaware of the findings.

4. Many nurses may doubt the validity or generalizability of the findings and are unwilling to try new techniques in their clinical settings. (NINR, 2012)

Role by Setting

Gerontological nurses are employed in most healthcare settings. In the United States, the term *long-term healthcare delivery system* is now used to designate several types of non–acute-care settings in which gerontological nurses have opportunities for practice. Patients requiring long-term care (LTC) have varying degrees of difficulty in performing ADLs. They may have a mental impairment such as Alzheimer's disease, be physically frail, or both.

About 64% of older adults requiring assistance for a disability rely on unpaid care from family members or other informal caregivers (Age in Place, 2012). Others rely on formal assistance from the LTC system. These sites of care include:

▶ *Skilled nursing facilities:* Skilled care is delivered by nurses and others to residents. Care may be subacute (e.g., Medicare-reimbursed, short stay) or chronic (e.g., private pay, Medicaid) for frail older residents requiring help with ADLs.

▶ *Retirement communities:* Older adult retirement communities range in size and scope of services. Some life-care communities offer coordinated independent living in apartments, assisted-living apartments, and nursing home care. Residents can move from one level of care to another as their situations demand. Some retirement communities offer a narrower range of services, such as independent apartments only. Others have clubhouses with activities; some have indoor or outdoor pools, dining rooms with optional meal services, healthcare facilities, and a range of housekeeping services. Some communities have 24-hour supervision and concierge services. Usually, a resident pays an admission fee and then a monthly fee for rent and services.

▶ *Adult daycare:* Adult daycare is an option for frail older adults who require daytime supervision and activities. Sometimes an older adult lives with an adult child who may have to work or otherwise be absent from the home during the day. Some daycare centers offer transportation, and others do not. Usually the older adult and family are offered options for attendance ranging from 1 or 2 days per week to daily. Daycare usually is paid for privately and not covered by insurance. Often meals are served, planned activities are provided, and some health services (e.g., podiatry, immunizations, monitoring of blood pressure, blood glucose testing) may be offered on a private-pay basis.

▶ *Residential care facilities:* Previously called "rest homes," these facilities sometimes are large private homes that have been converted to provide rooms for residents who can provide most of their own personal care but may need help with laundry, meals, and housekeeping. Supervision and health monitoring usually are provided.

▶ *Transitional care units:* Many acute care hospitals have established transitional care units to provide subacute care, rehabilitation, and palliative care health services to patients who no longer require acute care. Most of these patients are recuperating from major illness or surgery, have complex health-monitoring needs, or require palliative care with pain and symptom control. Diagnostic and support services of the acute care facility support the care given on transitional care units as needed.

▶ *Rehabilitation hospitals or facilities:* Special facilities exist to provide subacute care to patients with complex health needs. These patients may have head injuries or use ventilators, require aggressive rehabilitation after injury or surgery, or require the services and intensive treatments from specialists such as physical therapists, occupational therapists, dietitians, and physiatrists. Rehabilitation in these facilities is usually covered by the patient's private insurance or Medicare.

▶ *Community nursing care:* Visiting nurse services are an option for many older adults requiring skilled care in the home. Nurses may visit a patient regularly to monitor vital signs, provide education or counseling, administer intramuscular injections, change dressings and deliver wound care, and provide supervision to home health aides or homemakers. Such home care usually is covered by Medicare for the time period when the need for skilled nursing services exists under the direction of a physician.

Many of these LTC options are considered private-pay and are not covered by insurance. Nationally, spending from all public and private sources for LTC totaled about $230 billion in 2008, with an average cost of approximately $75,000 per year for a room in a nursing home (Commonwealth Fund, 2010).

Medicaid, the joint federal and state program for low-income individuals, funds approximately 43% of the cost of long-term care and is the largest source of LTC funding (Commonwealth Fund, 2010). To qualify for Medicaid, older people must "spend down" their assets to cover the costs of LTC. To become eligible, people must effectively impoverish themselves. In most states, an unmarried individual must "spend down" financial assets to $2,000 to qualify, and must fall within severe income limits. Another 28% of the cost of LTC is out of pocket; 18% is funded by Medicare, 7% by private insurance, and 4% from other sources (Commonwealth Fund, 2010).

Medicare is a federal program for older people and for younger people with certain chronic conditions or disabilities. After paying a monthly fee, Medicare D now offers a limited prescription drug benefit under which Medicare recipients can purchase drugs with a copay up to the limit of $2,930 per year in 2012. At that point, the older person enters the coverage gap (donut hole) and receives a 50% discount on the cost of brand-name drugs and must pay a maximum of 86% of the cost of generic drugs until total spending reaches $4,700. The older person then qualifies for catastrophic coverage and will pay about 5% of the monthly cost of the drug for the remainder of the benefit period (Medicare.com, 2012). Although Medicare primarily covers acute care, it also can pay for limited stays in subacute care units, rehabilitation hospitals, and home health care.

Currently, as a general requirement, an older adult must have a 3-day qualifying stay in a hospital and require ongoing skilled care to receive Medicare reimbursement in an LTC facility. With periodic recertification that documents the continued need for skilled care and the resident's progress toward established goals, 100 days of skilled care can be reimbursed per year.

Gerontological nurses and others will face a changing healthcare system in the future that is likely to be:

▶ More managed with better integration of services and financing;

▶ More accountable to those who purchase and use health care;

▶ More aware of and responsive to the needs of the enrolled populations;

▶ Able to use fewer resources more efficiently;

▶ More innovative and diverse in how it provides health services;

▶ Incorporating a more inclusive definition of health;

▶ More concerned with education, prevention, and care management and less focused on treatment;

▶ More oriented toward improving the health of the entire population; and

▶ More reliant on outcome data and evidence.

SUMMARY

Nurses are in a pivotal position to encourage health and wellness behaviors and care for older people who have healthcare deficits. ANA's *Scope and Standards of Practice* (2010) defines the necessary competencies and the care to be given at each step of the nursing process. Comprehensive geriatric assessment forms the basis of the individualized nursing care plan and guides the formation of measurable outcome objectives. As the number of older people continues to grow and funding for health care becomes more strained, it is important that nurses advocate for safe and effective health care across the healthcare delivery system.

REFERENCES

Age in Place. (2012). *Living at home with a chronic condition.* Retrieved from http://www.ageinplace.org/practical_advice/living_at_home_with_a_chronic_condition.aspx

American Nurses Association. (2010a). *ANCC certification package: Gerontological nursing.* Washington, DC: Author.

American Nurses Association. (2010b). *Nursing: Scope and standards of practice* (2nd ed.). Silver Spring, MD: Author.

Borson, S., Scanlan, J., Chen, P., & Ganguli, M. (2003). The Mini-Cog as a screen for dementia: Validation in a population-based sample. *Journal of the American Geriatrics Society, 51,* 1451–1454.

Carpenito, L. J. (2009). *Nursing diagnosis: Application to clinical practice.* Philadelphia: Lippincott Williams & Wilkins.

Commonwealth Fund. (2010). *Long-term care financial reform: Lessons from the U.S. and abroad.* Retrieved from http://www.commonwealthfund.org/~/media/Files/Publications/Fund%20Report/2010/Feb/1368_Gleckman_longterm_care_financing_reform_lessons_US_abroad.pdf

Doerflinger, D. (2007). *Mental status of older adults: The Mini-Cog. Try this: Best practices in care of older adults.* Retrieved from http://consultgerirn.org/uploads/File/trythis/try_this_3.pdf

Folstein, M., Folstein, S. E., & McHugh, P. R. (1975). "Mini-Mental State": A practical method for grading the cognitive state of patients for the clinician. *Journal of Psychiatric Research, 12*(3), 189–198.

Kurlowicz, L., & Greenberg, S. (2007). *The Geriatric Depression Scale (GDS). Try this: Best practices in nursing care for older adults.* New York: Hartford Institute of Geriatric Nursing. Retrieved http://consultgerirn.org/uploads/File/trythis/try_this_4.pdf

Medicare.com (2012). *2012 Medicare D outlook.* Retrieved from http://www.q1medicare.com/PartD-The-2012-Medicare-Part-D-Outlook.php

National Institute of Nursing Research. (2012). *NINR Strategic Plan: Bringing science to life.* Retrieved from http://www.ninr.nih.gov/NR/rdonlyres/8BE21801-0C52-44C2-9EEA-142483657FB1/0/NINR_StratPlan_F2_508.pdf

Reuben, D., Herr, K., Pacala, J., Pollock, B., Potter, J., & Semla, T. (2011). *Geriatrics at your fingertips* (13th ed.). New York: American Geriatrics Society.

Spector, R. (2008). *Cultural diversity in health and illness* (7th ed.). Upper Saddle River, NJ: Pearson Prentice Hall.

Strumpf, L., & Evans, L. (2008). *Individualized restraint-free care.* Philadelphia: University of Pennsylvania, Hartford Center for Geriatric Nursing Excellence. Retrieved from http://www.nursing.upenn.edu/centers/hcgne/restraints.htm

Yesavage, J. A., & Brink, T. L. (1983). Development and validation of a geriatric depression screening scale: A preliminary report. *Journal of Psychiatric Research, 17,* 37–49.

MENTAL HEALTH

An older person who is mentally healthy is one who is usually happy, enjoys life, accepts failures and disappointments, and has good coping abilities. Undiagnosed and untreated psychological or cognitive problems can lead to loss of function, premature institutionalization, decreased quality of life, and even death.

Most older adults have had considerable experience in problem-solving and dealing with crises. Older adults can experience a variety of healthcare problems, including almost all of those experienced by younger adults. Some problems may be new in onset and result from changes in life circumstances, physical illness, or medications or medical treatments. Others may be the recurrence of psychological problems that occurred earlier in life.

Key points to remember about mental health include:

- ▶ Mental health is fundamental to health.
- ▶ Mental illnesses are legitimate health problems.
- ▶ The efficacy of mental health treatments in older adults is well documented.
- ▶ Mind and body are inseparable.
- ▶ Stigma is a major obstacle that prevents many older people from seeking help.

It is important to assess psychological and cognitive function at the initial healthcare encounter and at regular intervals while older patients are receiving health care. The assessment should include screening for:

► Mood disorders

► Suicidal thoughts

► Cognitive function

► Delirium or acute confusional state

► Adjustment disorders

► Psychotic disorders

► Stress/anxiety

► Alcohol use/abuse

MOOD DISORDERS

Depression, the mental health problem of greatest frequency in the older population, is a mood disorder characterized by low mood tone, appetitite and sleep changes, difficulty with thinking and problem-solving, and bodily complaints related to feelings of loss or guilt. Some people have the mistaken idea that depression is a normal result of aging in older adults; however, most older people feel satisfied with their lives (National Institute of Mental Health [NIMH], 2010).

Mild depression often is called *dysthymia* and involves long-term chronic symptoms of sadness or irritability that do not disable someone, but keep the older person from functioning well or enjoying life to the fullest. Depression often is associated with chronic illness and pain, and it is estimated that 15% of community-residing elders and 50% of those in nursing homes have symptoms of depression (NIMH, 2010).

Women experience depression about twice as often as men. Marriage has been shown to protect against the development of depression, and married older people have a lower suicide rate than others (NIMH, 2010).

Depression can have many triggers or precipitating factors , including:

► Significant losses

► Forced retirement or other major life change over which the older person has no control

► Medical illness such as stroke, cancer, Alzheimer's disease, Parkinson's disease, epilepsy, hypothyroidism, congestive heart failure, vitamin B_{12} deficiency, or viral illness

► Drug interactions or side effects (see Table 6–1)

► Social isolation

The criteria for a diagnosis of major depression include:

▶ Depressed mood or loss of interest or pleasure

▶ Duration of symptoms for at least 2 consecutive weeks that represent a change from previous functioning

▶ Problems in at least five of the following (**SIG E CAPS**):

  ▸ *Sleep*—Insomnia or hypersomnia (excessive sleepiness)

  ▸ *Interest*—Diminished interest or pleasure (anhedonia)

  ▸ *Guilt*—Feelings of guilt or worthlessness

  ▸ *Energy*—Energy loss or fatigue

  ▸ *Concentration*—Lack of ability to concentrate

  ▸ *Appetite*—Appetite or unintentional weight gain or loss

  ▸ *Psychomotor*—Movement retardation or agitation

  ▸ *Suicide*—Suicidal thoughts or attempts, or recurrent thoughts of or desire for death with or without a plan

TABLE 6-1.
DRUGS THAT CAN CAUSE DEPRESSION IN OLDER ADULTS

TYPE	EXAMPLES
Antihypertensives/cardiac	Beta-blockers, digoxin, procainamide, guanethidine, clonidine, resperpine, methyldopa, spironolactone, thiazide diuretics
Hormones	Corticosteroids, corticotrophin, estrogen
Central nervous system depressants	Anti-anxiety agents, psychotropics, alcohol, haloperidol, flurazepam, barbiturates, benzodiazepines
Analgesics	Narcotics, nonsteroidal antiinflammatory agents
Others	Cimetidine, L-dopa, tamoxifen

Adapted from *Geriatrics at Your Fingertips* (13th ed.) by D. Reuben, K. Herr, J. Pacala, B. Pollock, J. Potter, & T. Semla, 2011, New York: American Geriatrics Society; and *Depression: Medicines That Cause Depression* by MedicineNet.com, 2012, retrieved from http://www.medicinenet.com/script/main/art.asp?articlekey=55169.

Various instruments are used to assess depression in older adults. For example, the Geriatric Depression Scale (GDS; Yesavage et al., 1983) is used in many clinical settings and can be used over time to monitor the effect of treatment. There is a long (30 question) and short (15 question) version, and both have been found to discriminate between depressed and nondepressed older adults (Yesavage et al., 1983).

No single intervention is preferred by or for older adults with depression. The treatment is guided by the nature of the problem and the goals and preferences of the patients. Individual, group, or family counseling or a combination often is effective and can be combined with pharmacological interventions. Geriatric social workers, geropsychiatrists, and psychiatric–mental health nurses can provide guidance and counseling when appropriate. Exercise, light therapy, recreational therapy, and attendance at support groups have all proven useful for older adults.

When pharmacological treatment is indicated, antidepressants may be prescribed to improve the quality of the older person's life. It takes between 6 and 12 weeks for many antidepressants to achieve therapeutic effects and ease depression. Antidepressants can interact with other classes of medications (e.g., antihypertensives, anticonvulsants), so it is important to obtain a complete drug history and investigate carefully for possible drug interactions before suggesting that these be prescribed. Postural blood pressure should be carefully monitored during the first few weeks of therapy to prevent postural hypotension. Many antidepressants can cause syndrome of inappropriate antidiuretic hormone (SIADH), so sodium should be carefully monitored (Kirkepar & Joshi, 2005). Older patients should be strongly urged to avoid alcohol while taking antidepressant medications. Divided dosages can help minimize side effects.

The major classes of antidepressants include:

▶ *Tricyclic antidepressants (TCAs):* Major side effects include constipation, dry mouth, hypotension, urinary retention, and tachycardia. Contraindicated in those with heart conduction defects, ischemic heart disease, benign prostatic hypertrophy, and glaucoma.

▶ *Selective serotonin reuptake inhibitors (SSRIs):* Major side effects include gastrointestinal problems, sleep disturbances, headache, and sexual dysfunction.

▶ *Llithium carbonate and monoamine oxidase inhibitors (MAOIs):* Sometimes used for older people who have not responded to other drug therapies and have serious side effects and interactions with other drugs and foods; therefore, careful monitoring is needed to ensure safe administration.

▶ *Buprion:* Use with caution in those with renal and hepatic impairment. Contraindicated in those with past or current seizure disorders. Interacts with alcohol, levodopa, and amantadine.

▶ *Mirtazepine:* Major side effects include potentiation with benzodiazepines, alcohol, and MAOIs (can be fatal), somnolence, weight gain, edema, and constipation.

Electroconvulsive therapy (ECT) is sometimes used for patients who have severe depression that does not respond to other treatments. ECT involves the use of a brief, controlled electrical current to produce a seizure within the brain. Usually a series of treatments (commonly 6–12) over a period of several weeks is required to produce a therapeutic effect.

SUICIDE

Older people age 65 or older have the highest suicide rates of all age groups, with the highest incidence in men ages 75 to 85. Depression is a major risk factor for suicide.

Gerontological nurses should identify and refer all older patients who are depressed and at risk for suicide. Risk factors for suicide include:

▶ Recent significant loss

▶ Age 75 or older

▶ Male gender

▶ Substance abuse or alcoholism

▶ Family history of suicide

▶ Chronic insomnia

▶ Chronic pain

▶ Social isolation

▶ Diagnosis of psychiatric illness

Nurses should question all patients who appear depressed by asking, "Have you ever thought of hurting yourself or ending your life?" Any patient who says "yes" should be further questioned by asking, "Do you have a plan?" Patients who respond "yes" to these questions need immediate emergency mental health intervention, protection from themselves, medication, and social intervention.

COGNITIVE FUNCTION

Dementia is a symptom of several acquired, progressive, life-limiting disorders that erase memory and personality. Growing older is the biggest risk factor for developing dementia, in particular Alzheimer's disease, for which currently there is no prevention or cure. People with dementia are cared for in a variety of settings, including their own homes, hospitals, nursing homes, congregate-living facilities, and hospices.

Types of progressive dementia include:

▶ *Alzheimer's disease:* Caused by genetic and environmental factors, resulting in neurofibrillary plaques and tangles because of the accumulation of abnormal proteins in the brain. Often predisposes people to develop secondary behavioral and psychiatric symptoms, including pacing, yelling, wandering, refusing care, aggressive behavior, depression, delusions, and paranoia.

▶ *Vascular dementia:* Usually abrupt in onset and caused by disruption of normal circulation to the brain, such as the presence of multiple small strokes. People with vascular dementia suffer from abrupt loss of cognitive function, sensation, language, or motor strength.

▶ *Lewy body disease:* Sometimes associated with Parkinson's disease and confirmed by the presence of round structures, or Lewy bodies, in the brain stem. In dementia with Lewy bodies, symptoms are similar to those seen in Alzheimer's disease and other progressive dementias; however, hallucinations may occur earlier in dementia with Lewy bodies than with other progressive dementias.

The Mini-Mental State Examination (MMSE; Folstein, Folstein, & McHugh, 1975) is the most widely recognized measure of cognitive function. This instrument includes 10 questions to assess orientation to time and place, word registration, attention and calculation, recall, and language. Scoring ranges from 0 to 30, with 30 representing the best score. In general, scores of 23–26 indicate mild dementia, scores of 15–23 are indicative of moderate dementia, and scores below 14 indicate severe dementia.

It is important to remember that dementia is a diagnosis of exclusion, with all other physical and psychological causes eliminated, such as profound depression, thyroid disease, infection, malignancy, or drug toxicity.

A safe environment is needed for the person with Alzheimer's disease or other dementias. Because a hallmark symptom is memory loss, careful planning and a predictable and supportive care environment are needed. Environmental cues such as family pictures and familiar objects are helpful for orienting patients with spatial disorientation. Treatment of underlying symptoms, such as pain and underlying anxiety, can improve the quality of life.

Cholinesterase inhibitors (ChEIs) prevent the destruction of neurotransmitters that are necessary for normal brain function and, thus, may delay the progression of Alzheimer's disease and allow the person to function at a higher level for 3 to 12 months. The newer N-methyl-d-aspartate (NMDA) receptor drugs prevent degeneration induced by beta-amyloid proteins. This class of drugs prevents deterioration in patients with moderate to severe Alzheimer's disease.

Additional nursing interventions include establishing advance directives and a healthcare proxy to prepare for progressive decline. This facilitates later treatment decisions such as conversations regarding use of feeding tubes, acute care hospitalization for treatment of infections or health emergencies not related to the disease, and attitudes toward aggressive medical interventions at the end of life, including the use of cardiopulmonary resuscitation.

DELIRIUM

Delirium, or acute confusional state, can exist in older adults. Delirium is often rapid in onset and can include impaired intellectual function, disorientation as to time and place, excessive drowsiness, altered level of consciousness, restlessness, extreme agitation, or a combination of these. Delirium is a nursing emergency and requires immediate assessment and treatment to prevent irreversible and progressive damage to the older person's cognitive function.

Potential risk factors for delirium include:

▶ Protein malnourishment

▶ Unstable or poorly managed disease

▶ Metabolic disturbance

▶ Advanced age (80 or older)

▶ Traumatic injury, including fracture

▶ Fever or hypothermia

▶ Drug toxicity or withdrawal

▶ Frailty

▶ Social isolation

Causes of delirium in the older adult include:

▶ Dehydration or overhydration

▶ Decreased cardiac function (e.g., acute myocardial infarction, congestive heart failure)

▶ Hypo- or hyperglycemia

▶ Hypo- or hyperthermia

▶ Hypo- or hypercalcemia

▶ Decreased respiratory function (e.g., chronic obstructive pulmonary disease, pneumonia)

▶ Decreased renal function (e.g., acute or chronic renal failure)

▶ Emotional stress

▶ Malnutrition

▶ Anemia

▶ Infection

▶ Trauma

▶ Polypharmacy

▶ Untreated pain

Because the onset of delirium is sudden, the nurse should notify the physician and conduct an immediate assessment to diagnose and improve the underlying cause of the problem. To rate delirium and distinguish it from other types of cognitive impairment, the Confusion Assessment Method (CAM) is recommended (Inouye, van Dyck, Allessi, Balkin, Siegal, & Horwitz, 1990). The first part of the CAM rates overall cognitive function, and the second part rates four features associated with delirium. This instrument can be administered in about 5 minutes and is highly accurate in older patients with delirium.

ADJUSTMENT DISORDERS

The most common stressor that leads to adjustment disorders in late life is physical illness. Other stressors that can trigger adjustment disorders include forced relocation, financial difficulties, death of a loved one, and family problems. A supportive social network can be an asset to an older person experiencing an adjustment disorder.

For more than 25 years, the World Health Organization has recognized that preventing social isolation is necessary to maintain good health. Supportive social relationships enhance physical and mental health among older adults, while social isolation, loneliness, and negative social relationships contribute to higher risk of disability, poor recovery from illness, and early death (Lubben et al., 2006).

Some older adults become socially isolated as they age, because of the deaths of friends and relatives, changes in vision and hearing that make social interactions more difficult, and physical illness, which can result in their having less energy to engage in social interactions. Older adults, like people of any age, vary in their needs for social interaction. Some older adults have never been "joiners" and may prefer to spend time alone, while others have always had a greater need to be with others. The older adult who chooses to be alone differs from the older adult who wishes to engage in social activity but does not have the resources or opportunity to do so.

Loneliness is a feeling of being apart from others and can occur even when the older person is in the presence of others. Older people who feel lonely should be carefully evaluated for additional signs and symptoms of depression, undergo a complete physical examination to rule out physical illness, and be offered encouragement and the opportunity to make new friends and engage in new recreational activities. Enjoyable social interactions can help the older person improve his or her self-esteem and feel wanted. Those who maintain caring relationships with others enjoy a buffer against social losses and are more likely to maintain good mental health and higher levels of morale. A good network of supportive friends and family can give meaning to life and provide stability.

About 23% of older men and 51% of older women have become widowed or widowers by age 70 (U.S. Census Bureau, 2011). Because there are many more older women than older men, the older man will have opportunities to remarry or enter new relationships, while the older woman may not.

Strains on relationships in later life include:

▶ Poor physical or mental health

▶ Economic strain

▶ Family strain (e.g., poor health, financial needs of adult children)

▶ Differing needs for intimacy

▶ Rekindling of past conflicts (including sibling rivalry) resulting from increased contact with family because of dependency

The nurse can assess the older person's social network to help the older person mobilize and use resources that may help him or her to recover from health threats and remain as independent as possible. Areas to consider include:

▶ Size of the social network (e.g., family, friends, significant others who are accessible to the older person)

▶ Ability to help (e.g., financial, emotional, physical resources)

▶ Willingness (i.e., How often can support be offered? Will it be offered easily and willingly?)

▶ Possible barriers to helping (e.g., competing demands such as work and family obligations, travel time)

▶ Recent changes that may alter the need for support

Nurses and other members of the healthcare team can educate and support older people as they try to remain socially engaged at appropriate levels. Possible suggestions for the older person include:

▶ Engage in volunteer activities.

▶ Seek mental health services if depression is suspected.

▶ Join a support group if a significant loss has occurred.

▶ Take up a new hobby or recreational pursuit.

▶ Engage in senior community activities or take classes at a local college.

▶ Identify and prepare for possible role transitions (e.g., make a living will, do estate planning).

PSYCHOTIC DISORDERS

The first episode of schizophrenia usually occurs before age 40, so it is likely that the older person with symptoms of this disease has a long history of hospitalization and psychotropic drug use. Some symptoms of schizophrenia, such as hallucinations and delusions, appear to decline with age, but other symptoms, such as apathy and withdrawal, may place the older person at a higher risk for social isolation or elder mistreatment.

The essential features of bipolar disorder are the experience of one or more manic episodes that may be followed by a period of depression. Mania in old age may be caused by drug therapy (e.g., steroids), recurrence of a previous psychiatric disorder, head trauma, or delirium. Because mania may resemble an agitated depression in the older person, it is often difficult to diagnose. A thorough physical examination and medical history are needed to rule out physical causes of the mania. Consultation with a mental health expert should be sought to prevent the older person from harming him- or herself or others. Older people who express suicidal ideation or verbalize a desire to harm others and have the means to carry out such a plan need immediate referral to emergency mental health services. To protect the patient and others, many of these patients will be hospitalized and observed while counseling and medications are initiated. (See the suicide assessment guidelines described on p. 95.)

Treatment of psychotic disorders in late life may require institutionalization to thoroughly assess the patient's unique situation, provide safety and support, and prescribe and monitor appropriate medications. Medications for psychotic symptoms in manic episodes include mood-stabilizing agents, such as lithium, carbamazepine, or valproic acid, in combination with other antipsychotic medications. These medications must be carefully prescribed, monitored, and adjusted to minimize toxicity and side effects.

Nonpharmacological interventions include patient and family education and support, the provision of sufficient food and fluids to support life and function, social interactions such as group therapy and peer support, and a schedule that allows adequate rest and activity.

STRESS AND ANXIETY

Stress and anxiety can have negative effects on the physical functioning of an older person, including increases in pulse, blood pressure, blood glucose, and muscle tension. Persistent high levels of stress can result in exhaustion, adrenal cortex hormone depletion, and even death. Positive coping mechanisms, such as exercise, meditation, listening to music, and reaching out to friends and family, can reduce stress levels and improve function. Negative coping mechanisms, such as use of drugs, tobacco, or alcohol or avoiding family and friends, can further exacerbate the problem and lead to higher rates of heart disease, cancer, and other illnesses.

Symptoms that indicate an older person is suffering negative effects of stress include:

- ▶ Sleep problems (e.g., sleeping too much, insomnia)
- ▶ Chronic high anxiety levels (easily startled, hypervigilant)
- ▶ Use and abuse of alcohol, prescription drugs, or tobacco
- ▶ New-onset tachycardia, tremors, irregular heartbeat, or hypertension
- ▶ New-onset pain or worsening of chronic pain levels
- ▶ Chronic fatigue, lack of pleasure in life, and new or worsening depression (Tabloski, 2006)

Older people with high stress levels should be referred to mental health experts for assessment and counseling. Anti-anxiety medications may be used for short-term treatment of anxiety, but many negative side effects are associated with some of these drugs, including somnolence, constipation, interactions with other medications, and increased risk of falls. Nursing interventions include:

- ▶ Assisting the older person to identify stressors
- ▶ Identifying successful positive coping mechanisms that have been used in the past
- ▶ Investigating community resources, support groups, stress reduction clinics, and other potential stress relievers

ALCOHOL USE AND ABUSE

The exact prevalence of alcohol abuse is unknown. However, because of age-related physical changes and the potential for interaction with prescribed medications, relatively low levels of alcohol can have negative effects on the health and function of the older person. Risk factors for alcohol abuse include genetic predisposition, male gender, limited education, poverty, and a history of depression.

Problems related to chronic or excessive alcohol intake include:

► Malnutrition (failure to prepare and eat an adequate diet)

► Cirrhosis of the liver (a leading cause of death for older people)

► Osteomalacia (thinning of the bones)

► Decrease in gastric absorption

► Falls

► Decline in cognitive function (impaired memory and information processing)

► Interactions with medications (over-the-counter and prescription)

Screening for alcohol use and abuse in the older adult includes use of the Short Michigan Alcoholism Screening Test–Geriatric Version (SMAST–G) or similar questionnaire (Regents of the University of Michigan, 1991). Some sample questions from the SMAST–G include:

► Do you ever underestimate to others the amount that you drink?

► Do you usually take a drink to relax or calm your nerves?

► Do you sometimes skip a meal because you have had a few drinks and don't feel hungry?

► When you feel lonely, does drinking help?

Of the 10 questions in the SMAST–G, two or more positive answers indicate an alcohol problem. More than two drinks per day for women or three for men is considered potentially harmful, depending on the older person's tolerance, physical health, medication use, and living situation.

Older people who are dependent on or abusing alcohol should be referred for further evaluation and treatment. Self-help groups such as Alcoholics Anonymous, professional counseling, social support, and drug therapy all have been shown to be effective in treating alcohol problems in older people. Hospitalization and careful monitoring may be needed in heavy long-term users, because acute agitation and hallucination may occur (delirium tremens) during the withdrawal process.

SUMMARY

Although mental health issues are not necessarily more common in older people, functional disabilities, numerous losses, and diagnosis of comorbidities are all risk factors that can lead to the development of serious illness, slow down rehabilitation after illness, and detract from quality of life. Many older people and their families will benefit from education about mental health problems in aging and the options for addressing these problems. Systematic assessment of mental health problems, careful documentation, and referral to mental health experts when appropriate are nursing interventions that can improve the social, intellectual, and emotional well-being of older adults.

REFERENCES

Folstein, M., Folstein, S., & McHugh, P. E. (1975). Mini-Mental State: A practical method for grading the cognitive state of patients for the clinician. *Journal of Psychiatric Research, 12,* 189–198.

Inouye, S., van Dyck, C., Allessi, C., Balkin, S., Siegal, A., & Horwitz, R. (1990). Clarifying confusion: The confusion assessment method. A new method for the detection of delirium. *Annals of Internal Medicine, 113*(12), 941–948.

Kirkepar, V., & Joshi, P. (2005). Syndrome of inappropriate ADH secretion (SIADH) associated with citalopram use. *Indian Journal of Psychiatry, 47*(2), 119–120.

Lubben, J., Blozik, E., Gillmann, G., Iliffe, S., von Renteln Kruse, W., Beck, J., et al. (2006). Performance of an abbreviated version of the Lubben Social Network Scale among three European community-dwelling older adult populations. *The Gerontologist, 46,* 503–513.

MedicineNet.com. (2012). *Depression: Medicines that cause depression.* Retrieved from http://www.medicinenet.com/script/main/art.asp?articlekey=55169

National Institutes of Mental Health. (2012). *Depression.* Retrieved from http://www.nimh.nih.gov/health/publications/depression/complete-index.shtml

Regents of the University of Michigan. (1991). *The University of Michigan Alcohol Research Center, Ann Arbor, Michigan.* Retrieved from http://consultgerirn.org/uploads/File/trythis/try_this_17.pdf

Reuben, D., Herr, K., Pacala, J., Pollock, B., Potter, J., & Semla, T. (2011). *Geriatrics at your fingertips* (13th ed.). New York: American Geriatrics Society.

Tabloski, P. (2006). *Gerontological nursing.* Upper Saddle River, NJ: Prentice-Hall.

U.S. Census Bureau. (2011). *Census Bureau reports 55 percent have married one time.* Retrieved from http://www.census.gov/newsroom/releases/archives/marital_status_living_arrangements/cb11-90.html

Yesavage, J., Brink, T., Rose, T., Lum, O., Huang, V. Adey, M., et al. (1983). Development and validation of a geriatric depression screening scale: A preliminary report. *Journal of Psychiatric Research, 17,* 37–49.

ADDITIONAL RESOURCES

Alzheimer's Association: www.alz.org/

American Geriatric Society: www.americangeriatrics.org/

Hartford Institute for Geriatric Nursing: www.consultgerirn.org/

John A. Hartford Institute for Geriatric Nursing: www.hartfordign.org/

MEDICATIONS

Among older adults, polypharmacy—taking more than one drug (see Chapter 6)—is a common problem. Currently, 44% of men and 57% of women older than age 65 take 5 or more medications per week; about 12% of both men and women take 10 or more medications per week (Woodruff, 2010). In addition, they consume 40%–50% of over-the-counter (OTC) medications—many of which are not disclosed to their primary care providers (Woodruff, 2010).

The use of multiple drugs places older adults at risk for adverse drug reactions and interactions, which can have serious consequences. It is reported that adverse drug reactions are two to three times greater in older adults and cause 10% to 35% of their hospital admissions. The reasons for these reactions are multiple and include the higher number of medications taken by older adults; impaired drug metabolism due to decreases in glomerular filtration rate and hepatic clearance; changes in volume distribution of drugs, with fat-soluble drugs having longer half-lives and water-soluble drugs becoming more concentrated; and individual variation in sensitivity to drugs (McPhee & Papadakis, 2011).

As adults age, pharmacodynamics and pharmacokinetics are altered, and drugs may exhibit an entirely different outcome from the therapeutic effect intended—absorption, distribution, metabolism, and excretion may be altered in the older adult. In addition, older adults may consume multiple medications, which often contributes to drug–drug interactions or reactions. Because of frailty and memory loss, which often accompany old age, noncompliance and/or inappropriate drug use may occur. Therefore, provider visits, whether to an office, ambulatory care clinic, or emergency room, should include a review of current drugs being taken—both prescribed and OTC. The nurse should ask questions to ascertain if there are any changes in medications, new medical diagnoses, or changes in overall health or function.

The kinds of medications used by the elderly population vary according to living situation, medical diagnoses, functional status, and quality of life. Healthcare providers use the 2012 AGS BEERS list as a guide to assist them in improving medication safety and to inform clinical decision making concerning the quality of care (American Geriatrics Society, 2012). The AGS BEERS lists drugs in categories and evidence-based recommendations for use, and provides dosing for each drug. A printable pocket guide is available at http://www.americangeriatrics. org/files/documents/beers/PrintableBeersPocketCard.pdf. Table 7–1 reflects some of the more commonly used agents that appear on the BEERS list.

Although the drugs on the BEERS list may be used at times, they are never first-line agents. Furthermore, if these drugs are given, there should be a clear indication in the patient's record as to the reason, and the patient should be monitored carefully.

TABLE 7-1.
COMMONLY USED MEDICATIONS AND THEIR RISKS AND CONCERNS

MEDICATION	REASON FOR CONCERN	POTENTIAL FOR RISK
Antipsychotics in dementia	Increased risk of CVA (stroke) and mortality those with dementia	High
Pentazocine (Talwin)	Can cause confusion and hallucinations more commonly than in other opioids	High
Trimethobenzamide (Tigan)	Very ineffective anti-emetic; can cause extrapyramidal effects	High
Muscle relaxants/Antispasmodics ▶ Methocarbamol (Robaxin) ▶ Carisoprodol (Soma) ▶ Metaxalone (Skelaxin) ▶ Cyclobenzaprine (Flexeril) ▶ Oxybutynin (Ditropan)	Many anticholinergic effects; can cause sedation	High
Flurazepam (Dalmane)	Half-life can exceed 24 hours; can cause sedation and increase risk of falls and fractures	High
Amitriptyline (Elavil) Chlordiazepoxide-amitriptyline (Limbitrol) Perphenazine–amitriptyline (Triavil)	Strong anticholinergic effects; very sedating	High
Long-acting benzodiazepines ▶ Chlordiazepoxide (Librium) ▶ Chlordiazepoxide-amitriptyline (Libritrol) ▶ Clindinium-chlordiazepoxide (Librax) ▶ Diazepam (Valium) ▶ Quazepam (Doral) ▶ Chlorazepate (Tranxene)	Half-life often can exceed 24 hours; can cause sedation and increase risk of falls and fractures	High
Digoxin (Lanoxin; Digi-Tek)	Decreased renal clearance, so doses should not exceed 0.125 mg/day	Low

MEDICATION	REASON FOR CONCERN	POTENTIAL FOR RISK
Chlopropamide (Diabenase)	Long half-life in older adults; can cause prolonged hypoglycemia; only antiglycemic drug that can cause syndrome of inappropriate antidiuretic hormone (SIADH)	High
GI antispasmodics ▸ Dicyclomine (Bentyl) ▸ Hyoscyamine (Levsin) ▸ Propantheline (Pro-Banthine) ▸ Belladonna alkaloids (Donnatol)	High anticholinergic effects; can produce toxic effects in older adults	High
Diphenhydramine (Benadryl)	Anticholinergic and sedating; should not be used as a hypnotic in older adults	High
Merperidine (Demerol)	Not effective orally; can produce toxic metabolite that can cause confusion and seizures in older adults	High
Ketorolac (Toradol)	Can cause prolonged renal and GI side effects in older adults	High
Long-term use of full dose, long half-life non-COX selective NSAIDs ▸ Naproxen (Naprosyn, Anaprox, Aleve) ▸ Oxaprozin (Daypro) ▸ Piroxicam (Feldene)	May cause GI bleeding, renal failure, hypertension, and congestive heart failure	High
Daily Fluoxetine (Prozac)	Long half-life and increased risk for excess stimulation (e.g., insomnia, agitation)	High
Doxazosin (Cardura)	Can cause dry mouth, orthostatic hypotension, and urinary problems	Low
Thioridazine (Mellaril)	Great potential for CNS and extrapyramidal effects	High
Short-acting Nifedipine (Procardia)	Can cause reflex tachycardia, hypotension, and constipation	High
Clonidine (Catapres)	Can cause sedation, orthostatic hypotension, and CNS effects	Low
Cimetidine (Tagamet)	Can cause CNS effects, including confusion and visual hallucinations	High
Armour Thyroid	Much concern about cardiac effects; safer alternatives are available	High

Note. CNS = central nervous system; GI = gastrointestinal.

Adapted from *AGS BEERS Criteria for Potentially Inappropriate Medication Use in Older Adults,* by American Geriatrics Society, 2012, retrieved from http://www.americangeriatrics.org/files/documents/beers/PrintableBeersPocketCard.pdf.

CHANGES IN PHARMACOKINETICS

Pharmacokinetics is what the body does to the drug; it is the impact of absorption, distribution, metabolism, and elimination of drugs. Age-related changes can occur that affect pharmacokinetics in older adults (see Table 7–2).

Drug levels often can provide needed information about drug absorption, drug distribution, and renal and liver function (protein binding, hepatic metabolism, and renal excretion). If the drug levels reveal excess serum amounts, at doses similar to those used in younger adults, drug toxicity can occur, unless the dosage or frequency of dosing is adjusted. The degree of variation depends on multiple factors, such as age (young-old, 65–74 years vs. old-old, age 85 or older); other medications being taken; nutritional state; and use of tobacco, alcohol, and caffeine (Reuben et al., 2011).

Drug Absorption

Age-related changes in drug absorption usually do not have a major impact on drug response in older adults. Other factors—presence of pain; use of other medications (such as anticholinergics); and concurrent metabolic disease, such as diabetes, pernicious anemia, or thyroid disease—can have some effect on absorption. Gerontological nurses should keep this in mind as they assess patient medication profiles.

Drug Distribution

Drug distribution alters with age. Decreased albumin levels result in decreased binding of certain drugs that are mainly bound to albumin. Because the unbound fragment of the drug is needed to give the desired effect, or may produce toxicity, an increase in the unbound fragment (as a result of less albumin to bind to) can cause untoward effects or side effects. Drug distribution also is affected by body water, body fat, and lean body mass.

As human beings age, they have less body water and intercellular water. These changes can lead to increased concentrations of water-soluble drugs (lithium or alcohol). Other body changes include increased body fat and decreased lean body mass. The added body fat may increase the distribution of fat-soluble drugs, such as benzodiazepines, causing prolonged half-lives and accumulation of the drug in the fat stores of the body. The decreased lean body mass can cause an increase in serum concentration of protein-bound drugs, such as warfarin (Coumadin) or lanoxin (Digi-Tek). Nurses should pay particular attention to protein-bound drug use in malnourished older patients.

Drug distribution also is affected by the *bioavailability* of the drug, which is the amount that reaches the systemic circulation. This amount may be altered by route of administration, drug solubility, and general circulation to the site where the drug is given (McPhee & Papadakis, 2011).

Renal and Liver Function

Age-related changes to the liver and kidney are important to recognize in the pharmacokinetics of aging. Biotransformation of drugs to more active forms occurs in all tissues of the body, but the main site of transformation is the liver. Through *biotransformation,* the liver detoxifies drugs and prepares them for excretion. This process takes place through complex enzyme activity that occurs in the cytochrome P450 system.

Metabolism of drugs in the liver is influenced by concomitant diseases; gender; genetics; nutrition; activity levels; and caffeine, tobacco, and alcohol ingestion. The liver metabolizes drugs in one of two ways: (1) oxidation or reduction *(Phase I metabolism)* or (2) conjugation *(Phase II metabolism;* Schonbom, 2010).

Phase I metabolism is oxidation or reduction to more-polar compounds. Drugs such as long-acting benzodiazepines or tricyclic antidepressants are more likely to have reduced hepatic clearance and, thus, a longer effect in older adults.

Phase II metabolism is the conjugation of a drug to a more water-soluble molecule. Drugs that are metabolized in this fashion are usually cleared as in younger people and, thus, no alteration in dosage for older adults is needed. Drugs that fit this profile include acetaminophen and short-acting benzodiazepines such as lorazepam or oxazepam.

However, because the hepatic metabolism of drugs is not entirely predictable, gerontological nurses must continually assess the effects of medications on their patients.

The last important factor to consider in pharmacokinetics is *renal excretion* of drugs. Because renal function declines with normal aging, significant changes may occur with drugs that are excreted via this pathway. The changes in this body system are so pronounced that this topic is discussed in the pharmacodynamics section.

TABLE 7-2.
IMPACT OF PHYSIOLOGICAL AGING ON PHARMACOKINETICS

FACTOR	PHYSIOLOGICAL EFFECT	PHARMACOLOGICAL EFFECTS AND DRUG INTERACTIONS
Absorption	▶ Decreased gastric emptying time, intestinal blood flow, and intestinal motility ▶ Increased gastric pH	▶ Decreased rate of absorption ▶ Extended length of absorption process ▶ Decreased gastric elimination ▶ Increased possibility of ulcer formation ▶ Oral antibiotics, salicylates, nonsteroidal antiinflammatory drugs, histamine 2 blockers, oral antipsychotics
Distribution	▶ Decreased lean body mass, total body water, and albumin ▶ Increased fatty tissue	▶ Decreased distribution to receptors ▶ Higher concentration of water-soluble drugs ▶ Lower concentration/extended release of fat-soluble drugs ▶ Beta blockers, diazepam, flurazepam, digoxin, warfarin, phenytoin
Metabolism	▶ Decreased liver mass, liver blood flow, and liver enzyme activity	▶ Decreased liver metabolism or elimination ▶ Propanolol, phenytoin, meperidine, benzodiazepines, verapamil, warfarin, nitrates, acetaminophen, tricyclics
Elimination	▶ Decreased renal mass, functioning nephrons, glomerular filtration rate, tubular secretion, creatinine clearance, and reabsorption ▶ Decreased air exchange	▶ Decreased renal clearance/elimination of any drug and drug metabolites eliminated via renal route ▶ Decreased/extended elimination of aerosol and inhalation drugs ▶ All drugs and drug metabolites eliminated via kidneys ▶ Inhaled anesthetics, respiratory inhalants

Adapted from *Preventing Polypharmacy in Older Adults* by K. Woodruff, 2010, retrieved from http://www.americannursetoday.com/article.aspx?id=7132&fid=6852.

CHANGES IN PHARMACODYNAMICS

Pharmacodynamics refers to the specific action of a drug at the tissue level. The pharmacodynamic effect of a given drug may be enhanced or decreased in older adults. This effect is due to physiological and pathological changes in both target and nontarget organs. Beta-receptor sensitivity may be reduced in late life, leading to diminished response to both beta antagonists and agonists (Tonner, Kampen, & Scholz, 2003). More commonly, pharmacodynamic effects of drugs are enhanced—or appear to be enhanced—in older adults. Multiple drugs affect the central nervous system, causing confusion. Cognitive impairment can occur suddenly and may not be recognized as a side effect of and attributed to medication.

When a variety of drugs are taken and an acute confusional state (delirium) is exhibited, consider addressing drugs taken. Some of the drugs that can have exaggerated effects and may cause delirium include:

► Sedatives

► Opioid analgesic agents

► Hypnotics

► Antidepressants

► Anticonvulsants

► Central-acting antihypertensives

► Lidocaine

► Digoxin

► Isoniazid

► Corticosteroids

► Theophylline

► Anticholinergic agents

► Nonsteroidal antiinflammatory drugs

► Histamine 2 blockers

Renal Function

As mentioned in the section on pharmacokinetics, the most significant change with relation to drug use and effects in older adults is the age-related changes in the kidney. Beginning between the ages of 35 and 40, the glomerular filtration rate (GFR) begins to fall approximately 1% per year, based on age alone. Older adults who also have hypertension, diabetes, or other chronic medical problems are especially at risk when given medications that are excreted renally. This information is important in regard to drugs with a narrow therapeutic index, such as digoxin, vancomycin, and imipenem.

Creatinine clearance is an indirect measure of glomerular filtration rate. As stated earlier, the GFR decreases with normal aging. Therefore, even if the older adult has a normal serum creatinine, this does not mean that the creatinine clearance is normal. The creatinine clearance is best measured indirectly with the following Cockroft–Gault formula:

Creatinine Clearance (mL/minute) = 140 – Age (in years) x Weight (in kilograms) 72 x Serum creatinine (For women, multiply the final result by 0.85.) (mg/dL)

This example shows how the serum creatinine can be misleading: Mrs. Grace is 90 years old and weighs 40 kilograms. She has a serum creatinine of 0.9 mg/dL. Her calculated creatinine clearance is 26 mL/minute. Given that information, drugs such as quinolone antibiotics, digoxin, and histamine blockers would require reduction in drug doses because of this marked change in renal status.

This scenario is quite common for both inpatient and outpatient older adults. Nurses must be aware of the normal renal changes of aging when administering medications and monitor patients for untoward effects as a result of these changes.

POLYPHARMACY

Polypharmacy is common in the older adult and, in addition to taking more than six medications daily on a routine basis, may also be defined as:

▶ Taking medication for a specific condition without diagnosis of that condition (for instance, taking an antidepressant without a diagnosis of depression)

▶ Taking a brand-name medication and a generic form of that same medication simultaneously (for example, both Coumadin and warfarin)

▶ Taking multiple medications that interact with each other

▶ Taking medications to control the side effects of other medications (Lorenz, 2012; Tabloski, 2010)

End results of polypharmacy can range from mild annoyance to life-threatening symptoms. These symptoms can be the result of:

▶ Nonadherence

▶ Adverse drug reactions (ADRs)

▶ Drug–drug interactions

▶ Medication errors

▶ Hospitalization related to an ADR

▶ Potential underuse of needed medications

▶ Financial burden

People who are at risk for adverse effects from polypharmacy often are faced with expensive, complicated regimens that can result in nonadherence, perhaps even unintentional omission of medications. *ADRs*—a negative, unexpected response to a medication at a recommended dosage—have been shown to increase the risk of mortality and long-term-care placement (Cowley, Diebold, Gross, & Hardin-Fanning, 2006).

The likelihood of a drug–drug interaction markedly increases in the person taking multiple medications, and taking multiple medicines can lead to medication errors by patients, family, and healthcare providers.

According to Cowley and colleagues (2006), ADRs are the cause of 28% of all hospitalizations in older adults. Other complications of ADRs include electrolyte imbalances, gastrointestinal bleeding, falls, and fractures. Any of these scenarios can lead to a hospitalization.

Although great strides have been made to reduce polypharmacy in older adults, underuse of needed therapies sometimes results from "preventing polypharmacy." Examples include beta-blockers not being prescribed to an older adult who has had a heart attack; inadequately treated pain; and lack of treatment to prevent or delay progression of osteoporosis. Nurses are critical in helping prescribers reach appropriate treatment of needed conditions without giving a pill for every symptom.

Risk factors for polypharmacy include:

► Multiple medical problems

► Having prescriptions filled at multiple pharmacies

► Receiving care from multiple healthcare providers

► Inadequate communication among providers

► Duplicate medications from providers

► Providers writing prescriptions because that is "what the patient wants"

► Medications ordered to treat side effects of other medications

To address and reduce the problems of polypharmacy, nurses first can become familiar with medications that are known to cause problems in older adults. Next, nurses should be vigilant in monitoring patients for untoward effects of medications, and, finally, nurses should have a high index of suspicion—if an elderly patient has a new symptom, consider that it might be an ADR.

Some key points to remember to reduce polypharmacy include:

► Use medications that have once- or twice-daily dosing.

► Only use medications with known efficacy.

► Use medications with half-lives of 24 hours or less to avoid toxicity.

► Avoid alternate-day therapies if possible.

► Review medicine regimens often.

► Use nonpharmacological options, when possible, to reduce or eliminate drug doses.

► Help ensure that patients and caregivers are informed.

► Recognize that new symptoms may stem from drugs that patients are taking.

▶ Encourage patients to get all medications (prescription and OTC) from the same pharmacy.

▶ Encourage patients to know their pharmacists.

▶ Review every medicine at every healthcare provider visit.

▶ Discourage pill sharing and hoarding.

▶ Advise patients to check medicine cabinets at least once a year and throw away all old and outdated medications (Cowley et al., 2006; Reuben et al., 2011).

Gerontological nurses should be aware that *rational polypharmacy* is sometimes indicated, given an older person's diagnosis of multiple comorbidities. For instance, an older person receiving chemotherapy for metastatic cancer may be prescribed anti-neoplastic drugs, antinausea drugs, bowel stimulants, antidepressants, opioid and nonopioid pain medications, and vitamins and nutritional supplements. In these cases, nurses must closely monitor patients to ensure that adverse drug effects do not occur and that the intended effects of the medications are achieved.

It also is important to older adults' functional and cognitive abilities that they manage their medication regimens themselves. Older adults with cognitive impairments may completely forget to take a medication or, conversely, may take it too many times because they are unsure whether they have taken it. Discontinued medications or old medications that have been mixed in with current medications may be refilled in error. To avoid major reactions or interactions, including falls, hospitalization, or even death, attention to drug safety is imperative for all healthcare providers, including home care nurses, family caregivers, and providers.

The guiding principle when prescribing medications for the older person is to "start low and go slow"; conversely, medications should be discontinued when the desired effect is not attained, the medications are causing troublesome side effects, or the medical diagnosis for which the drug has been prescribed is no longer valid. Medications can be discontinued under the following circumstances:

▶ The potential harm of the drug outweighs the benefit.

▶ The older person did not take the drug, and no ill effect resulted.

▶ A new medication or diagnosis has been added, making the risk of an adverse drug reaction greater.

If possible, gradually taper the dose of all psychotropic drugs to prevent withdrawal reactions resulting from abrupt discontinuation (Reuben et al., 2011).

Herbal Remedies
One popular healthcare practice in the United States is that of alternative therapies. *Complementary and alternative medicine (CAM)* is the name given to diverse medical and healthcare therapies and products that are not considered part of conventional medical treatments. CAMs include:

▶ *Alternative medical systems:* Homeopathy, naturopathic medicine, ayurveda, and traditional Chinese medicine

▶ *Mind–body intervention:* Prayer, deep breathing, meditation, yoga, biofeedback, tai chi chuan, and guided imagery

▶ *Manipulative and body-based therapies:* Chiropractic, osteopathic manipulation, massage, reflexology, and rolfing

▶ *Energy therapies:* Veritable and putative energy field treatments, therapeutic touch, healing touch, Reiki, magnet therapy, sound and light therapy

▶ *Biologically based therapies:* Therapy using substances found in nature, including herbs, vitamins, and foods. Can include use of elk horn; shark cartilage; and diets such as macrobiotic, Atkins, Ornish, Pritikin, The Zone, and all types of vegetarianism. Chelation and folk medicine. The most popular therapy is the use of herbals, often referred to as *botanicals.*

Herbals are considered dietary supplements by the Federal Drug Administration (FDA) and, as a result, do not require FDA approval. The CAM industry is quite popular with older adults, because these supplements promise to rejuvenate people, eliminate ailments, and prevent further aging. Unfortunately, much of the advertising for these products is not reliable or truthful, and the labels for herbals often do not warn about possible drug–drug interactions.

Herbal supplements are manufactured in several forms—capsules, extracts, oils, pills, salves, teas, and tinctures. Their efficacy varies depending on the form of the herb used. Herbal teas appeal to consumers, and people spend millions of dollars annually on this form of botanical. Because there are few reports of untoward effects of teas, consumers believe that they are harmless. They may, in fact, be safe, if the tea is consumed in moderation. However, liver disease was reported with frequent to constant use of comfrey, causing it to be removed from the market in 2002.

More than 50% of Americans use herbal remedies and do not report these to their healthcare provider (National Center for Complementary and Alternative Medicine, 2007). Some considerations regarding botanicals include:

▶ Botanicals are not regulated or approved by the FDA (i.e., not subject to clinical trials).

▶ Manufacturers describe only product effects on structure and function.

▶ Toxicity and carcinogenicity have been reported.

▶ Synergistic effects may occur with prescribed medications; the more herbs a patient takes, the more likely it is that a drug–drug interaction will occur.

Common herbals used by Americans (see Table 7–3 for side effects and precautions) include:

▶ *Psychoactive:* St. John's wort, kava kava, valerian root, chamomile

▶ *Weight loss:* Ma huang, guarana, hydroxy citric acid, bitter orange

▶ *Sports enhancement:* Yohimbe, Asian ginseng

▶ *Miscellaneous:* Cranberry, echinacea, feverfew, garlic, ginkgo, saw palmetto

TABLE 7-3.
COMMON HERBALS AND THEIR SIDE EFFECTS AND PRECAUTIONS

HERB	BOTANICAL OR CHEMICAL NAME	USE	MECHANISM OF ACTION	SIDE EFFECTS	PRECAUTIONS
St. John's wort	*Hypericum perforatum*	Wound healing; depression	Serotonin reuptake is primary mechanism, perhaps MAOI and catechol-O-methyltransferase activity, along with modulation of melatonin and norepinephrine uptake	Photosensitivity; possible serotonin syndrome if used with SSRI	Lack of product standardization
Kava kava	*Piper methysticum*	Calming effects; ceremonial drink in South Pacific and Fiji; natural alternative to sedatives and anxiolytics	Thought to inhibit GABA receptor binding, yet may have effects other than on GABA	Eye irritation; yellow scaly rash with heavy chronic use; cases of hepatitis, fulminant hepatitis, and death reported (rare and idiosyncratic)	Regular monitoring of liver function indicated
Valerian root	Valerian root	Sedative agent; sleep aid	Effects on GABA receptors	Headache; cardiac disturbances	Exercise care when combining with other sedatives and ETOH
Chamomile	Chamomile	GI discomfort; PUD; pediatric colic; mild anxiety	Binding to central benzodiazepine receptors	No significant toxicities reported	No reported drug–drug interactions
Ma huang, guarana	Ma huang and guarana	Weight loss	Ma huang—source of ephedrine; guarana—source of caffeine; ephedrine stimulates metabolic rate through norepinephrine release from sympathetic nerve endings, causing anorectic thermogenic effects by increasing metabolism	Deaths reported from hypertension and arrhythmias	Banned by FDA in 2004; available from Canada and other foreign distributors through the Internet
Hydroxy citric acid	*Garcinia cambogia*	Weight loss	Thought to increase fat oxidation by inhibiting citrate lyase, an enzyme that plays a critical role in energy metabolism during novo lipogenesis	High doses can cause abdominal pain, vomiting, and a laxative effect	

HERB	BOTANICAL OR CHEMICAL NAME	USE	MECHANISM OF ACTION	SIDE EFFECTS	PRECAUTIONS
Bitter orange (also known as zhi shi)	*Citrus aurantium*	Weight loss	Contains synephrine, a sympathomimetic amine that can suppress appetite and theoretically can raise pulse and blood pressure	Case reports have linked it to myocardial infarction, syncope, and ischemic stroke	
Yohimbe	*Pausinystalia yohimbe*	Aphrodisiac ("natural Viagra"); hallucinogen (when smoked); body-building agent	Stimulates release of norepinephrine, decreases cholinergic activity, and increases adrenergic activity	Agitation, tremors, insomnia, hypertension, tachycardia	Should not be used with tyrosine, antidepressants, sedatives, or amphetamines; clonidine can reverse effects
Asian ginseng	*Panax ginseng*	Strengthens mental and physical capacity; adaptogenic (stress-protective) agent	Affects nitric oxide synthesis in endothelial cells of lung, heart, and kidney; effects serotonin and dopamine; ginsengs are thought to contain ginsenosides, which act as antioxidants	Nervousness; insomnia	Generally thought to be safe
Cranberry	Cranberry	Treatment of urinary tract infection	Proanthocyanidins present in cranberries may inhibit adherence of *Escherichia coli* to urinary tract epithelium	Renal stones	Literature suggests that it is effective
Echinacea	*Echinacea purpurea, Echinacea angustifolia, Echinacea pallida*	Colds; analgesic effects	Protects the integrity of hyaluronic acid matrix by stimulating an alternative complement pathway in the immune system; promotes nonspecific T-cell activation by binding to T-cells and increasing Interferon production	Skin rash, GI upset, diarrhea	Should not be given to people with autoimmune disease, those taking immuno-suppressive agents, or those with HIV/AIDS

CONTINUED ▶

◀ **TABLE 7-3 CONTINUED**

HERB	BOTANICAL OR CHEMICAL NAME	USE	MECHANISM OF ACTION	SIDE EFFECTS	PRECAUTIONS
Feverfew	*Tanacetum parthenium*	Prevention and treatment of migraine	Inhibits prostaglandin, thromboxane, and leukotriene synthesis; inhibits histamine release from mast cells and degranulation of platelets; also decreases serotonin release from thrombocytes and polymorphonuclear leukocytes	Chewing plant leaves can cause mouth ulcers	Use with caution in persons with sensitivity to aspirin or those on aspirin therapy
Garlic	*Allium sativum*	Natural cholesterol-lowering agent; effective only short-term	Sulfur-containing substances in garlic may inhibit 3-hydroxy-3-methylglutaryl coenzyme-A reductase; decreases platelet aggregation	Generally considered safe; can cause GI distress and gas	No good long-term efficacy in clinical trials
Ginkgo	*Ginkgo biloba*	Improving memory; treating dementia, peripheral vascular disease, and tinnitus	Increases blood flow; inhibits platelet-activating factors; alters neuronal metabolism; works as an antioxidant	Rare; can cause GI complaints or headache; case reports of spontaneous bleeding	Do not use in patients on anticoagulant therapy
Saw palmetto	*Serenoa repens*	Treat symptoms of BPH	Exact mechanism is unknown; may be related to inhibition of 5-alpha reductase; now thought to change PSA level; has few sexual side effects	Rare	Male patients should obtain baseline PSA and check level 8 weeks after starting therapy to assess for a reduction in the baseline PSA
Coenzyme Q10	Ubiquinone	Cardiac conditions; suggested to prevent statin-induced myotoxicity	Substance produced by the body that is structurally similar to vitamins E and K; considered to be an antioxidant and plays a role in mitochondrial oxidative phosphorylation	Considered safe; used in high doses (> 1,000 mg/day) in Parkinson's disease; will decrease the effect of Coumadin when given concurrently; cardiac dose is 50–200 mg/day	Very expensive

HERB	BOTANICAL OR CHEMICAL NAME	USE	MECHANISM OF ACTION	SIDE EFFECTS	PRECAUTIONS
Glucosamine, chondroitin (e.g., Osteo Bi-flex)		Symptomatic and functional benefits for patients with osteoarthritis of knees or hips; may slow disease progression	Glucosamine is amino sugar that is a substrate for production of glycosaminoglycans and proteoglycans (building blocks of connective tissue); chondroitin is a glycosaminoglycan that may inhibit enzymatic destruction of synovial tissue and have an antiinflammatory role (in addition to its role in cartilage formation)	Considered safe; dose is 500/400 mg, respectively, t.i.d.; may take 8 weeks before treatment response is seen	Expensive ($30–$50 per month)
SAMe	S-adenosylmethionine	To improve symptoms of osteoarthritis (with potency equivalent to that of NSAIDs, but with fewer side effects); treatment of depression	Common metabolic intermediary produced in the body through interaction of methionine and ATP	Thought to interfere with TCAs	Dosage is 400–1,600 mg/day

Note: ATP = adenosine triphosphate, FDA = Food and Drug Administration, GABA = gamma-aminobutyric acid, GI = gastrointestinal, MAOI = monoamine oxidase inhibitor, NSAID = nonsteroidal antiinflammatory drug, PSA = prostate specific antigen, SSRI = selective serotonin reuptake inhibitor, TCA = tricyclic antidepressant, ETOH = ethanol, PUD = peptic ulcer disease, BPH = benign prostatic hyperplasia.

Education is imperative for all healthcare providers and caregivers, and asking questions regarding the use of herbal remedies is recommended when obtaining the health history. It is important to acquire accurate information to protect an older adult's health. The *Physicians' Desk Reference* now has information to alert healthcare providers about herbal remedies and their side effects, and the National Institutes of Health has a dedicated institute called the National Center for Complementary and Alternative Medicine (NCCAM). NCCAM sponsors research on alternative remedies and treatments, publishes evidence-based recommendations, and provides guidance for those seeking reliable practitioners of holistic medicine. (See http://nccam.nih.gov/ for further information.)

REFERENCES

American Geriatrics Society. (2012). *AGS BEERS criteria for potentially inappropriate medication use in older adults.* Retrieved from http://www.americangeriatrics.org/files/documents/beers/PrintableBeersPocketCard.pdf

Cowley, J., Diebold, C., Gross, J. C., & Hardin-Fanning, F. (2006). Management of common problems. In K. L. Mauk (Ed.), *Gerontological nursing: Competencies for care.* Sudbury, MA: Jones & Bartlett.

Lorenz, J. (2012). Polypharmacy in the elderly. *Advance for Nurses.* Retrieved from http://nursing.advanceweb.com/Continuing-Education/CE-Articles/Polypharmacy-in-the-Elderly.aspx

McPhee, S., & Papadakis, M. (2011). *Current medical diagnosis & treatment* (50th ed.). New York: McGraw Hill Medical.

National Center for Complementary and Alternative Medicine. (2007). *Older adults not discussing complementary and alternative medicine use with doctors.* Retrieved from http://nccam.nih.gov/news/2007/011807.htm

Reuben, D., Herr, K., Pacala, J., Pollock, B., Potter, J., & Semla, T. (2011). *Geriatrics at your fingertips* (13th ed.). New York: American Geriatrics Society.

Schonbom, J. (2010). *The role of liver in drug metabolism. Anesthesia tutorial.* Retrieved from http://totw.anaesthesiologists.org/wp-content/uploads/2010/05/179-The-role-of-the-liver-in-drug-metabolism.pdf

Tabloski, P. (2010). *Gerontological nursing.* Upper Saddle River, NJ: Prentice-Hall.

Tonner, P., Kampen, J., & Scholz, J. (2003). Physiologic changes in the elderly. *Best Practice and Research in Anaesthesiology.* Retrieved from http://www.scribd.com/doc/20266489/Physiological-Changes-Elderly-Bprca04

Woodruff, K. (2010). *Preventing polypharmacy in older adults.* Retrieved from http://www.americannursetoday.com/article.aspx?id=7132&fid=6852

ADDITIONAL RESOURCES

Alternative Medicine Foundation: www.amfoundation.org

Federal Drug Administration: www.fda.gov/medwatch

National Center for Complementary and Alternative Medicine: http://nccam.nih.gov

Office of Dietary Supplements, National Institutes of Health: http://dietary-supplements.info.nih.gov

NUTRITION, HYDRATION, ELECTROLYTES, AND ACID–BASE BALANCE

This chapter reviews important aspects of nutritional assessment, risks for malnourishment, and interventions in the older adult. It also discusses fluid balance and specific electrolyte derangements and their consequences. Finally, it explains acid–base balance, including identification and consequences of both respiratory and metabolic conditions.

NUTRITION

Nutrition, hydration, and electrolyte balance are related and can have profound effects on a person's functional status, immune competence, and well-being. Beyond physiological survival, food has social and cultural significance. This complex view of food often is enhanced in older adults who survived the Great Depression in the 1930s or other hardships when food was scarce.

Poor nutrition is not a natural concomitant of aging, but older adults who are diagnosed with multiple comorbidities are at higher risk for under- or malnutrition. The term *malnourished* can refer to individuals who are undernourished or even those who are obese. Either problem can lead to chronic illnesses and contribute to morbidity and mortality. Persons who are underweight (body mass index [BMI] < 22) and those who are overweight (BMI > 25) often have loss of muscle mass, compromised immune systems, and increased complications and premature death. The progression to malnutrition is often insidious, and is often undetected. The nurse plays a key role in prevention of and early intervention in nutritional problems (Amella, 2007).

When assessing nutritional status, the gerontological nurse must remember that caloric requirements are a function of basal metabolic rate (BMR) and activity level. BMR is calculated as follows:

> **Women:** BMR = 655 + (4.35 x weight in pounds) + (4.7 x height in inches) – (4.7 x age in years)
> **Men:** BMR = 655 + (6.23 x weight in pounds) + (12.7 x height in inches) – (6.8 x age in years)

This calculation accounts for the gradual decline in BMR that occurs with age. Because activity level for most older adults decreases with time, caloric requirements drop accordingly. Older adults who do not reduce their caloric intakes or maintain their caloric expenditures will notice an increase in body weight. However, extreme dietary restrictions may lead to excessive weight loss, depression, anxiety, postural hypotension, or skin problems. The chronic diseases that affect many older adults (e.g., hypertension; congestive heart failure; renal, liver, and pulmonary diseases) often require dietary interventions for disease management.

Early identification and intervention of at-risk persons or those with nutritional deficiencies can result in improved health and quality of life for older adults.

Nutritional Screening

Nutritional screening is the first step to identifying people who are at risk for poor nutrition and its complications. Several screening tools are available, but the instrument recommended by the Hartford Institute of Geriatric Nursing is the Mini Nutritional Assessment (MNA), developed by the Nestle Nutrition Institute (http://consulgerirn.org). The Mini Nutritional Assessment (MNA®) is an assessment tool that can be used to identify older adults (> 65 years) who are at risk of malnutrition. It is a clinician-completed instrument with two components: screening and assessment. A score of 11 or less on the screen indicates a problem and the need to complete the assessment portion. The assessment score is then added to the screen score; if the total score is 17–23.5, there is a risk of malnutrition, while a score of < 17 indicates existing malnutrition. The test also can be used as a self-evaluation or completed by a caregiver or healthcare professional.

Cultural and personal preferences of the older adult and family should be considered when scoring the MNA, and laboratory data such as a serum albumin, transferrin, total lymphocytic count, and hemoglobin and hematocrit supplement the score on the MNA. Consult http://consultgerirn.org/uploads/File/trythis/try_this_9.pdf to view the instrument and further scoring recommendations.

Nutrition Assessment

A nutrition assessment is more comprehensive than a screening and usually is completed by a registered dietitian or as a collaborative effort among the dietitian, nurses, or other members of the healthcare team. The components of a comprehensive nutrition assessment are:

Dietary History and Intake

- ► Food preferences and eating habits
- ► Cultural or religious food practices
- ► Meal schedule
- ► Fluid intake (types)
- ► Alcohol intake
- ► Special diets
- ► Vitamin or supplement use

Social and Cognitive Factors

- ► Functional limitations
- ► Control over food choices and preparation
- ► Financial status
- ► Cognitive changes affecting appetite and self-feeding
- ► Psychosocial issues, such as depression or isolation

Clinical Evaluation

- ► Chronic illnesses
- ► Physical exam
- ► Oral health
- ► Chewing and swallowing
- ► Cognitive or psychological assessment
- ► Medications
- ► Lab work (e.g., CBC, electrolytes, BUN, creatinine, serum proteins, pre-albumin, lipids)

Anthropometric Assessment

- ► BMI
- ► Skinfold measurements
- ► Waist circumference (fat distribution)
- ► Weight changes (usual vs. current weight)

Physiological Changes Affecting Nutrition

The physiological changes of aging that affect nutritional status include:

► Declining sensory function (e.g., vision, smell, taste, hearing)

► Declining gastrointestinal function, inhibiting digestion and excretion

► Delayed gastric emptying, leading to early satiety

► Changes in oral cavity, particularly dentition and taste buds

► Mouth dryness

► Decreased metabolic rate

► Decreased hepatic and renal reserves

► Diminished thirst

► Declining functional status.

Not only does declining sensory function affect appetite, desirability of food, and interest in food, but these changes also may affect the older adult's ability to detect foods that have spoiled. Altered smell and taste can increase the risk of foodborne illness.

Changes in body composition occur with the aging process. A decrease in lean body mass begins in the third decade of life, although, because of a simultaneous increase in body fat, there often is little change in weight. Loss of lean body mass can be attenuated by exercise, which has been shown to improve functional status by 10–20 years (McPhee & Papadakis, 2011).

Older adults in different living situations may demonstrate different risk factors for malnutrition. Malnutrition in older persons living in the community is defined as:

► Involuntary weight loss of more than 10 lbs. over 6 months, or more than 4% over 1 year

► BMI < 22 kg/m²

► Hypoalbuminemia (< 3.8 g/dL)

► Hypocholesterolemia (< 160 mg/dL)

► Overweight (BMI 25–29.9 kg/m²)

► Obesity (BMI > 30 kg/m²)

► Specific vitamin or micronutrient deficiencies (e.g., vitamin B_{12})

► Cancer-related anorexia/cachexia syndrome

► Sarcopenia (age-related loss of muscle mass)

Malnutrition in the hospitalized older person is defined as:

▶ Dietary intake of less than 50% of daily requirement

▶ Hypoalbuminemia (< 3.5 g/dL)

▶ Hypocholesterolemia (< 160 mg/dL)

Malnutrition in the nursing home resident is defined as:

▶ Weight loss of > 5% in past 30 days or > 10% in 180 days

▶ Dietary intake of < 75% of most meals (Reuben et al., 2011)

Psychosocial Factors Affecting Nutrition

Psychosocial aspects play an important role in the desire to eat, as well as in acquiring nutritious foods. Older adults who live alone may have little motivation to prepare and consume balanced meals. People who no longer drive may not be able to get to the grocery store to obtain food. Some older adults lack adequate financial and motivational resources to buy and prepare healthy foods. Less-expensive foods tend to be those with the least nutritional value. Federal programs only reach about one-third of the population in need.

Psychosocial factors that adversely affect nutrition are:

▶ Poverty

▶ Culture

▶ Social isolation

▶ Depression

▶ Dementia

▶ Inability to access programs or transportation

▶ Lack of education or information

Food Guide Plate

The U.S. Department of Agriculture (USDA) developed the Food Plate in 2010 to replace the Food Pyramid. The purpose of the Food Plate (Figure 8–1) is to simplify current dietary recommendations and improve the nutritional status of all U.S. citizens. General recommendations include eating smaller portions, replacing whole milk with fat-free, substituting water for sugary drinks, and eating whole-grain products when possible.

The USDA Web site also provides additional information for older adults, as well as a way to create individualized meal plans, at http://www. choosemyplate.gov.

FIGURE 8-1.
THE FOOD PLATE

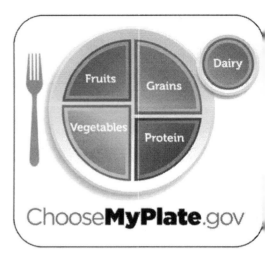

Reprinted from *10 Tips to a Great Plate*, by U.S. Department of Agriculture, 2011, retrieved from http://www.choosemyplate.gov/ groups/downloads/TenTips/DGTipsheet1ChooseMyPlate.pdf.

Oral, Dental, and Swallowing Conditions

The following oral and swallowing problems may affect a person's ability to consume a well-balanced diet:

▶ Tooth decay

▶ Missing teeth or ill-fitting dentures

▶ Periodontal disease

▶ Xerostomia (dry mouth)

▶ Taste disorders

▶ Oral infections or lesions

▶ Drugs affecting taste, appetite, and level of consciousness, or causing nausea or dry mouth

▶ Dysphagia related to aging, central nervous system difficulties, or neuromuscular diseases

About half of all cancers occur in people ages 65 or older, with an average survival rate of 5 years. Alcohol and tobacco use are the greatest risk factors. Treatment of these cancers may result in pain, swallowing difficulties, and immunosuppression, all of which can affect nutritional status.

Failure to Thrive

Older adults who are losing weight often are diagnosed with "failure to thrive." These persons have a decreased appetite, poor nutritional status, and declining functional status, and often are clinically depressed, putting them at risk for dehydration, falls, and impaired immune function. Survival depends on detection and reversal of the cause when possible, or any intervention that improves nutritional status, such as medications that stimulate appetite. Possible causes of failure to thrive are:

▶ Infection (e.g., HIV/AIDs, tuberculosis)

▶ Cancer

▶ Inflammatory disease (e.g., polymyalgia rheumatica, rheumatoid arthritis)

▶ Endocrine disorders (e.g., diabetes mellitus, thyroid disease)

▶ Organ failure (e.g., heart failure, end-stage lung disease, renal failure)

▶ Medications (any)

▶ Psychosocial problems (e.g., depression, grief, intentional starvation)

▶ Neurological disorders (e.g., Parkinson's disease, stroke)

▶ Cognitive problems (e.g., Alzheimer's dementia, vascular dementia)

▶ Neglect and abuse

Nutrition Interventions

Treatment of undernutrition is initially aimed at correcting reversible causes when possible. For example, treating depression or periodontal disease may improve intake without other interventions. Avoiding restrictive diets without exacerbating underlying disease is another strategy to improve food intake. For example, low-fat foods may not be palatable to some people or may be too calorie-restrictive for others. In such situations, it may be wise to choose to liberalize the diet while giving cholesterol-lowering medications. Foods also can be made more calorie-dense without increasing the volume of feeding. Examples are using whole milk instead of low-fat milk; adding protein powder to cereals, soups, sauces, or beverages; adding butter to hot foods; or adding sugar, corn syrup, or honey to sweet foods. Combining powdered breakfast drink, whole milk, and ice cream can make a delicious, relatively inexpensive calorie-dense milkshake. Other interventions include the following:

▶ Time oral supplements so they do not interfere with meals.

▶ Refer patients with dysphagia to a speech–language therapist.

▶ Assist clients with eating problems.

▶ Monitor bowel function and treat constipation.

FLUID BALANCE

Body fluid is located primarily in the intracellular (ICF; 60%) or extracellular (ECF; 40%) compartments of the body. The ECF compartment is composed of the blood volume (one-third) and the interstitial space (two-thirds).

Total body water decreases with age. A young adult's body is approximately 60% water, while an older adult has only 40% total body water. This decrease in total body water, combined with decreased thirst leading to decreased intake, increased sodium loss, and increased insensible fluid losses (through the bowel, skin, and respiratory systems), greatly increases the risk of dehydration in older adults. Altered cognitive status also may increase risk (e.g., failure to recognize the thirst sensation or need to drink), as can physical limitations and diuretic use. Alterations in fluid balance, in turn, affect electrolyte balance (Huether & McCance, 2012). The types and causes of dehydration are listed in Table 8–1.

TABLE 8-1.
TYPES AND CAUSES OF DEHYDRATION

TYPE	DESCRIPTION AND CAUSES	
Isotonic	▸ Equal loss of sodium and water ▸ Gastrointestinal illness	
Hypertonic	▸ Most common cause ▸ Water loss exceeds sodium loss ▸ Fever ▸ Limited fluid intake	
Hypotonic	▸ Sodium loss exceeds water loss ▸ Diuretic use	

Adapted from *Current Medical Diagnosis and Treatment* (50th ed.), by S. McPhee & M. Papadakis, 2011, New York: McGraw Hill Medical, p. 842.

Movement of Fluid

Fluid movement in the body occurs by:

▸ *Filtration:* Fluid moves through a semipermeable membrane from an area of higher hydrostatic pressure to one of lower pressure.

▸ *Diffusion:* Solutes (particles) move across a semipermeable membrane from an area of higher concentration to one of lower concentration.

▸ *Osmosis:* Water moves across a semipermeable membrane from an area of lower particle concentration to one of higher concentration.

▸ *Active transport:* Particles move against a pressure gradient, which requires energy.

Osmotic pressure is created by the particle concentrations on either side of a semipermeable membrane. Sodium is the major contributor to osmotic pressure. *Oncotic pressure* is the "pulling" force created by the concentration of particles that cannot pass through a membrane. Proteins in the bloodstream are major contributors to oncotic pressure.

Fluid Regulation

The kidneys are the main organs involved in regulating bodily fluids. In states of dehydration (hypovolemia), the posterior pituitary secretes aldosterone and antidiuretic hormone (ADH), causing the kidney to retain more sodium and fluid. Excessive volume causes suppression of these hormones, leading to increased urine output.

Dehydration

In addition to age-related physiological changes in the kidneys, many other factors may lead to dehydration in older adults:

► Infections (e.g., pneumonia, cystitis)

► Disease states (e.g., congestive heart failure, diabetes, chronic obstructive pulmonary disease, depression)

► Environmental conditions

► Decreases in thirst sensation

► Decreases in functional and cognitive ability, or both

► Restraint use

► Limited intake caused by fear of incontinence

The following interventions can prevent dehydration:

► Encourage patient fluid intake of 1,000–3,000 mL daily (e.g., filling a pitcher each day and making sure it is empty at the end of the day).

► Monitor patient lab values for increased BUN/creatinine, serum sodium, serum osmolarity, or hematocrit.

► Monitor patient urine output.

► Monitor patient for constipation or diarrhea.

► Weigh patient daily.

► Teach patient to drink despite not feeling thirsty, particularly if taking diuretics.

► Advise patient to avoid alcoholic, carbonated, and caffeinated beverages, which can increase diuresis.

Fluid Imbalances

Table 8–2 summarizes three types of fluid imbalances.

TABLE 8-2.
TYPES OF FLUID IMBALANCES

	HYPOVOLEMIA	HYPERVOLEMIA	HYPOPROTEINEMIA
Definition	▶ Extracellular fluid deficit	▶ Extracellular fluid excess	▶ Loss of oncotic pressure leads to hypovolemia
Causes	▶ Hemorrhage ▶ Overdiuresis ▶ Vomiting/diarrhea ▶ Third-spacing (ascites, burns)	▶ Congestive heart failure ▶ Renal failure ▶ Liver disease ▶ Overzealous IV fluids ▶ Sodium overload	▶ Decreased protein intake ▶ Increased protein loss ▶ Liver/kidney disease ▶ Burns ▶ Infection ▶ Hemorrhage
Clinical findings	▶ Dry mucous membranes ▶ Sudden weight loss ▶ Oliguria ▶ Tachycardia ▶ Orthostatic hypotension	▶ Sudden weight gain ▶ Pitting edema ▶ Tachycardia ▶ Tachypnea ▶ Elevated blood pressure ▶ Elevated jugular venous ▶ pressure	▶ Weight loss ▶ Impaired healing ▶ Edema ▶ Compromised immunity
Interventions	▶ Correct underlying conditions ▶ IV volume replacement ▶ Isotonic fluid (0.9% NS, lactated ringers) ▶ Whole blood, PC, plasma	▶ Correct underlying conditions ▶ Semi-Fowler's position ▶ Administer diuretics ▶ Limit sodium ▶ Assess for S/S of pulmonary edema ▶ Crackles in lungs ▶ Cough ▶ Increased respiratory effort	▶ Complete nutritional assessment ▶ High-protein diet ▶ IV replacement ▶ Whole blood ▶ Albumin ▶ Plasma

Adapted from *Current Medical Diagnosis and Treatment* (50th ed.), by S. McPhee & M. Papadakis, 2011, New York: McGraw Hill Medical.

ELECTROLYTES

Electrolyte imbalance can lead to serious consequences in older adults. Dehydration is the most common precipitant of electrolyte disturbances. Because the causes of dehydration are numerous (see above), electrolyte imbalances are common in older adults.

Electrolytes are inorganic substances (e.g., acids, bases, salts) that break up into ions in solution. Ions may be positively charged (*cations*) or negatively charged (*anions*). Blood testing measures the concentration of various electrolytes in the ECF fluid. Because many electrolytes (e.g., potassium, magnesium) are most abundant in the ICF compartment, the amount in the ECF compartment is but a small portion of the amount in the whole body.

The most common electrolytes are: sodium (Na+), potassium (K+), chloride (Cl–), phosphorus (PO^4–), calcium (Ca++), and magnesium (Mg+).

Sodium (Na+)

Sodium balance is an index of body water excess or deficit. Hyponatremia (low sodium; see Table 8–3) may result from a loss of sodium in excess of water (primary salt depletion) or from an excess of water, which dilutes the sodium level (dilutional hyponatremia). Most hyponatremia occurs in older adults because of the kidney's inability to excrete free water. With age, the renin–angiotension–aldosterone response is less vigorous, leading to less efficient resorption of sodium. Congestive heart failure and liver failure can add to this problem. Older adults often have hyponatremia as a result of inappropriate secretion of ADH (SIADH), which causes water retention and dilutes the sodium.

Hypernatremia (see Table 8–4) results from excess ingestion or administration of sodium or, more commonly, from a water deficit due to diarrhea or decreased intake. Key points about sodium include:

▶ It is the most abundant electrolyte in ECF contributing to osmotic pressure.

▶ It is not permeable to the cell membrane.

▶ It is absorbed from the gastrointestinal tract and excreted in urine.

▶ Chloride loss follows sodium loss.

▶ Aldosterone maintains sodium balance in the body by promoting renal tubular resorption.

▶ Antidiuretic hormone (ADH) reduces sodium concentration by stimulating water retention.

TABLE 8-3.
HYPONATREMIA: CAUSES, ASSESSMENTS, AND INTERVENTIONS

CAUSES	ASSESSMENTS	INTERVENTIONS
Loss of sodium ▸ Vomiting ▸ Diarrhea ▸ Burns ▸ Hemorrhage ▸ Adrenal insufficiency ▸ Diuretics **Gains of water** **Increased fluid intake** ▸ Excessive D5W ▸ Psychogenic polydipsia ▸ Hypotonic/Isotonic tube feedings with excessive H_2O **Decreased renal function** **CHF/liver failure** **Impaired renal H_2O excretion** ▸ Antidepressants (e.g., selected serotonin reuptake inhibitors [SSRIs], tricyclic antidepressants [TCAs]) ▸ Carbamazepine (Tegretol) ▸ Thioridazine (Mellaril) **Diseases associated with SIADH** **Certain cancers** ▸ Oat cell of lung ▸ Duodenal ▸ Pancreas **HIV/AIDS** **Head trauma** **Stroke** **Tuberculosis**	Anorexia Nausea/abdominal cramps Vomiting Lethargy Confusion Muscle twitching Seizures Coma Serum Na < 135 mEq/L Serum osmolality < 285m Osm/kg	**Review medications** **Monitor laboratory data** ▸ Daily weights ▸ Intake and output ▸ Encourage high-sodium foods ▸ Skin care ▸ Isotonic IV fluid replacement ▸ 3% NaCl solution **Water excess** **Daily weights** **Intake and output** **Water restriction** **Possible medications** ▸ Demeclocycline ▸ Lithium ▸ Furosemide with increased Na–K intake **Safety precautions**

Adapted from *Current Medical Diagnosis and Treatment* (50th ed.), by S. McPhee & M. Papadakis, 2011, New York: McGraw Hill Medical, p. 844.

TABLE 8–4.
HYPERNATREMIA: CAUSES, ASSESSMENTS, AND INTERVENTIONS

CAUSES	ASSESSMENTS	INTERVENTIONS
Decreased water intake	Thirst (earliest)	Encourage fluid intake
Diminished functional capacity	Dry mucous membranes	Decrease Na+ intake
Dementia	Tachycardia	Administer hypotonic IV fluidss
Altered thirst sensation	Oliguria	
High Na+ IV fluids	Confusion	
Vomiting	Lethargy	
Watery diarrhea	Delirium	
Excessive sweating	Stupor	
Fever	Coma	
Excess sodium ingestion	Serum sodium > 145 mEq/L	
Diabetes insipidus		

Adapted from *Current Medical Diagnosis and Treatment* (50th ed.), by S. McPhee & M. Papadakis, 2011, New York: McGraw Hill Medical, p. 844.

Potassium (K+)

Potassium is most abundant in the ICF, where 98% of total body potassium is located. Only 2% of the body's potassium is in the ECF. The high concentration of intracellular potassium is maintained by the Na^+–K^+ pump, which controls potassium flux across the cell membrane according to the body's needs. The kidneys excrete 80% of the potassium lost each day, with the other 20% being lost through the bowels (15%) and skin (5%). Imbalances in potassium can cause life-threatening cardiac arrhythmias, including ventricular tachycardia, ventricular fibrillation, and asystole.

Common causes of hypokalemia can be divided into renal, gastrointestinal, shifts into the cell, and sweat losses. Inadequate dietary intake of potassium rarely causes deficiency, unless there are concomitant causes of increased loss (e.g., diuretics, diarrhea). Clinical manifestations of hypokalemia are usually not apparent until the serum potassium falls below 3.0 mEq/L. However, patients who are taking digitalis may be more susceptible to arrhythmias at only minor reductions. Symptoms of hypokalemia may include fatigue, cardiac arrhythmias, EKG changes, skeletal or respiratory muscle weakness, muscle cramps, adynamic ileus, impaired insulin release, and sensitivity (see Table 8–5).

Hyperkalemia is uncommon in people with normal renal function, but may occur if over-replacement exceeds the kidney's ability to excrete potassium. Also, potassium supplementation given in combination with drugs that interfere with potassium elimination (e.g., angiotensin-coverting enzyme inhibitors [ACEI], nonsteroidal antiinflammatory drugs [NSAIDs], potassium-sparing diuretics) can lead to severe hyperkalemia. Other causes are shifts in potassium out of the cells in states of acidosis and decreased aldosterone production, which causes potassium retention. Clinical manifestations of high potassium are cardiac arrhythmias, EKG changes, muscle weakness or paralysis, nausea, diarrhea, or intestinal colic (see Table 8–6). Key points about potassium include the following:

▶ It is the most abundant electrolyte (cation) in the ICF.

▶ Balance is maintained by the Na^+–K^+ pump.

▶ Aldosterone is the most important hormone regulating potassium homeostasis.

▶ Low magnesium levels can lead to hypokalemia (these must be corrected together).

▶ High glucocorticoid levels (Cushing's syndrome or exogenous administration) cause potassium depletion.

▶ Catecholamines promote movement of potassium into the cells.

TABLE 8-5.
HYPOKALEMIA: CAUSES, ASSESSMENTS, AND INTERVENTIONS

CAUSES	ASSESSMENTS	INTERVENTIONS
Renal losses ▶ Potassium-wasting diuretics ▶ Excess aldosterone ▶ High glucocorticoid levels ▶ Licorice ingestion (contains enzyme that acts like aldosterone) ▶ Osmotic diuresis ▶ Hypomagnesemia **Gastrointestinal losses** ▶ Vomiting ▶ Gastric suction ▶ Diarrhea ▶ Ileostomy ▶ Villous adenoma **Intracellular shifts** ▶ Alkalosis ▶ Hyperinsulinemia ▶ Beta adrenergic agonists (albuterol) ▶ Hypothermia **Poor dietary intake** ▶ Anorexia nervosa ▶ Alcoholism ▶ Sweat losses in people acclimated to heat	**Skeletal muscle** ▶ Weakness ▶ Fatigue ▶ Diminished reflexes ▶ Pain or cramps ▶ Paralysis **Cardiovascular** ▶ Problems with blood pressure regulation ▶ Postural hypotension ▶ Increased digitalis sensitivity ▶ Arrhythmias **Gastrointestinal** ▶ Decreased bowel sounds **Respiratory** ▶ Shortness of breath with shallow respirations **Central nervous system** ▶ Confusion **Renal** ▶ Impaired concentrating ability causing polyuria ▶ Serum $K^+ < 3.5$ mEq/L ▶ Alkalosis common	▶ Identify patients at risk (especially those taking digitalis) ▶ Give oral supplements with food to decrease gastrointestinal side effects ▶ Educate about dietary sources of potassium (e.g., dried fruit, bananas, orange juice) ▶ Salt substitutes contain 50–60 mEq per teaspoon and may be dangerous for people on potassium-sparing diuretics or other medications that cause potassium retention (e.g., angiotensin-converting enzyme inhibitors [ACEIs], angiotensin II receptor antagonists [ARBs], nonsteroidal antiinflammatory drugs [NSAIDs])

Adapted from *Current Medical Diagnosis and Treatment* (50th ed.), by S. McPhee & M. Papadakis, 2011, New York: McGraw Hill Medical.

TABLE 8-6.
HYPERKALEMIA: CAUSES, ASSESSMENTS, AND INTERVENTIONS

CAUSES	ASSESSMENTS	INTERVENTIONS
Pseudohyperkalemia from clenching fist during blood draw or specimen hemolysis	**Cardiovascular** ▶ EKG changes = narrow, peaked T waves, shortened QT interval, prolonged PR interval ▶ Ventricular arrhythmias ▶ Cardiac arrest	▶ Identify patients at risk (especially those with renal disease) ▶ Avoid salt substitutes, potassium supplements, or potassium-sparing diuretics in patients with renal disease
Decreased renal excretion ▶ Chronic kidney disease (CKD) ▶ Potassium-sparing diuretics ▶ Trimethoprim (antibiotic) ▶ Nonsteroidal antiinflammatory drugs (NSAIDs); (with CKD) ▶ Angiotensin-converting enzyme inhibitors (ACEIs); (inhibit aldosterone secretion) ▶ Adrenal insufficiency (Addison's disease) ▶ Excessive oral or parenteral intake	**Neuromuscular** ▶ Muscle weakness ▶ Parasthesias ▶ Paralysis **Gastrointestinal** ▶ Diarrhea ▶ Intestinal colic ▶ Serum $K^+ > 5.0$ mEq/L ▶ Acidosis common	▶ Advise patients to avoid high-potassium foods (e.g., coffee, tea, cocoa, oranges, bananas, dried beans, dried fruits, whole-grain breads, meat, eggs) ▶ Administer the following treatments as ordered: ▶ Sodium polystyrene (enema, oral, NG)
Intracellular shifts ▶ Acidosis ▶ Burns ▶ Crush injuries ▶ Catabolic states ▶ Chemolysis of malignant cells ▶ Beta-blockers		▶ IV glucose and insulin ▶ Calcium gluconate ▶ Sodium bicarbonate

Adapted from *Current Medical Diagnosis and Treatment* (50th ed.), by S. McPhee & M. Papadakis, 2011, New York: McGraw Hill Medical, p. 850.

Calcium (Ca++)

The bones and teeth hold 99% of the body's calcium. The 1% of calcium that is circulating is partly ionized (47%) and partly bound to protein (53%). Calcium is important for the following body functions:

▶ Transmission of nerve impulses

▶ Skeletal and cardiac muscle contraction and relaxation

▶ Cardiac conduction and automaticity

▶ Blood clotting

▶ Hormone secretion

Total calcium levels reflect both the ionized and non-ionized calcium in the blood. As long as pH and albumin levels are normal, total calcium is a reliable marker of active (ionized) calcium levels. However, when the albumin is abnormal, the total calcium must be mathematically "corrected" (see formula next page). Changes in the blood pH also affect calcium levels. Alkalosis (increased pH) will increase the amount of calcium that is bound to protein, and acidosis will decrease protein binding. Ionized calcium, which is the physiologically active form, also can be measured directly (normal: 4.6–5.1 mg/dL).

Corrected Calcium

Normal albumin (4) – Patient albumin x 0.8 + Ca

Regulation of calcium is controlled primarily through the action of parathyroid hormone (PTH), calcitonin, and calcitriol, which is the most active metabolite of vitamin D. Table 8–7 summarizes the effect that each has on calcium regulation. Calcium enters the body through intestinal absorption. About 30%–50% of ingested calcium is absorbed under the influence of vitamin D.

TABLE 8-7.
EFFECTS OF PARATHYROID HORMONE, CALCITONIN, AND CALCITRIOL ON CALCIUM REGULATION

PARATHYROID HORMONE (PTH)	CALCITONIN	CALCITRIOL (1,25-DIHYDROXYVITAMIN D3)
Promotes transfer from bone to plasma	Antagonizes PTH	Promotes intestinal absorption
Increases intestinal absorption	Released when calcium levels are high	Enhances bone resorption
Increases renal reabsorption	Decreases calcium release from bone	Stimulates renal reabsorption

Adapted from *Current Medical Diagnosis and Treatment* (50th ed.), by S. McPhee & M. Papadakis, 2011, New York: McGraw Hill Medical.

Hypocalcemia (see Table 8–8) may occur in response to low albumin levels, but this generally does not affect the ionized or active calcium level. However, a patient with an alkalotic blood pH may have a low ionized calcium (more bound to protein) and show signs of hypocalcemia, despite a total serum calcium level in normal range. Abnormally low calcium levels may also be seen with:

► Parathyroid or thyroidectomy

► Radical neck surgery for cancer

► Acute pancreatitis

► Elevated serum phosphate (hyperphosphatemia)

► Low magnesium level (hypomagnesemia), which inhibits PTH secretion

► Vitamin D deficiency/inadequate sunlight

► Malabsorption syndromes

► Citrate from rapid blood transfusions

► Alcoholism

► Renal failure

Ninety percent of hypercalcemia (Table 8–9) is attributed to primary hyperparathyroidism or malignancy. The remainder of cases usually occur as result of:

▶ Thiazide diuretics

▶ Immobilization

▶ Lithium use

▶ Vitamin D or A overdose

▶ Renal transplantation (due to parathyroid hyperplasia)

TABLE 8-8.
HYPOCALCEMIA: CAUSES, ASSESSMENTS, AND INTERVENTIONS

CAUSES	ASSESSMENT	INTERVENTIONS
Primary hypoparathyroidism	**Neuromuscular**	Identify patients at risk
Surgical removal of parathyroid tissue	▶ Circumoral or peripheral numbness or tingling	Monitor airway
Acute pancreatitis	▶ Muscle cramps	Safety precautions with confusion
Malabsorption	▶ Carpopedal spasm	Seizure precautions when severe
Alkalotic states	▶ Tetany or neuromuscular irritability	Educate patients about reducing risk of osteoporosis:
Hyperphosphatemia	▶ Laryngeal stridor	▶ Adequate calcium and vitamin D intake
Hypomagnesemia	▶ Hyperactive deep tendon reflexes	▶ Regular weight-bearing exercise
Excessive transfusion of citrated blood	▶ Chvostek's sign	▶ Smoking cessation
Sepsis	▶ Trousseau's sign	Calcium chloride should be diluted and given through a central vein if possible due to risk for venous sclerosis or soft-tissue damage with extravasation
Hypoalbuminemia	**Cardiac**	
	▶ Decreased ventricular contractility	
	▶ Prolonged QT interval	
	▶ Arrhythmias	
	Central nervous system	
	▶ Altered mental status	
	▶ Depression/psychosis	
	Total serum Ca^{++} < 8.9 mg/dL	
	Ionized Ca^{++} < 4.6 mg/dL	

Adapted from *Current Medical Diagnosis and Treatment* (50th ed.), by S. McPhee & M. Papadakis, 2011, New York: McGraw Hill Medical.

TABLE 8–9.
HYPERCALCEMIA: CAUSES, ASSESSMENTS, AND INTERVENTIONS

CAUSES	ASSESSMENT	INTERVENTIONS
Hyperparathyroidism Malignant disease **Drugs** ▶ Thiazide diuretics ▶ Lithium ▶ Excessive calcium ▶ Excessive vitamin D or A ▶ Excessive calcium-containing antacids ▶ Theophylline Prolonged immobilization Renal disease	**Neuromuscular** ▶ Muscle weakness ▶ Decreased deep tendon reflexes ▶ Muscle hypotonicity **Gastrointestinal** ▶ Nausea, vomiting ▶ Anorexia ▶ Constipation **Central nervous system** ▶ Confusion ▶ Lethargy ▶ Depression ▶ Psychosis ▶ Stupor, coma Total serum Ca^{++} > 10.3 mg/dL Ionized Ca^{++} > 5.1 mg/dL	Identify patients at risk Increase mobilization Encourage oral fluids Possible restriction of high-calcium foods Safety precautions with confusion Monitor for digoxin intoxication, if on medication Note medications that might cause hypercalcemia Administer bisphosphanates, as directed Administer phospates, if low

Adapted from *Current Medical Diagnosis and Treatment* (50th ed.), by S. McPhee & M. Papadakis, 2011, New York: McGraw Hill Medical.

Phosphorus (PO⁴–)

Phosphorus is regulated by PTH hormone and has an inverse relationship with calcium. Phosphorus is an abundant intracellular anion and is found in all tissues of the body. Of the phosphorus circulating in the blood, 45% is either complexed or bound to protein, and the other 55% is ionized or in the active form. Phosphate is found in most foods, including red meat, fish, chicken, legumes, eggs, and milk products. It is efficiently absorbed in the jejunum in the absence of malabsorption disorders or antacids that block absorption. The kidneys are the primary route for phosphorus excretion, so they play an important role in regulation.

Phosphorus serves many functions. One is the formation of adenosine triphosphate (ATP), the major source for cellular energy facilitating muscle contraction, transmission of nerve impulses, and transport of electrolytes. Phosphorus also is important for:

▶ Intracellular messages

▶ Muscle function

▶ Red blood cell function

▶ Metabolism of protein, carbohydrate, and fat

Low serum phosphorus levels may reflect a true body deficit or may be due to shifting of phosphorus into the cells. Measurement of urinary phosphorus excretion can help differentiate these two states. In cases of a total body deficit, urinary excretion will drop to less than 50–100 mg/day (Huether & McCance, 2012).

The causes of hypophosphatemia are listed in Table 8–10, but nutritional recovery syndrome deserves further explanation. Debilitated older adults are at particular risk, as are alcoholics and persons with anorexia nervosa. A malnourished patient will be in a catabolic state, causing depletion of intracellular phosphorus stores, although serum levels remain normal. Administering a large glucose load, usually as total parenteral nutrition (TPN), causes the pancreas to release insulin, moving glucose and phosphorus into the cells. If replacement phospates are insufficient, this situation leads to severe phosphate depletion.

Hyperphosphatemia (Table 8–11) may be the result of decreased renal phosphate excretion, increased intake or absorption, or a shift of phosphorus out of the cells into the ECF. Renal excretion of phospates is dependent on the glomerular filtration rate and will decrease in acute and chronic renal failure. Cases of intoxication from phosphosoda enemas have been documented. Shifts in phosphorus to the ECF may be seen in any condition that causes muscle or tissue breakdown, such as sepsis, burns, or rhabdomyolysis. Tumor lysis that results from administration of chemotherapy can cause large shifts in phosphorus.

TABLE 8–10.
HYPOPHOSPATEMIA: CAUSES, ASSESSMENTS, AND INTERVENTIONS

CAUSES	ASSESSMENTS	INTERVENTIONS
Glucose/insulin administration	**Neuromuscular**	**Identify patients at risk**
Refeeding after starvation	▸ Muscle pain/tenderness	▸ Malnourished on
Hyperalimentation	▸ Muscle weakness	triphosphopyridine nucleotide
Respiratory alkalosis	▸ Parasthesias	▸ Alcoholics
Alcohol withdrawal		▸ Diabetic ketoacidosis
Phosphate-binding antacids	**Cardiac**	Monitor for signs of hypocalcemia
	▸ Decreased contractility	while replacing phosphorus
	Central nervous system	
	▸ Altered mental status	
	▸ Seizures	
	▸ Respiratory failure	
	Serum $PO^{4-} < 2.5$ mg/dL	

Adapted from *Current Medical Diagnosis and Treatment* (50th ed.), by S. McPhee & M. Papadakis, 2011, New York: McGraw Hill Medical.

TABLE 8-11.
HYPERPHOSPATEMIA: CAUSES, ASSESSMENTS, AND INTERVENTIONS

CAUSES	ASSESSMENTS	INTERVENTIONS
Renal failure	**Signs of hypocalcemia**	Identify patients at risk
Chemotherapy	► Tetany	Observe for signs of hypocalcemia
Overdose of supplementation	► Fingertip and circumoral parasthesias	Cautious use of phosphate-containing enemas and laxatives
Excessive Fleet's phosphosoda	► Muscle pain/spasm	
Large vitamin D intake		
	Long-term precipitation of phosphate	
	► Skin	
	► Cornea	
	► Kidney	
	► Heart	
	► Arteries	
	Serum PO^{4}– > 4.5 mg/dL	

Adapted from *Current Medical Diagnosis and Treatment* (50th ed.), by S. McPhee & M. Papadakis, 2011, New York: McGraw Hill Medical.

Magnesium (Mg++)

The majority of magnesium is located in bones (two-thirds) and inside the cells (one-third). Only 1% is in the ECF space, and only 0.3% is in the serum. Of the serum magnesium, two-thirds is ionized (active form), and one-third is bound to proteins. This distribution (very small amount in the serum) makes testing magnesium levels problematic. A serum test represents only a very small portion of the body's total stores of magnesium. Elevated levels are good predictors of magnesium excess, but a normal level does not preclude a total body deficit. Tables 8–12 and 8–13 outline the causes, assessments, and interventions of low and elevated magnesium levels.

Magnesium stores decrease about 15% between the ages of 30 and 80. The balance of magnesium depends on dietary intake and renal excretion. Magnesium is absorbed in the jejunum and ileum, and is found in green vegetables, seafood, nuts, and grains. The kidneys are very efficient at conserving magnesium or excreting excess amounts, as needed. Magnesium is closely coupled with calcium and phosphorus, as well as potassium.

Several factors increase the risk of elevated magnesium levels in older adults, including:

► Age-related decline in renal function

► Increased consumption of magnesium-containing antacids or mineral supplements

► Possible increased absorption due to altered gastrointestinal mucosa (Huether & McCance, 2012)

Magnesium plays a role in:

► ATP production and use

► Neuromuscular control

► Neuronal control

► Cardiovascular tone

► More than 300 enzymatic reactions

TABLE 8–12.
HYPOMAGNESEMIA: CAUSES, ASSESSMENTS, AND INTERVENTIONS

CAUSES	ASSESSMENTS	INTERVENTIONS
Chronic alcoholism	**Neuromuscular**	Identify patients at risk
Refeeding after starvation	► Parasthesias	Safety precautions for confusion and seizures
Diarrhea or laxative abuse	► Muscle cramps or twitching	
NG suction/vomiting	► Chvostek's sign	Monitor swallowing (can cause dysphagia)
Malabsorption	► Trousseau's sign	
	Cardiac	Encourage increased dietary intake
Drugs increasing renal wasting	► Increased digoxin sensitivity	
► Loop and thiazide diuretics	► Hypertension	Ensure complete detailed orders for magnesium replacement, because various concentrations exist
► Aminoglycosides	► Arrhythmias	
► Amphotericin B	► Coronary artery spasm	
► Cisplatinin		
► Cyclosporine	**Central nervous system**	
	► Altered mental status	Monitor DTRs (knee jerks) during magnesium administration and hold infusion if absent
Drugs causing intracellular shift	► Depression/psychosis	
► Glucose	► Seizures	
► Insulin		
► Catecholamines	**Metabolic**	
Uncontrolled diabetes mellitus	► Low potassium	
	► Low calcium	
Citrated blood products	► Low phosphorus	
	► Insulin resistance	
	Serum Mg++ < 1.3 mEq/L	

Adapted from *Current Medical Diagnosis and Treatment* (50th ed.), by S. McPhee & M. Papadakis, 2011, New York: McGraw Hill Medical.

TABLE 8–13.
HYPERMAGNESEMIA: CAUSES, ASSESSMENTS, AND INTERVENTIONS

CAUSES	ASSESSMENTS	INTERVENTIONS
Renal failure	Peripheral vasodilation/flushing	Identify patients at risk
Overdose of supplementation	Nausea/vomiting	Observe for assessment signs
Adrenal insufficiency	Hypotension	Avoid magnesium-containing medications in patients with renal insufficiency
Excessive magnesium-containing antacids or laxatives	Bradycardia	
	Decreased DTRs	
	Respiratory depression	
	Coma	
	Cardiac arrest	
	Serum Mg^{++} > 2.1 mEq/L	

Adapted from *Current Medical Diagnosis and Treatment* (50th ed.), by S. McPhee & M. Papadakis, 2011, New York: McGraw Hill Medical.

ACID–BASE BALANCE

Disturbances of acid–base balance can be classified as either acidosis or alkalosis, with the primary disorder being either respiratory or metabolic. This section reviews acid–base regulation and the method for classifying these derangements.

Regulation of Acid–Base Balance

The body maintains the internal pH within a very narrow range—between 7.35 and 7.45. This balance is maintained through various buffering systems. A buffer is able to rapidly take up or release a hydrogen (H+) ion to change the pH of the blood. An increase in hydrogen ions reduces the pH *(acidosis),* and a decrease increases the pH *(alkalosis).* Most buffering is provided by the kidneys *(metabolic)* and the lungs *(respiratory).* In addition, several less important buffering systems are at work in the ECF and ICF:

▶ Organic and inorganic phosphates

▶ Plasma proteins

▶ Red blood cells

▶ Hemoglobin

The lungs eliminate "acid" by blowing off CO_2 or can compensate for a metabolic alkalosis by retaining more CO_2. The kidneys either eliminate or retain bicarbonate ions (base), depending on the blood pH. The carbonic anhydrase equation describes the transport:

> **In the lungs, carbonic acid dissociates into CO_2 (exhaled) and water:**
>
> $H_2CO_3 = CO_2 + H_2O$
>
> **In the kidneys, carbonic acid can dissociate into bicarbonate ions (either reabsorbed or eliminated) and hydrogen ions:**
>
> $H_2CO_3 = HCO_3- + H+$

Lungs

With normal lung function, the respiratory center in the brain responds to the arterial pressure of carbon dioxide ($PaCO_2$) by increasing the rate and depth of breathing (ventilation). In people with chronic CO_2 elevations, the drive to breathe is stimulated by a fall in the arterial pressure of oxygen (PaO_2).

The lungs provide rapid compensation for acid–base disturbances, usually responding within minutes to hours. Alterations in the rate and depth of ventilation influence the amount of CO_2 that is eliminated. For example, in the case of diabetic ketoacidosis (metabolic acidosis), the rate and depth of ventilation are increased, leading to elimination of maximal CO_2 to increase the pH.

Kidneys

The kidneys compensate by eliminating or retaining bicarbonate ions (HCO_3) and hydrogen ions (H^+). This compensation is slower than compensation by the lungs and takes hours to days. The body will not compensate for acute respiratory disturbances, but it will for chronic conditions. For example, a patient with COPD will develop a respiratory acidosis because of chronic CO_2 retention. To compensate, the kidneys will eliminate H^+ ions and retain HCO_3 to maintain the blood pH within the normal range.

Electrolytes

Conditions of alkalosis are generally associated with hypokalemia. The release of H^+ into the ECF causes the movement of potassium from the ECF into the ICF (to maintain electroneutrality), resulting in low levels of potassium in the ECF. This alteration is much more pronounced with metabolic alkalosis than with respiratory alkalosis.

In contrast, acidosis leads to hyperkalemia. In this scenario, H^+ ions move into the ICF to raise the plasma pH, in exchange for a potassium ion moving into the ECF. This movement of potassium leads to a relative hyperkalemia. Again, this shift is much more pronounced with metabolic acidosis than with respiratory acidosis.

Arterial Blood Gas Interpretation

Arterial blood gas (ABG) samples are used to determine acid–base balance. Table 8–14 lists the components and significance of the information reported from this blood sample.

TABLE 8-14.
ARTERIAL BLOOD GAS INTERPRETATION FOR ACID-BASE BALANCE

TEST	NORMAL VALUE	SIGNIFICANCE OF CHANGE
pH	7.35–7.45	Low = acidosis High = alkalosis
$PaCO_2$	35–45 mm Hg	Low = respiratory alkalosis High = respiratory acidosis
HCO_3	21–28 mmol/L	Low = metabolic acidosis High = metabolic alkalosis
PaO_2	35–45 mm Hg	Low = impaired gas exchange
O_2 saturation	95%–100%	Low = impaired gas exchange

Adapted from *Current Medical Diagnosis and Treatment* (50th ed.), by S. McPhee & M. Papadakis, 2011, New York: McGraw Hill Medical, p. 860.

CO_2 reported on the chemistry panel (venous blood) reflects primarily the bicarbonate level and is, therefore, a marker of metabolic status. This can be confusing, because the $PaCO_2$ in the arterial blood reflects respiratory acid.

The four major acid–base derangements and their causes are listed in Table 8–15.

TABLE 8-15.
ACID-BASE DERANGEMENTS AND CAUSES

METABOLIC ACIDOSIS	METABOLIC ALKALOSIS
High anion gap ▶ Diabetic ketoacidosis ▶ Lactic acidosis ▶ Toxic ingestion (e.g., aspirin, methanol) ▶ Renal failure Normal or low anion gap ▶ Diarrhea ▶ Excess chloride	▶ Vomiting ▶ Gastric suction ▶ Excessive alkali ingestion ▶ Diuretics ▶ Hypokalemia ▶ Hypoaldosteronism

RESPIRATORY ACIDOSIS	RESPIRATORY ALKALOSIS
▶ Respiratory depression or hypoventilation ▶ Chronic lung disease	Hyperventilation due to any cause ▶ Anxiety ▶ Hyperthermia ▶ Thyrotoxicosis ▶ Excessive mechanical ventilation ▶ Pregnancy ▶ Sepsis ▶ Early salicylate intoxication

Adapted from *Current Medical Diagnosis and Treatment* (50th ed.), by S. McPhee & M. Papadakis, 2011, New York: McGraw Hill Medical, p. 860.

To determine the acid–base disturbance for a given blood gas, one must follow these steps (see Table 8–16):

1. Identify whether the derangement is an acidosis (low pH) or alkalosis (high pH).

2. Examine the CO_2 to determine if this value explains the abnormal pH. If yes, the problem is respiratory in origin.

3. Examine the HCO_3 to determine if this value explains the abnormal pH. If yes, the problem is metabolic in origin.

TABLE 8-16.
CLASSIFICATION OF ACID-BASE IMBALANCES

	pH	CO$_2$	HCO$_3$
Metabolic acidosis	< 7.35	Normal	< 22
Respiratory acidosis	< 7.35	> 45	Normal
Metabolic alkalosis	> 7.45	Normal	> 26
Respiratory alkalosis	> 7.45	< 35	Normal

Adapted from *ABG Interpreter*, by Manuelsweb.com, 2012, retrieved from http://www.manuelsweb.com/abg.htm.

Compensation

As discussed above, the lungs and kidneys will attempt to compensate for acid–base imbalances caused by the other system. The lungs act rapidly to compensate, and the kidneys take longer. Successful compensation will bring the pH back to normal range (7.35–7.45).

The steps for interpreting compensated blood gases are the same, except that the pH (Step 1) will be within normal range. In this case, consider 7.40 to be the "normal" level for pH. Any higher value represents a primary alkalosis, and a pH below 7.40 represents a primary acidosis. Then follow Steps 2 and 3 to determine if the primary derangement is a respiratory or metabolic disorder.

It also is possible to have a mixed acid–base disorder. It's possible to have more than one disorder influencing blood gas values. For example, ABGs with an alkalemic pH may exhibit respiratory acidosis and metabolic alkalosis. These disorders are termed *complex acid–base* or *mixed disorders* (manuelsweb.com, 2012).

SUMMARY

This chapter reviewed the basic tenets of nutrition, fluid, and electrolyte and acid–base balance. Adequate nutritional screening and assessment are needed to prevent the complications of under- or overnutrition. Derangements of fluid, electrolyes, and acid–base balance are common in older adults and can have lethal consequences. Nurses should remain vigilant and seek to prevent imbalances, but, when these do occur, it is vital that nurses promptly identify and seek treatment for the disorder.

REFERENCES

Amella, E. (2007). *Assessing nutrition in older adults: Try this: Best practices—Hartford Institute of Geriatric Nursing.* Retrieved from http://consultgerirn.org/uploads/File/trythis/try_this_9.pdf

Manuelsweb.com. (2012). *ABG interpreter.* Retrieved from http://www.manuelsweb.com/abg.htm

McPhee, S., & Papadakis, M. (2011). *Current medical diagnosis and treatment* (50th ed.). New York: McGraw Hill Medical.

Reuben, D., Herr, K., Pacala, J., Pollock, B., Potter, J., & Semla, T. (2011). *Geriatrics at your fingertips* (13th ed.). New York: American Geriatrics Society.

U.S. Department of Agriculture. (2011). *10 tips to a great plate.* Retrieved from http://www.choosemyplate.gov/food-groups/downloads/TenTips/DGTipsheet1ChooseMyPlate.pdf

ADDITIONAL RESOURCES

Nutrition Needs for the Older Adult: http://fcs.tamu.edu/food_and_nutrition/

HEALTH PROMOTION AND WELLNESS

Appropriate health promotion, wellness, and screening in older adults requires knowledge of current recommendations, as well as the older adult's functional status, approximate life expectancy, desire and willingness to participate in screenings and therapies, and quality of life. The process of health promotion in older adults is complex, and the gerontological nurse cannot rely on a "one size fits all" approach. Furthermore, the context of some healthcare settings for older adults is not conducive to addressing health promotion activities. Unfortunately, fiscal reimbursement is tied to managing or treating acute or chronic illness, and not to prevention. Another barrier is the time constraint; once attention has been devoted to acute problems and chronic illnesses, there is little or no time to focus on prevention.

HEALTH PROMOTION MODELS AND THEORIES

Nurses use many theories and models to identify health promotion deficits and develop plans and interventions for patients. However, none is specific to older adults. Some of the most common theories or models are outlined below.

Pender's Model of Health Promotion

Nola Pender developed an interest in health promotion early in her nursing career, when she noted that health care focused more on treating patients with major illness than on trying to prevent health problems. The major tenets of Pender's model are:

▶ Adoption and maintenance of health promotion behaviors depend on cognitive–perceptual factors, modifying factors, and cues to action.

▶ Cognitive–perceptual factors include perceived health, perceived self-efficacy, and perceived barriers and benefits.

▶ Modifying factors include demographic, biological, and interpersonal influences.

▶ Cues to action (internal or external) include media, peer support, and enhanced well-being (Pender, 1996).

Health Belief Model

The Health Belief Model was originally developed by Rosenstock in 1966 in response to the failure of a free tuberculosis screening program. Several years later, the model was advanced and refined by Becker. The model attempts to explain and predict health behaviors.

▶ The model attempts to explain why healthy people do or do not take advantage of screenings.

▶ Variables affecting these decisions include perceptions of susceptibility to and seriousness of disease, benefits of treatment, perceived barriers to change, and expectations of efficacy (Becker, 1972).

Transtheoretical Model of Change

The Transtheoretical Model is an integrative model of intentional behavioral change and the decision-making process of the individual, rather than social and biological influences on behavior.

▶ The model includes six stages of change:

1. *Pre-contemplation:* Having no interest in or intent to change in the near future

2. *Contemplation:* Acknowledging problem and need for change

3. *Preparation:* Preparing to make change

4. *Action:* Modifying behavior or environment to make change

5. *Maintenance:* Working to prevent relapse

6. *Termination:* End of process (Prochaska & DiClemente, 1984)

Self-Efficacy or Social–Cognitive Theory Model

The concept of self-efficacy is the central tenet of psychologist Albert Bandura's Social–Cognitive theory. According to Bandura's theory, persons with high self-efficacy are more likely to view challenges as opportunities for mastery than as something to avoid.

▶ *Self-efficacy* is one's perception of his or her ability to perform a task at a given level of accomplishment.

▶ *Outcome expectations* are the beliefs that certain behaviors result in specific outcomes.

▶ Self-efficacy and outcome expectations are influenced by four sources:

- » Mastery experience: This is the most important; achieving success raises self-efficacy.

- » Modeling or vicarious experience: When someone sees a peer succeeding at something, it increases the person's own self-efficacy or belief that success is possible.

- » Social persuasions: These are the encouragement or discouragement that one receives.

- » Physiological responses: One's interpretation of responses such as nausea, shakes, and fear also influences performance. Someone who interprets jitters before public speaking as normal and unrelated to his or her ability to do a job has higher self-efficacy (Bandura, 1986).

PREVENTION

The concepts of health promotion and specific prevention activities are closely related. Various health promotion activities can be classified according to levels of prevention. Secondary prevention activities also are referred to as "screening" tests. Both primary and secondary prevention activities are called "health maintenance."

Levels of Prevention

There are three levels of prevention: primary, secondary, and tertiary. Most available prevention data and recommendations are based on young and middle-aged adults. When these recommendations are applied to older adults, who may be four or five decades older than the people studied, clinical judgment and patient desire must always be considered.

Primary Prevention

Primary prevention refers to an action that is taken to prevent disease or make an environment less harmful. Immunizations are one example; others include safety education regarding the use of sunscreen, information on fall prevention, and education about nutrition and exercise interventions to prevent cardiovascular disease. Primary prevention is cost-effective, because it reduces prevalence of a health problem or disease, which eliminates the associated cost of treating that problem.

Secondary Prevention

Secondary prevention involves detecting the presence of a disease in its asymptomatic state to favorably alter the outcome. Secondary prevention is synonymous with *screening*, which is discussed further in the next section. Examples of secondary prevention include cholesterol screening, blood pressure screening, prostate-specific antigen (PSA) screening, mammography, colonoscopy, and testing stool for fecal occult blood.

Tertiary Prevention

Tertiary prevention involves intervention to prevent late complications of disease. Because of the high prevalence of health problems in older adults, tertiary prevention is very important. Examples include a comprehensive diabetes education program or cardiac rehabilitation for someone who is post–myocardial-infarction.

Health Promotion Interventions (Primary Prevention)

A variety of behaviors and actions promote health and well-being and help prevent disease or illness from developing.

Exercise

Exercise has beneficial health effects at any age, but its benefit is probably most profound in older adults. Benefits of regular exercise include:

▶ Decreased falls and related injuries

▶ Improved functional status

▶ Improved conditioning

▶ Reduced risk of cardiovascular disease, hypertension, obesity, type 2 diabetes mellitus, osteoporosis, colon and breast cancers, anxiety, depression, and cognitive decline

▶ Effective therapy for chronic pain, constipation, sleep and mood disorders, dementia, congestive heart failure, and stroke (National Institutes of Health, 2012)

The American Heart Association and the American College of Sports Medicine recommend four types of exercise (Nelson et al., 2007):

1. *Aerobic:* Minimum of 30 minutes of moderate-intensity exercise 5 days each week, or a minimum of 20 minutes of vigorous activity 3 days a week, or some combination of these

2. *Muscle strengthening:* May include weight training, resistance training, or weight-bearing calisthenics

3. *Flexibility:* 10 minutes of static stretching of major muscle groups on days when other exercise is performed

4. *Balance training:* Dynamic balance training, such as tai chi, has been shown to reduce the risk of falls.

Smoking Cessation

Cigarette smoking is the most preventable cause of premature death in the United States (Centers for Disease Control and Prevention [CDC], 2008). According to a U.S. Surgeon General's report, cigarette smoking accounts for approximately 30% of all cancer deaths, with lung cancer accounting for 80% of the smoking-attributable cancer deaths. Smoking also causes cancers of the oral cavity, pharynx, larynx, esophagus, stomach, bladder, pancreas, liver, kidney, and uterine cervix, as well as myeloid leukemia. Tobacco use is lower in the population age 65 or older than in the younger population; however, many older adults have long histories of smoking, leading to death from cardiovascular disease, lung cancer, and chronic obstructive pulmonary disease. Smoking deaths are significantly reduced within 5 years of smoking cessation (CDC, 2008).

Various smoking cessation therapies are available. Not every therapy is effective or appropriate for everyone, and none has been studied specifically in older adults. Therapies include:

▶ Health professional recommendation

▶ Formal counseling

▶ Nicotine replacement

▶ Bupropion (Zyban)

▶ Varenicline (Chantix)

All healthcare workers play an important role in smoking cessation for patients. Three key steps are:

1. *Ask* if a person uses tobacco.

2. *Advise* the person to quit.

3. *Refer* the person for cessation assistance (CDC, 2008)

Alcohol

Alcohol use in older adults can lead to chronic health problems, increased risk of falling or other accidents, drug–substance interactions, malnutrition, and social and cognitive decline. Although alcohol and substance abuse is statistically at epidemic proportions among the elderly, it remains for the most part unreported, undiagnosed, or ignored. The National Institute of Alcohol Abuse and Alcoholism (NIAAA, 2005) recommends that alcohol consumption for adults age 65 and older be limited to one standard drink (12 ounces of beer, 4–5 ounces of wine, or 1½ ounces of distilled spirits) per day, or seven standard drinks per week, and no more than three drinks on one occasion.

Substance abuse by older adults goes undetected for a variety of reasons, but most have to do with the fact that older adults are no longer active in mainstream society and no one notices if they abuse drugs or alcohol. It is estimated that older Americans drink less alcohol than other age groups, but, with the numbers of older adults increasing rapidly, an increase in alcohol-related problems is likely to occur over the next decade (Naegle, 2012). Risk factors include:

- ▶ Depression
- ▶ Anxiety
- ▶ Pain
- ▶ Bereavement
- ▶ Disability
- ▶ Social isolation
- ▶ Family history of alcoholism
- ▶ Previous use of alcohol

The Hartford Institute for Geriatric Nursing recommends the Short Michigan Alcoholism Screening Test–Geriatric Version (SMAST–G; Regents of the University of Michigan, 1991) for use in the clinical setting to assess alcohol abuse problems (Hartford Institute for Geriatric Nursing, 2012). See Chapter 6 for further information on the use and scoring of this instrument.

Immunizations (Primary Prevention)

Annual guidelines for adult immunizations are available from the Centers for Disease Control and Prevention:

- ▶ *Td booster:* Every 10 years (Tdap replaces 1 dose in adults ages 65 or older)
- ▶ *Influenza:* 1 dose annually
- ▶ *Pneumococcal:* 1 dose for adults age 65 or older; or repeat 1 time if initial vaccine occurs at younger than age 65; also revaccinate for those with renal disease or immunosuppression
- ▶ *Hepatitis A:* 2 doses for adults with chronic liver or renal disease or other chronic illness such as diabetes, COPD, heart disease, or immunodeficiency
- ▶ *Hepatitis B:* 3 doses (same as Hepatitis A)
- ▶ *Varicella:* 2 doses for all adults who lack evidence of immunity (history of herpes zoster diagnosed by healthcare professional is evidence of immunity)

► *Zoster:* 1 dose for adults age 50 or older regardless of history of disease. In 2011, the Food and Drug Administration expanded the age indication for Zostavax® to include adults 50 through 59 years of age for preventing herpes zoster in select groups of patients, such as those with chronic pain and comorbidities, those with hypersensitivity to medications, and those with special extenuating employment circumstances, such as close contact with those with severe varicella (CDC, 2011b).

Screening (Secondary Prevention)

Screening for disease is useful when the disease can be detected before there are clinical manifestations and at a reasonable cost. The value of various screening tests is expressed as the sensitivity and specificity of the test. The "best" screening tests have a high sensitivity and specificity.

► *Sensitivity:* Ability of a test to detect persons *with* the disease (limited false-negative results)

► *Specificity:* Ability of a test to detect persons *without* the disease (limited false-positive results)

The value of a screening test in patients age 65 or older must be determined on the basis of these variables and many others. Some factors to consider include:

► Life expectancy; unlikely to be of benefit if life expectancy is less than 10 years

► Patient desire to know if something is wrong

► Patient desire to undergo treatment if a problem is identified

► Potential morbidity, mortality, or discomfort associated with testing

► Cognitive status; ability of patient to understand testing and possible treatment

Cancer Screening

Although there is a lack of evidence to guide nurses and healthcare providers about the benefits and risks of cancer screenings in older adults, a "common sense" approach is recommended. In other words, if an older adult is functional (no matter what the chronologic age), is enjoying his or her life, and is a candidate for antineoplastic treatment should something be detected, then cancer screening is logical. However, if the older adult is frail, cognitively impaired, and diagnosed with multiple comorbid illnesses, the risks and benefits of cancer screening must be considered. Some screening tests pose more risk (colonoscopy) than others (stool for fecal occult blood), but even low-risk tests can have several potentially negative outcomes:

► False-positive results, which lead to more risky testing, unpleasant interventions, and anxiety

► Increased cost

► Discomfort

► Embarrassment

► Overdiagnosis of conditions that, if left undetected, would not have altered quality or length of life

Recommended Screening Tests

Recommendations for screening are published by multiple organizations and expert panels. The 2012 recommendations of the U.S. Preventive Services Task Force (USPSTF) are primarily:

▶ *Colon cancer:* Appropriate for anyone with a life expectancy of at least 5 years beginning at age 50 and continuing to age 75. Sigmoidoscopy every 5 years (usually in combination with stool cards for fecal occult blood) or colonoscopy every 10 years. Routine screening after age 75 is not recommended.

▶ *Breast cancer:* Mammography every 1–2 years for women between the ages of 50 and 74 with life expectancy of 4 or more years. There is insufficient evidence to support screen at the age of 75 or older.

▶ *Cervical cancer:* Cytology (Pap smear) every 3 years for women age 21 to 65 years. Screening for cervical cancer in women older than age 65 who have had adequate prior screening and are not otherwise at high risk for cervical cancer is not recommended. Screening is also not recommended in women who have had a hysterectomy with removal of the cervix and do not have a history of a high-grade precancerous lesion (i.e., cervical intraepithelial neoplasia [CIN] grade 2 or 3) or cervical cancer.

▶ *Prostate cancer:* Current evidence is insufficient to assess the balance of benefits and harms of prostate cancer screening in men younger than age 75. The USPSTF recommends against screening for prostate cancer in men age 75 or older. Some experts think that screening is appropriate in men who have a life expectancy of at least 10 years.

▶ *Blood pressure screening:* Hypertension is very common among older adults, affecting 60%–80% of the population, and is the most important risk factor for ischemic heart disease and stroke. Recommended screening intervals vary from 1 to 2 years.

▶ *Lipid screening:* Older adults have the highest risk of atherosclerotic cardiovascular disease, and hyperlipidemia remains one of the most important risk factors for this disease. People with a 10% or greater risk of atherosclerotic cardiovascular disease over the next 10 years probably benefit from screening and treatment of elevated cholesterol. The current guideline recommends testing a fasting lipid panel every 5 years in people age 20 or older.

▶ *Osteoporosis:* Low bone mineral density is a common problem in older adults. The USPSTF recommends screening for osteoporosis in women age 65 or older and in younger women whose fracture risk is equal to or greater than that of a 65-year-old White woman who has no additional risk factors. Current evidence is insufficient to assess the balance of benefits and harms of screening for osteoporosis in men.

▶ *Abdominal aortic aneurysm:* One-time screening for abdominal aortic aneurysm (AAA) by ultrasonography in men age 65 to 75 who have ever smoked is recommended. No recommendation is made for or against screening for AAA in men age 65 to 75 who have never smoked. Routine screening for AAA in women is not recommended. (U.S. Preventive Services Task Force [USPSTF], 2012)

SAFETY

There are many safety issues facing older adults. This section discusses the safety concerns that may have the biggest effect on morbidity and mortality.

Falls

Falls are an increasingly prevalent and serious problem among older adults. According to the CDC (2011a):

▶ More than one-third of adults age 65 or older fall each year.

▶ 5% of these falls result in fracture or hospitalization.

▶ Falls are the leading cause of injury-related deaths.

▶ Falls are the most common cause of nonfatal injury and trauma resulting in hospitalization.

▶ In 2009, 15,800 people age 65 or older died from fall-related injuries; 1.8 million were treated in emergency rooms, and 582,000 were hospitalized.

▶ One in three adults age 65 and over falls each year.

▶ Men are more likely to die from a fall than women.

▶ In 2010, the direct medical cost to the U.S. healthcare system for treatment of falls was $28.2 billion.

▶ More than 90% of hip fractures are caused by falls.

▶ About one-fifth of people with a hip fracture die within 1 year of the injury.

▶ Most fractures in older adults are caused by falls, with the most common sites for fracture being the spine, hip, forearm, leg, ankle, pelvis, upper arm, and hand.

▶ Rates of fracture are 2 times higher in women than in men.

▶ Many older adults who fall (even without injuries) develop a fear of falling and limit their activities to reduce the risk; such action leads to decreased mobility and balance, and actually increases the risk of falling.

Falling is defined as unintentionally coming to rest on a lower level, not as the result of loss of consciousness or a violent blow. Many older adults have varying definitions or descriptions of what constitutes a fall, making obtaining an accurate history difficult. They often do not regard "slipping" or "tripping" as falling. Older adults may often blame perceived environmental hazards for their falls instead of their own limitations.

Risk Factors for Falling

The following risk factors increase the likelihood that an older adult will fall:

▶ Past history of a fall

▶ Age

▶ Female gender

▶ Decreased vision

▶ Cognitive impairment

▶ Medications (e.g., polypharmacy; anticholinergic, psychotropic, and cardiovascular medications)

▶ Diseases affecting muscle strength and coordination

▶ Orthostatic hypotension

▶ Dizziness

▶ Anemia

Many medical conditions can present as a fall in older adults:

▶ Myocardial infarction

▶ Stroke

▶ Infection (e.g., pneumonia, urinary tract)

▶ Low blood pressure

▶ Arrhythmias

▶ Electrolyte derangements

▶ Other acute medical illness

Most falls in older adults are multifactorial, meaning that several issues may have led to the fall. These problems may occur in any of the following systems: sensory, cardiovascular, central integrative, or musculoskeletal. The sensation of "dizziness" may result from dysfunction in any of these areas.

Assessment of Falls

Older adults should be asked about recent falls. Assessment of those who fall should include:

▶ Circumstances of the fall(s)

▶ Orthostatic vital signs

▶ Testing visual acuity

▶ Cognitive evaluation

▶ Medication review

▶ Inquiry about home safety

▶ Gait-and-balance assessment (Ganz, Bao, Shekelle, & Rubenstein, 2007)

One evaluation of gait and balance is the Timed Up and Go (TUG; Podsaidlo & Richardson, 1991). For this test, a person is asked to rise from a chair and walk 3 meters (10 ft.), then turn and return to a seated position in the chair. The maneuver is timed for two trials and then averaged. People who use assistive devices (canes, wheelchairs) should have those with them. People completing this test in < 10 seconds are considered freely mobile, and those taking more than 29 seconds have impaired mobility. Other gait-and-balance assessment tools are available at http://www.hospitalmedicine.org/geriresource/toolbox/howto.htm.

Resnick (2003) has published the guideline "Preventing Falls in Acute Care," which states that falls can be prevented by a four-step approach:

1. Evaluate and identify risk factors.

2. Develop an appropriate plan of care for prevention.

3. Perform a comprehensive evaluation of falls that occur in the hospital.

4. Revise the plan of care as needed after a fall.

Risk Factors for Injury

Not all falls by older adults result in injury. The risk factors that increase the chance of injury are:

▶ Antiplatelet drugs

▶ Anticoagulants (e.g., warfarin)

▶ Osteoporosis

▶ Malnourishment

Fall Prevention

According to Resnick (2003), several interventions for fall prevention are considered standard for older adults:

▶ Familiarize the patient with the environment (e.g., call light, bathroom).

▶ Maintain the call light in reach, and have the patient demonstrate correct use.

▶ Lock the bed, and place the patient in a low position.

▶ Ensure that the patient has well-fitted, nonskid footwear.

▶ Determine if side rails should be used, on the basis of the patient's functional and cognitive status.

▶ Use a night-light.

▶ Keep the floor clean and dry.

▶ Ensure that the room is free of clutter, and that furniture is in good condition.

▶ Have adequate handrails in room, bathroom, and hallways.

▶ Establish a care plan for bowel and bladder incontinence.

▶ Evaluate the effects of medications that can increase risk of falling.

▶ Encourage exercise at the patient's highest physical level, and refer to physical therapy as appropriate.

▶ Monitor the patient regularly.

▶ Educate the patient and family about fall prevention.

▶ Make sure there are no loose throw rugs or floormats.

Other specific interventions may apply to certain patients. For example, a patient with cognitive impairment may require a bed or chair alarm for safety. For patients with dizziness, one may need to monitor blood pressure, both seated and standing.

Hyperthermia and Hypothermia

Extremes of temperature resulting in altered body function are serious problems in older adults.

Risk Factors for Hyperthermia

Both normal age-related changes and other chronic health conditions can impair heat regulation abilities in older adults. Conditions of overheating may be classified as either heat exhaustion or heat stroke. Heat exhaustion, which is caused by heat exposure, may be associated with symptoms such as nausea, dizziness, or weakness. It is not life-threatening and may not be associated with an elevation in core body temperature. Heat stroke is associated with impaired thermoregulation (core body temp > 104° F) and a systemic inflammatory response that leads to organ dysfunction and often death (Mayo Clinic, 2012a). Rapid intervention is necessary to reduce complications (see Table 9–1). Several factors are known to increase the risk of heat stroke:

▶ Heart failure (reducing ability to increase blood flow to the skin to facilitate cooling)

▶ Medications that reduce sweating ability (e.g., diuretics, tranquilizers, some heart and blood pressure medications)

▶ Loss of subcutaneous fat

▶ Alcohol use

▶ Obesity

▶ Social issues preventing cooling of home

▶ "Misinterpretation" of environmental temperature due to age-related changes in brain

TABLE 9-1.
COMPLICATIONS OF HYPERTHERMIA AND INTERVENTIONS

COMPLICATION	INTERVENTION
Hypotension	500 cc bolus normal saline to maintain urine output and SBP over 90 mm Hg
Shivering/seizures	Chlorpromazine 25–50 mg IV for shivering Diazepam 5–10 mg IV for seizures
Acidosis	No specific intervention beyond hydration and cooling
Hypoglycemia	D5W IV and monitor blood glucose q 30 minutes
Acute renal failure	Mannitol infusions to increase volume Furosemide to maintain urine output Dialysis may be needed
Hypercoagulable state	Monitor prothrombin time (PT), partial thromboplastin time (PTT), fibrin degradation products, and platelet count

Adapted from "Hypothermia and hyperthermia," by R. Slevenski, 2007, in R. J. Ham, P. D. Sloane, G.A. Warshaw, M.A. Bernard, & E. Flaherty (Eds.), *Primary Care Geriatrics: A Case-Based Approach* (5th ed., pp. 385–390). Philadelphia: Mosby.

Risk Factors for Hypothermia (Core Body Temperature < 95° F)

Hypothermia results from exposure to environmental cold. As with hyperthermia, prompt intervention is necessary to prevent complications (see Table 9–2). Several risk factors increase the risk of a significant drop in body temperature during times of exposure:

► Age

► Health

► Nutrition

► Mental status

► Body size

► Dehydration

► Wind speed

► Environmental temperature

► Humidity

► Medications

► Alcohol (Mayo Clinic, 2012b)

TABLE 9-2.
COMPLICATIONS OF HYPOTHERMIA AND INTERVENTIONS

COMPLICATION	INTERVENTION	
Hyperkalemia	Administer the following as ordered: ▸ Calcium chloride IV ▸ Sodium bicarbonate IV ▸ D5W plus insulin ▸ Kayexalate enema	
Hemoconcentration	Administer D5NS 250–500 cc bolus IV Must avoid Lactated Ringer's (liver cannot metabolize during hypothermic states)	
Myoglobinuria	Maintain urine output at 2 ml/kg/h by administering the following as ordered: ▸ 20% mannitol ▸ Furosemide ▸ Sodium bicarbonate	
Acute tubular necrosis	Referral to nephrologist	
Hypercoagulable state (DIC)	Monitor prothrombin time, partial thromboplastin time, fibrin degradation products, and platelet count	

Adapted from "Hypothermia and hyperthermia," by R. Slevenski, 2007, in R. J. Ham, P. D. Sloane, G. A. Warshaw, M. A. Bernard, & E. Flaherty (Eds.), *Primary Care Geriatrics: A Case-Based Approach* (5th ed., pp. 385–390). Philadelphia: Mosby.

Living Alone

Mentally competent older adults usually can live alone safely. Risk increases for older adults who are frail or at risk for falling.

"Call" or "alert" systems can be purchased to increase safety for older adults who spend much time alone unsupervised. The systems usually require that the person wear a bracelet or necklace that contains a button to be pressed in case of emergency. These call systems may alert designated family members or local rescue services.

Cell phones are another option for obtaining help, but people must carry them. Special cell phones and services designed to meet the needs of older adults are available. Some examples include special phones with large number pads, a large font menu, and 911 pads; roadside assistance; and lower monthly rates for those over 65.

Older adults who experience cognitive impairment require careful assessment for home safety. Those with early dementia can live alone with a few modifications to habits. These suggestions are from the Alzheimer's Association (www.alz.org):

▸ Arrange for help with daily chores.

▸ Arrange for direct deposit of income and automatic payments for routine bills.

▸ Give a trusted person the authority to handle money matters.

▸ Plan for home meal delivery, if available.

▶ Give a trusted neighbor a key to the house.

▶ Arrange for someone to regularly check smoke detectors.

▶ Have family, neighbors, or a community service program check in daily.

For older adults with cognitive impairments, cooking can be a potential hazard, because forgetfulness and distractibility can lead to burns or fires. Early use of microwave ovens is helpful, especially if the person will have to learn this new skill.

Driving

The ability to drive and maintain one's independence often is critical to the self-esteem of older adults. Depending on others for transportation leads to frustration, decrease in social activities, and depression in many people.

There are more than 30 million licensed drivers age 65 and over in the United States. In the next 20 years, the number of drivers age 70 and over is predicted to triple. Normal aging causes declines in visual acuity, hearing, and psychomotor skills, which may lead to driving impairment. Although drivers 65 and older account for 8% of all miles driven, they account for 17% of all traffic fatalities (Council of State Governments, 2012). In fact, only teenage boys have more accidents than older drivers.

People do change some driving habits as they get older, which probably helps to reduce accidents:

▶ Driving only during daylight hours and in good weather

▶ Avoiding rush hour

▶ Avoiding freeways

▶ Driving shorter distances

▶ Avoiding left turns during peak traffic hours

▶ Driving more slowly

Several factors have been noted to lead to adverse driving events:

▶ History of prior motor vehicle accidents

▶ History of falls in past 1–2 years

▶ Current use of benzodiazepines, tricyclic antidepressants, or alcohol

▶ Visual and cognitive deficits (Council of State Governments, 2012)

Persons with dementia pose an increased risk on the road. Those with an early diagnosis can often drive safely for a short period of time. However, older adults with dementia are usually unaware of their deficits and become defensive at suggestions that they should stop driving. Often, family members must take the keys or vehicle when an individual continues to drive despite deficits, because there is potential liability for accidents. Reporting of drivers with dementia and other neurologic diseases is mandatory in some states (Drazkowski & Sirven, 2011). Most metropolitan areas offer programs to evaluate drivers by means of neuropsychological and roadside tests. Departments of motor vehicles will give roadside tests when requested. Such testing may be appropriate or necessary for older adults without dementia who have other medical illnesses that impair their ability to drive, such as a history of stroke or neuromuscular disease.

Firearms

Firearms are the most common method of suicide in men and women age 65 or older. Access to firearms (particularly handguns) should be routinely assessed in older adults, especially those with symptoms of depression. Those who have a handgun in the home are more than twice as likely to commit suicide as those without one (Harvard School of Public Health, 2012). Another safety concern involves access to firearms by people with dementia who lack impulse control and judgment. Should any nurse have concerns about gun safety in the home or any clinical setting, the police and facility security guards should be notified immediately of the situation.

COMPLEMENTARY AND ALTERNATIVE MEDICINE

Complementary and alternative medicine (CAM) describes a group of diverse healthcare practices that are outside "conventional medicine" as defined in the United States. The National Center for Complementary and Alternative Medicine (NCCAM, 2012), which is a component of the National Institutes of Health, groups CAM into five categories:

1. *Whole medical systems:* Homeopathic and naturopathic medicine

2. *Mind-body medicine:* Prayer, meditation, mental healing, music, art, and dance

3. *Biologically based practices:* Herbs, foods, and vitamins

4. *Manipulative and body-based practices:* Chiropractic manipulation and massage

5. *Energy-based therapies:* Therapeutic touch and Reiki

A survey by NCCAM and AARP determined that two-thirds of adults age 50 or older use some form of CAM, but fewer than one-third speak with their medical providers about it. Older adults may be more likely to turn to CAM when conventional medical therapy fails to improve chronic or life-threatening medical conditions. The NCCAM Web site (see "Additional Resources" at end of chapter) is an excellent reference for scientific information on various therapies.

Gerontological nurses must warn patients to avoid unsafe, unproven, potentially harmful therapies that often are marketed to older adults. For example, there are herbal products that are marketed for treatment of cancer, liver and kidney disease, and memory loss, but it would never be advisable for a patient to use unproven herbal therapies for such conditions in lieu of conventional medical treatment. (Specific herbal therapies are discussed elsewhere; see Chapter 7.)

SUMMARY

Health in older adults emerges from a complex interaction among physical, functional, and psychosocial factors. The gerontological nurse can play a key role in the implementation of the goals of Healthy People 2020. Assisting older adults to avail themselves of the recommended health screenings and interventions can help them to stay active and healthy and enjoy a higher quality of life. Healthcare providers must make health promotion assessment and recommendations part of every encounter with all older patients, regardless of their level of health, to ensure that the activities discussed in this chapter are accomplished and older adults have safe living environments.

REFERENCES

Alzheimer's Association. (2008). *Coping with changes.* Retrieved from http://www.alz.org/living_with_ alzheimers_coping_with_changes.asp

Bandura, A. (1986). *Social foundations of thought and action.* Englewood Cliffs, NJ: Prentice-Hall.

Becker, M. (1972). The Health Belief Model and personal health behavior. *Health Education Monographs, 2,* 326–327.

Centers for Disease Control and Prevention. (2011a). *Cost of falls among older adults.* Retrieved from http:// www.cdc.gov/HomeandRecreationalSafety/Falls/fallcost.html

Centers for Disease Control and Prevention. (2011b). *Herpes zoster vaccination for health care professionals.* Retrieved from http://www.cdc.gov/vaccines/vpd-vac/shingles/hcp-vaccination.htm

Council of State Governments. (2012). *State licensing policies on older drivers. Knowledge Center.* Retrieved from http://knowledgecenter.csg.org/drupal/content/state-licensing-policies-older-drivers

Drazkowski, J., & Sirven, J. (2011). Driving and neurologic disorders. *Neurology, 76*(7), S44–S49.

Ganz, D. A., Bao, Y., Shekelle, P. G., & Rubenstein, L. Z. (2007). Will my patient fall? *JAMA, 297,* 77–86.

Hartford Institute for Geriatric Nursing. (2012). *Alcohol use screening and assessment for older adults. Try this: Best practices in nursing care to older adults.* Retrieved from http://consultgerirn.org/uploads/File/ trythis/try_this_17.pdf

Harvard School of Public Health. (2012). *Firearms access is a risk factor for suicide. Means matters.* Retrieved from http://www.hsph.harvard.edu/means-matter/means-matter/risk/index.html

Mayo Clinic. (2012a). *Heat stroke.* Retrieved from http://www.mayoclinic.com/health/heat-stroke/DS01025

Mayo Clinic. (2012b). *Hypothermia: Risk factors.* Retrieved from http://www.mayoclinic.com/health/ hypothermia/ds00333/dsection=risk-factors

Naegel, M. (2012). *Alcohol use and screening for older adults. Try this: Best practices in nursing care to older adults. Hartford Institute for Geriatric Nursing.* Retrieved from http://consultgerirn.org/uploads/File/ trythis/try_this_17.pdf

National Institute of Alcohol Abuse and Alcoholism (NIAAA). (2005). *Helping patients who drink too much: A clinician's guide.* Rockville, MD: Author. Available at http://pubs.niaaa.nih.gov/publications/ Practitioner/CliniciansGuide2005/clinicians_guide.htm

National Institutes of Health. (2012). Benefits of exercise. *Senior Health.* Retrieved from http:// nihseniorhealth.gov/exerciseforolderadults/healthbenefits/01.html.

Nelson, M. E., Rejeski, J., Blair, S. N., Duncan, P. W., Judge, J. O., King, A. C., et al. (2007). Physical activity and public health in older adults: Recommendations from the American Colleges of Sports Medicine and the American Heart Association. *Circulation, 116,* 1094–1105.

Pender, N. (1996). *Health promotion in nursing practice* (3rd ed.). Norwalk, CT: Appleton & Lange.

Podsiadlo, D., & Richardson, S. (1991). The Timed "Up & Go": A test of basic functional mobility for frail elderly persons. *Journal of the American Geriatric Society, 39,* 142–148.

Prochaska, J. O., & DiClemente, C. C. (1984). *The trans-theoretical approach: Crossing traditional boundaries of change.* Homewood, IL: Dow Jones Irwin.

Resnick, B. (2003). Preventing falls in acute care. In M. Mezey, T. Fumer, I. Abraham, & D. A. Zwicker (Eds.), *Geriatric nursing protocols for best practice* (2nd ed., pp. 141–164). New York: Springer.

Slevenski, R. (2007). Hypothermia and hyperthermia. In R. J. Ham, P. D. Sloane, G. A. Warshaw, M. A. Bernard, & E. Flaherty (Eds.), *Primary care geriatrics: A case-based approach* (5th ed., pp. 385–390). Philadelphia: Mosby.

U.S. Preventive Services Task Force. (2012). *Preventive services.* Retrieved from http://www. uspreventiveservicestaskforce.org/uspstopics.htm

ADDITIONAL RESOURCES

Complementary and Alternative Medicine: http://nccam.nih.gov/

Information on Falls: http://www.cdc.gov/ncipc/factsheets/adultfalls.htm

Preventing Falls in Acute Care: http://www.guideline.gov/summary/summary.aspx?doc_id=12265&nbr=00 6349&string=Preventing+AND+Falls+AND+Acute+AND+care

LIFESTYLE, HEALTH CHANGES, AND VULNERABILITY IN THE OLDER ADULT

Nurses spend more time with patients and their families at the end of life than any other member of the healthcare team. Viewing the death of an older person as a natural process, and not a medical failure, can help nurses provide the highest quality of nursing care with important benefits to the patient and family:

► Attention to pain and symptom control

► Relief of psychosocial distress

► Coordinated care across settings, with high-quality communication between healthcare providers

► Assessing and treating pain, nausea, constipation, anxiety, insomnia, and fatigue to positively affect quality of life, costs, and survival

► Preparing the patient and family for death

► Clarification and communication of goals for treatment and values

► Support and education during the decision-making process, including the benefits and burdens of treatment (National Consensus Project for Quality Palliative Care, 2004: Spellman, 2012)

The top leading causes of death (accounting for 80% of all deaths in the United States) include heart disease, cancer, chronic lower respiratory disease, cerebrovascular disease, accidents and unintentional injury, Alzheimer's disease, diabetes mellitus, kidney disease, influenza, pneumonia, and intentional injury (Murphy, Xu, & Kochanek, 2012). Many of these causes are associated with high degrees of symptom distress; high use of burdensome and often nonbeneficial treatment; caregiver strain on families, and problems with communication among patients, families, and caregivers. Possible barriers to providing high-quality end-of-life care include failure of healthcare providers to acknowledge the limits of medical science, lack of training in effective means of controlling pain and symptoms, unwillingness of providers to be honest about a poor prognosis, discomfort in relaying bad news, and lack of understanding about the valuable contributions to be made by referral to and collaboration with comprehensive hospice or palliative care services (Murphy, Xu, & Kochanek, 2012).

PALLIATIVE CARE

The goals of palliative care are to prevent and relieve suffering and to support the best possible quality of life for patients and their families, regardless of the stage of the disease or the need for other therapies. Palliative care should be provided when older adults have:

▶ Acute, serious, life-threatening illness (e.g., stroke, trauma, acute myocardial infarction, renal disease, or cancer, where cure or reversibility may or may not be a realistic goal, but the burden of treatment is high)

▶ Progressive chronic illness (e.g., end-stage dementia, congestive heart failure, renal or liver failure, frailty)

Palliative care can take place in hospitals, long-term-care facilities, outpatient clinics, or the patient's home. The care provided emphasizes quality of life until the moment of death.

HOSPICE CARE

The goals of hospice care are to support and care for people in the last phase (usually the last 6 months) of an incurable disease. A multidisciplinary team of physicians, nurses, therapists, home health aides, pharmacists, pastoral counselors, social workers, and trained volunteers assists the family in providing care at home. Hospice nurses assume the role of specialist in the management of pain and symptom control.

According to Elizabeth Kübler-Ross (1969), there are five stages in the dying process:

1. *Denial:* "Not me. There must be some mistake."

2. *Anger:* "Why me? I always tried to be a good person and take care of myself."

3. *Bargaining:* "OK. I'll try one more round of chemotherapy if I can make it to my daughter's graduation in June."

4. *Depression:* "Why bother? I feel so sick, I should just give up."

5. *Acceptance:* "OK. I know my time to die is coming, so I think I'll get my affairs in order."

Not all patients will progress through or experience these stages in the same way or order, so nurses should remain objective and not expect a "one size fits all" reaction to the dying process.

PAIN RELIEF AT THE END OF LIFE

Pain is a distressing sensation that can be acute or chronic. Assessment of pain has been called the "fifth vital sign" and must be routinely carried out when other vital signs are assessed. Many older patients have difficulty communicating pain at the end of life because of delirium, dementia, aphasia, motor weakness, language barriers, and fear of being labeled a complainer. Additionally, there are cultural variations. Patients of some cultures are likely to be more verbal when communicating their pain, and those of other cultures may be more likely to "keep a stiff upper lip" and not offer any complaints.

Pain in the person with dementia often may be expressed as a change in baseline behavior. The family and the nurse may notice increased agitation, restlessness, grimacing, crying, withdrawal from normal activity, a change in function such as loss of appetite, moaning, calling out, or other signs. Nurses should acknowledge the importance of caregiver reports because they often are the first to notice subtle changes in behavior or function. When dealing with nonverbal patients, nurses should observe the following signs:

▶ Moaning or groaning at rest or with movement

▶ Failure to eat, drink, or respond to the presence of others

▶ Grimacing or strained facial expression

▶ Guarding or not moving parts of the body

▶ Resisting care or not cooperating with therapeutic interventions

▶ Rapid heartbeat, diaphoresis, or change in vital signs

For older patients who are verbal, standard pain assessment instruments should be used, including asking patients to rate their pain on a 1–10 scale (with 10 being the worst pain ever) or on the smiley-face scale. Additional helpful questions may include:

▶ Where does it hurt the most?

▶ How would you describe the pain (sharp, dull, shooting)?

▶ Do nausea, vomiting, or diarrhea accompany the pain?

▶ Can you sleep when you are having pain?

▶ What do you think is causing the pain?

▶ What makes the pain better or worse?

Once the baseline level of pain has been documented, ongoing pain assessment can document the effect of the intervention. Inadequate pain relief hastens death by increasing physiological stress, potentially diminishing immunocompetency, decreasing mobility, worsening the risk of pneumonia and thromboembolism, and increasing the work of breathing and myocardial oxygen requirements. Unrelieved pain also can cause psychological distress to the patient and family, because it is associated with suffering and spiritual distress (Institute of Medicine, 2011).

Pain Management

After conducting a complete pain assessment, nurses share information with other team members to collaborate for adequate pain control. Types of drugs used to control pain at the end of life are:

▶ *Nonopioids:* Including acetaminophen and nonsteriodal antiinflammatory drugs (NSAIDs). These drugs are helpful for mild to moderate pain and can be used alone or in combination with other medications to enhance their effect. Acetaminophen should be limited to less than 4 g daily for most older adults; those with hepatic insufficiency or current or history of alcohol abuse should have a 50%–75% daily dose reduction to avoid liver damage (Geriatric Pain, 2012). Current guidelines recommend 3 g daily for healthy older adults and 2 g daily for frail older adults with comorbidities. NSAIDs can cause gastrointestinal (GI) bleeding and should be avoided in patients with histories of GI bleeding or ulcers.

▶ *Opioids:* Including codeine, morphine, hydromorphone, fentanyl, methadone, and oxycodone. Morphine is considered the gold standard for the relief of cancer pain. Constipation and sedation are two troublesome symptoms that often are associated with opioid use. Avoid meperidine because it is associated with seizure, delirium, and tremor caused by the accumulation of toxic metabolites (American Geriatrics Society, 2012).

▶ *Adjuvant analgesics:* Usually given to enhance the effectiveness of other classes of drugs, allowing effective treatment of pain with lower doses and less chance of side effects. Medications in this class include muscle relaxers, corticosteroids, anticonvulsants, antidepressants, and topical medications.

Administration of Pain Medication

Usually the oral route is preferred because it is easiest and most comfortable for the patient; however, medications may be administered by other routes.

▶ *Oral:* Tablets, liquids, and sustained-release capsules can control pain for up to 24 hours. Usually a higher dose of medication is needed when given orally, because the medication must be deactivated in the liver (first pass effect).

▶ *Oral mucosa:* Concentrated liquids can be given by dropper into the oral or buccal mucosa. This route can be used even when the patient can no longer swallow.

▶ *Rectal:* Some medications come in suppository form; however, this route is invasive, and insertion may be difficult in patients who cannot move easily.

▶ *Transdermal:* A fentanyl patch can be placed on the skin every 72 hours for pain relief. Peak onset may be delayed up to 24 hours, and changes in blood flow, metabolism, and fat distribution may affect absorption.

▶ *Topical:* Topical capsaicin and local anesthetics (eutectic mixture of lidocaine and prilocaine; EMLA) can be used for pain relief from herpes or arthritis and before the insertion of intravenous medication or injections.

▶ *Parenteral:* The intravenous, intramuscular, and subcutaneous routes are used when the patient cannot swallow. If the IV route is used, try to deliver the smallest amount of fluid possible to minimize excessive secretions that can require suctioning and cause difficulty breathing.

▶ *Epidural or intrathecal:* Administration of drugs into or around the spinal cord can be used for those patients who cannot achieve pain relief in any other manner. There is increased cost and risk of infection when these techniques are used.

In general, avoid the use of p.r.n. medications to treat pain once the patient voices a complaint. It is more beneficial to achieve good baseline control of pain with long-acting medications, rather than waiting for pain to recur and then waiting further for medication to relieve the pain. If patients experience frequent breakthrough pain and require equally frequent p.r.n. dosing, the baseline dose of long-acting medication should be increased to prevent the breakthrough (Tabloski, 2010).

In rare occasions, a medication given for pain relief may have the unintended consequence of shortening the patient's life span. This is usually considered the merciful administration of pain medication at the end of life, and not mercy killing or euthanasia, because the intent is to relieve pain and not to hasten death (American Nurses Association, 2010).

Common symptom management strategies for older patients at the end of life are given in Table 10–1.

TABLE 10-1.
COMMON END-OF-LIFE PROBLEMS AND SUGGESTED NURSING INTERVENTIONS

PROBLEM	INTERVENTION AND MEDICATION
Constipation	Give stimulant laxatives and enema after 3 days without bowel movement.
Delirium	Treat pain, fever, social isolation; avoid restraints or excessive sedating medications.
Dyspnea	Administer opioids to slow rate, and provide humidified oxygen for comfort.
Cough	Use cough suppressants for comfort; elevate head of bed; suction as needed.
Anorexia	Provide careful mouth care; treat constipation, nausea, and vomiting; offer patient's favorite food and fluids as tolerated.
Nausea and vomiting	Use antinausea and anti-emetic drugs and complementary therapies (e.g., music, relaxation, hypnosis) as needed.
Fatigue	Treat anemia if needed; provide frequent rest periods.
Anxiety	Use antidepressants and benzodiazepines for sleep and relaxation; provide support, and encourage socialization.

Adapted from *Palliative Nursing* by B. Ferrell & N. Coyle, 2010, New York: Oxford University Press.

ADVANCE DIRECTIVES

A living will or healthcare proxy may help ensure that the older patient receives the level of care he or she wants at the end of life. Personal values, cultural beliefs, religious preferences, medical knowledge, and life experiences all determine end-of-life preferences. Most healthcare institutions have developed policies concerning advance directives, and nurses may become involved in the process. Be sure to address issues related to hospitalization for acute illness, use of feeding tubes, and administration of aggressive interventions such as CPR at the end of life.

Types of advance directives include:

▶ *Durable power of attorney and healthcare proxy:* A document naming a person to make decisions for another if the patient is no longer capable of making his or her wishes known. The proxy may be a family member, friend, or significant other.

▶ *Living will:* A personal statement of how one wishes to die, setting forth instructions for those providing end-of-life care.

Barriers to completion of advance directives include fear, procrastination, lack of family support, inability to understand the process, and deferring decisions to physicians or other healthcare providers.

GRIEF

Death of a loved one results in feelings of shock and grief in those left behind. *Grief* is the emotion felt after the loss, and *mourning* is the period of active grieving. Phases of grief include:

▶ *Phase 1: Numb shock.* The survivor cannot believe the death occurred. This phase is protective to blunt the feeling of loss.

▶ *Phase 2: Emotional turmoil.* Alarm or panic reactions occur. Anger, guilt, or longing for the deceased person takes place.

▶ *Phase 3: Loneliness.* When the full effects of the death set in, the survivor's life purpose may be unclear, and he or she may have mood swings.

▶ *Phase 4: Reorganization.* Coping begins, and the survivor begins to move on with his or her life. (Kübler-Ross, 1969)

Grief is active rather than reactive. Behaviors associated with grief and mourning are social and cultural. Grief in the older person may take longer than anticipated, and no normal grieving time can be described, because it is different for each person. Grief that fails to resolve over an extended time or results in self-neglect may have progressed to depression, indicating the need for counseling and perhaps antidepressant medications.

Grieving survivors should be urged to care for themselves, eat properly, rest and exercise as tolerated, plan social and family events so that they have something to look forward to, and reach out to others for support and encouragement. The art of healing requires knowing and nourishing oneself. Nurses can be a vital link in the healing process (Tabloski, 2010).

SEXUALITY

In our society, discussion of sexuality in the older adult has been considered taboo and embarrassing to both the older person and the nurse. Additionally, many older people and healthcare providers believe that sexual intercourse and other expressions of sexuality are strictly limited to youth and middle age, while older adults are asexual. Although sexual desire tends to decline with age, many older adults continue to enjoy sexual activity well into their later years, if they have interested and interesting partners.

Chronic pain and osteoarthritis are two common problems that can inhibit sexual activity and enjoyment. Appropriate use of pain medication, warm baths before sexual activity, and use of alternative sexual positions ("spoon" position) can be tried to alleviate pain and increase enjoyment. An older adult with cardiovascular disease is considered healthy enough for sexual activity if he or she can climb two flights of stairs without discomfort, or walk at a rate of two miles per hour without chest pain or shortness of breath. The older person should check with his or her doctor before engaging in sexual intercourse (Tabloski, 2010).

Normal changes of aging in the reproductive tract related to sexual function include:

▶ Male: Decreased sperm production; decreased testosterone levels; increased time to sexual arousal, ejaculation, and refractory period; decreased firmness of erection and force of ejaculation

▶ Female: Decreased estrogen levels; decreased thickness, elasticity, and lubrication of vaginal tissues; decreased glandular tissue in breasts; and increased time to arousal

Although menopause is a normal change of aging, not a disease, some older women experience problems during this period that persist into later life. These problems may include sleep disorders, decreased vaginal lubrication, atrophic vaginitis (thinning and atrophy of the vaginal wall due to decreased estrogen levels), more frequent urinary tract infections, hot flashes, and pain or discomfort with sexual activity. At one time, treatment for these problems included hormone replacement therapy (HRT); however, recent research has revealed that HRT is associated with higher rates of myocardial infarction, stroke, breast cancer, pulmonary embolism, and deep vein thrombosis (Womenshealth.gov, 2010). Current recommendations are that HRT should be used at the lowest dose for the shortest period of time to relieve severe hot flashes, help those at high risk for osteoporosis and fracture, and prevent colorectal cancer. The potential risk/benefit analysis should be thoroughly discussed with the older woman before beginning therapy.

Lifestyle modification may be beneficial for coping with severe hot flashes. Measures include dressing in layers, using fans for cooling, and lowering room temperatures. Atrophic vaginitis may be successfully treated with topical estrogen creams applied directly to the vaginal tissues. Topical estrogen creams have not been linked to adverse effects (Womenshealth.gov, 2010).

Male impotence, or erectile dysfunction (ED), affects nearly 70% of men over the age of 70 (Wessells, Joyce, Wise, & Wilt, 2007), and the rate increases with each decade of life. *Erectile dysfunction* is defined as the inability to achieve or maintain an erection sufficient for sexual satisfaction. ED may be caused by medications (antidepressants, antihypertensives, antipsychotics, diuretics), poor arterial blood flow, cigarette smoking, poor lifestyle habits (stress, excessive alcohol use, obesity), psychological factors (depression, anxiety), and diagnosed physical illness (diabetes mellitus, hypertension). Men who awaken with an erection are likely to have ED caused by psychological rather than physiological problems.

Treatment of ED depends on the cause and may include discontinuation of offending medication, psychological counseling, weight loss, surgical implants, or use of ED drugs such as sildenafil (Viagra). Nearly 6% of American men take oral ED drugs. These medications are generally well tolerated, although they should not be taken along with oral nitrates (Wessells et al., 2007).

Sexually active older adults are at risk for the same sexually transmitted infections that can affect younger and middle-age adults, including HIV/AIDS, genital herpes, gonorrhea, and syphilis. Older adults should be offered the same education about safe sex, including the use of condoms. In addition, many gay and lesbian older adults may avoid discussing their sexuality because they fear rejection or prejudice. An insensitive or judgmental nurse may easily compromise the sexual health of this group of older adults.

CULTURAL, ETHNIC, AND RELIGIOUS DIVERSITY

An older person's heritage is composed of background, ethnicity, and religion (Spector, 2009). *Culture* encompasses the thoughts, communications, actions, beliefs, values, and institutions of racial, ethnic, religious, or social groups (U.S. Department of Health and Human Services, 2012). Culture depends on many factors, including societal knowledge, belief, art, law, morals, and habits.

Ethnicity pertains to a social group that claims to possess variable traits, such as a common religion or language. Many diverse ethnic groups are represented in the United States.

Religion is the belief in a divine power to be obeyed and worshipped. The practice of religion is often associated with practices and rituals related to life, death, and illness. When these practices are not followed or are violated by well-meaning healthcare providers, spiritual distress can occur.

National standards for culturally and linguistically appropriate services in health care have been established and specify guidelines that must be followed by most healthcare-related agencies (U.S. Department of Health and Human Services, 2012). Some of these standards include:

▶ Respectful delivery of care compatible with cultural beliefs and practices and preferred language

▶ Recruitment and retention of diverse staff and leadership, representative of the demographics of the service area

▶ Ongoing staff education and training in culturally and linguistically appropriate service delivery

▶ Providing bilingual staff or interpreters in a timely manner

▶ Signs and pamphlets distributed in commonly understood languages in the service area

▶ Data on patient's ethnicity, race, and spoken and written languages collected and documented in the health record, and integrated into the organization's management information systems and periodically updated

▶ Formation of partnerships with community representatives to encourage participation in designing, implementing, and evaluating delivery of culturally appropriate health care

Questions the nurse can use to prepare to deliver culturally appropriate health care include:

▶ Respect: Does the older person have particular beliefs about roles, responsibilities, or care received from a person of a different gender?

▶ Death and dying: What are the perspectives and rituals surrounding death, life-sustaining treatment, treatment of the body after death, and burial?

▶ Pain: What are the beliefs about relief of pain, use of medications, and accepted behaviors of a person in pain?

▶ Medicine and nutrition: Are there home remedies, herbals, or special foods to be used to treat disease or bring relief of suffering?

▶ Role of the older person: How independent are older persons in this culture? Is truth valued, or is it believed that the older person should be protected?

▶ Manner: How is the older person to be addressed? Should the older person be touched?

▶ Space: Is privacy for prayer needed? Does the family or religious advisor need space for ceremony and ritual? (McBride, 2012)

Nurses are urged to discuss these issues with patients and families, and not make assumptions based on stereotypical thinking. Each older person and family is unique, and great diversity occurs with aging, so each person should be approached as an individual.

Common cultural conflicts can occur in the clinical setting. Table 11–2 describes these conflicts, consequences, and adverse patient outcomes.

TABLE 10-2.
CONSEQUENCES OF CULTURAL CONFLICTS

SITUATION	CONSEQUENCE	PATIENT OUTCOME
Language barriers	Inadequate assessment	Poor pain control, decreased quality of life
Dietary blunders	Refusal to eat	Malnutrition, weight loss, dehydration, anger
Violation of manners	Resistance to care	Avoidance, skin breakdown, fear

Adapted from *Gerontological Nursing: The Essential Guide to Clinical Practice* (2nd ed.), by P. Tabloski, 2010, Upper Saddle River, NJ: Prentice Hall.

Culturally appropriate nursing involves incorporating relevant cultural, ethnic, and religious customs into the care setting. Recognizing the older person's viewpoint requires excellent communication skills. Care must be taken to minimize conflict and prevent the development of a crisis. Culturally appropriate care is challenging and requires great understanding of the meaning of the older person's ethnocultural and religious heritage, along with the person's life trajectory. The gerontological nurse will benefit from each experience with a culturally diverse older patient.

ELDER MISTREATMENT

Each year, more than two million vulnerable older adults are victims of abuse, neglect, and exploitation. Research has shown that older adults who are abused, neglected, or exploited are three times more likely to die within 10 years of such experiences than those who are not. According to national statistics, elder abuse is grossly underreported because of vulnerable older adults who are being abused find it very difficult to tell anyone, because of shame and fear. Elder abuse affects men and women of all ethnic backgrounds and social status, and occurs in private residences and in facilities (North Carolina Division of Aging and Adult Services, 2011).

The National Center on Elder Abuse (2006) periodically reports data regarding elder mistreatment in the United States. Key findings from the 2006 report include:

▶ Total reported abuse and neglect increased by 19.7% since the 2000 survey.

▶ Proven elder abuse and neglect increased by 15.6% since the 2000 survey.

▶ The vast majority (89.3%) of abuse and neglect occurred in the home setting.

▶ The typically abused older person is a White woman over the age of 80.

▶ The typical abuser is an adult child (32.6%) or family member (21.5%); spouses accounted for only 11.3% of abuse.

The number of cases of elder mistreatment is overwhelming and warrants the attention of all healthcare providers, especially gerontological nurses. Every state has mechanisms for reporting elder mistreatment, and adult protective services exist in every state. The Nursing Home Reform Act of 1987 (OBRA) mandates reporting of abuse or mistreatment occurring in long-term-care settings. In most states, elder abuse or mistreatment must be reported by law, and reported cases will be aggressively investigated.

There are three categories of elder mistreatment:

▶ Domestic mistreatment occurring in the older adult's home

▶ Institutional mistreatment occurring in long-term-care facilities, rehabilitation settings, and acute care hospitals

▶ Self-neglect occurring when older adults who are mentally competent enough to understand their actions make decisions that threaten their lives and safety (Strasser, Dowling-Castronovo, & Fulmer, 2009).

Definitions of elder mistreatment include:

▶ *Physical abuse:* Intentional infliction of injury or pain such as hitting, shaking, or pushing. Look for bruising, fractures, and injuries in various stages of healing.

▶ *Emotional abuse:* Inflicting emotional distress or anguish by yelling, swearing, or name calling. Look for agitation or withdrawal.

▶ *Sexual abuse:* Any form of nonconsensual sexual intimacy, such as rape, molestation, and sexual harassment. Look for genital bruising, unexplained rectal or vaginal bleeding, and sexually transmitted infections.

▶ *Caregiver neglect:* Intentional or unintentional failure to meet the physical, social, or psychological needs of the older person, including not helping with hygiene, enforced social isolation, withholding food or fluids, and lack of attention to healthcare needs. Look for dehydration, malnutrition, pressure ulcers, untreated physical illness, and reports of being left alone for long periods of time.

▶ *Financial exploitation:* Diverting or withholding monetary funds, including taking Social Security checks or pension funds. Look for unexplained inability to pay for food, shelter, medications, or clothing.

▶ *Abandonment:* Purposefully deserting an older person, including taking him or her to a public place, such as a hospital emergency department or a bus station, and leaving him or her alone. Look for older patients who cannot describe the circumstances by which they came to be alone or how to contact friends or family to arrange for a safe return to their previous living arrangements.

If elder abuse or mistreatment is suspected, the nurse should conduct a careful assessment, with emphasis on identifying the factors listed above. The Hartford Institute for Geriatric Nursing recommends the use of the Elder Mistreatment Assessment (Fulmer, 2012). The older person should be completely undressed and all areas of the body inspected, because sometimes abusers will inflict injury in areas normally hidden by clothing. Laboratory and x-ray examinations may be necessary to document the extent of injuries and neglect. Laboratory testing may include markers of dehydration (blood urea nitrogen and creatinine) and nutritional status (serum albumin, red blood count, cholesterol). X-ray examinations may document fractures, displaced joints, and presence of pneumonia. If possible, the older person should be interviewed by the nurse and a social worker in a private setting. Pictures of physical abuse should be taken to document the extent of injury.

Once elder mistreatment is identified, an interdisciplinary team approach is needed for treatment. Educational interventions may be appropriate for caregiver neglect, if the caregiver is stressed and requires support and assistance. Hospital admission may be needed while a safety plan, which may include removing the older person from the home setting, is developed for older adults who are frail or have comorbidities. For mistreatment occurring in institutional settings, the abuser should be terminated immediately and charges pressed to document the crime and prevent the abuser from gaining employment in another healthcare setting. Criminal background checks are now required for all persons seeking employment in institutional settings.

Financial management assistance or legal help to establish a guardian may be needed for those older adults without appropriate advocates or conservators. There is a lack of evidence-based interventions to offer victims and their families (Fulmer, 2012). Community and professional education is needed at all levels, including local, state, and national initiatives. Ideally, future research will identify appropriate effective healthcare interventions.

SUMMARY

Many factors can affect lifestyle, health, and vulnerability in the older adult. Careful nursing care at the end of life, with meticulous pain and symptom control, is required and is an integral role of gerontological nurses. Providing culturally competent care at all stages of the health and illness spectrum is mandated and crucially important to older patients and their families. Careful assessment and recognition of each older person as a unique individual is needed to avoid stereotypical thinking and miscues in the clinical setting. Finally, recognition of elder abuse and mistreatment is needed to protect those frail elders who cannot advocate for themselves. Early identification of older adults at risk for mistreatment and aggressive intervention are needed to protect vulnerable older adults from further injury or exploitation.

REFERENCES

American Geriatrics Society. (2012). *Beers criteria: Potentially inappropriate medications for the elderly.* Retrieved from http://www.americangeriatrics.org/files/documents/beers/2012AGSBeersCriteriaCitations.pdf

American Nurses Association. (2010). *Registered nurses' roles and responsibilities in providing expert care and counseling at the end of life. Position statement.* Retrieved from http://www.nursingworld.org/MainMenuCategories/EthicsStandards/Ethics-Position-Statements/etpain14426.pdf

Ferrell, B., & Coyle, N. (2010). *Palliative nursing.* New York: Oxford University Press.

Fulmer, T. (2012). *Elder mistreatment assessment. Try this: Best practices in nursing care to older adults.* Retrieved from http://consultgerirn.org/uploads/File/trythis/try_this_15.pdf

Geriatric Pain. (2012). *FDA announcement regarding acetaminophen in prescription drugs.* Retrieved from http://www.geriatricpain.org/Pages/acetaminophen.aspx

Institute of Medicine. (2011). *Relieving pain in America.* Retrieved from http://iom.edu/~/media/Files/Report%20Files/2011/Relieving-Pain-in-America-A-Blueprint-for-Transforming-Prevention-Care-Education-Research/Pain%20Research%202011%20Report%20Brief.pdf

Kübler-Ross, E. (1969). *On death and dying. What the dying have to teach doctors, nurses, clergy, and their own families.* New York: MacMillan.

McBride, M. (2012). *Ethnogeriatrics and cultural competence for nursing practice.* Hartford Institute for Geriatric Nursing. Retrieved from http://consultgerirn.org/topics/ethnogeriatrics_and_cultural_competence_for_nursing_practice/want_to_know_more

Murphy, S., Xu, J., Kochanek, K. (2012). Deaths: Preliminary data for 2010. *National Vital Statistics Reports, 60*(4). Retrieved from http://www.cdc.gov/nchs/data/nvsr/nvsr60/nvsr60_04.pdf

National Center on Elder Abuse. (2006). *Elder abuse: Prevalence and incidence.* Retrieved from http://www.ncea.aoa.gov/Main_Site/pdf/publication/FinalStatistics050331.pdf

National Consensus Project for Quality Palliative Care. (2004). *Clinical practice guidelines for quality palliative care.* Retrieved from www.nationalconsensusproject.org

North Carolina Division of Aging and Adult Services (2011). *Vulnerable adult and elder abuse proclamation.* Retrieved from http://www.ncdhhs.gov/aging/eaday/index.htm

Spector, R. (2009). *Cultural diversity in health and illness* (7th ed). Upper Saddle River, NJ: Prentice Hall.

Spellman, C. (2012). Who benefits from palliative care? *ONS Connect: The Official Newsmagazine of the Oncology Nursing Society.* Retrieved from http://www.onsconnect.org/2012/02/reconnect/who-benefits-from-palliative-care

Strasser, S., Dowling-Castronovo, A., & Fulmer, T. (2010). Violence and elder mistreatment. In P. Tabloski (Ed.), *Gerontological nursing: The essential guide to clinical practice* (2nd ed., pp. 271–292). Upper Saddle River, NJ., Prentice Hall.

Tabloski, P. (2010). *Gerontological nursing: The essential guide to clinical practice* (2nd ed). Upper Saddle River, NJ: Prentice Hall.

U.S. Department of Health and Human Services. (2012). *Think cultural health: Advancing health equity at every point of contact.* Retrieved from https://www.thinkculturalhealth.hhs.gov/Content/communication_tools.asp

Womenshealth.gov (2010). *Menopause and menopause treatments fact sheet.* Retrieved from http://www.womenshealth.gov/publications/our-publications/fact-sheet/menopause-treatment.cfm#h

ADDITIONAL RESOURCES

End of Life Nursing Consortium: www.aacn.nche.edu/ELNEC/

Hartford Institute of Geriatric Nursing: www.hartfordign.org

Hospice and Palliative Nurses Association: www.hpna.org

National Hospice and Palliative Care Organization: www.nhpco.org

Pain Knowledge and Resource: www.painknowledge.org

CHRONIC ILLNESS AND PAIN

CHRONIC CONDITIONS

More than one in four Americans have multiple (two or more) concurrent chronic conditions (MCC), including arthritis, asthma, chronic respiratory issues, diabetes, heart disease, human immunodeficiency virus infection, hypertension, or a combination. Chronic illnesses are defined as conditions that last a year or more and require ongoing medical attention, limit activities of daily living, or both. In addition to comprising physical medical conditions, chronic conditions also include problems such as substance use and addiction disorders, mental illnesses, dementia and other cognitive impairment disorders, and developmental disabilities (U.S. Department of Health and Human Services [USDHHS], 2010).

Chronic conditions are a major cause of illness, disability, and death in the United States. It is projected that, by 2020, an estimated 157 million people in the United States will have at least one chronic illness. Almost three out of four people age 65 and older have multiple chronic conditions (Robert Wood Johnson Foundation [RWJ], 2010). Because of medical advances, many people with chronic illness survive today who, only a few decades ago, might have died much younger.

The resource implications for addressing multiple chronic conditions are immense: 66% of total healthcare spending is directed toward care for the approximately 27% of Americans with chronic illnesses. Increased spending on chronic diseases among Medicare beneficiaries is a key factor driving the overall growth in spending in the Medicare program. Older adults with chronic illness also face substantial challenges related to the out-of-pocket costs of their care, including higher costs for prescription drugs, uneven and confusing reimbursement for drugs under the Medicare D plan, and rising costs of Medi-Gap policies to cover Medicare copays (USDHHS, 2010).

Box 11–1 lists the most common chronic conditions for older people living in the United States.

> ## BOX 11–1.
> ## MAJOR CHRONIC CONDITIONS IN AMERICANS OVER 65 AND % DIAGNOSED WITH THE CONDITION
> ► Hypertension (60%)
> ► Cholesterol disorders (41%)
> ► Arthritis (28%)
> ► Heart disease (25%)
> ► Eye disorders (23%)

Adapted from *Chronic Care: Making the Case for Ongoing Care* by Robert Wood Johnson Foundation, 2010, retrieved from http://www.rwjf.org/files/research/50968chronic.care.chartbook.pdf.

Symptoms of chronic illness often are perceived as a "normal part of aging" and, thus, are underreported and undertreated. The advocacy role of nurses is important in addressing these conditions and encouraging appropriate treatment and follow-up. Nurses can greatly affect the quality of life of older adults. Although nurses may not be able to cure these diseases, they can provide a healing and therapeutic environment in which older adults can maximize their potential.

The approach to and goals of treating chronic illness are very different from those of acute illness. Unfortunately, health care has historically emphasized an acute care model in which diagnosis, treatment, and cure were the natural order of events. Managing chronic illness to maximize functionality, prevent complications, promote dignity, and limit suffering are the goals of chronic care and, thus, the essence of gerontological care. "Curing" disease is not an appropriate goal for most patients, except for a minority of people with acute, reversible conditions.

Some chronic conditions are more disabling than others and their impact varies, according to the potential of the diagnosis to decrease overall quality of life. In general, being chronically ill is associated with symptoms of depression, social isolation, and sometimes pain with loss of function. More than a quarter of the people with chronic conditions also have some type of functional disability, including difficulty walking, requiring assistance with activities of daily living, and inability to engage in social activities (Robert Wood Johnson Foundation, 2010). As symptoms of some chronic illnesses progress, many older adults may require skilled nursing care and nursing home placement.

The role of the gerontological nurse when caring for an older person includes:

► Obtain an accurate history and assessment (physical, cognitive, emotional, social, etc.).

► Educate older patients and their families that a cure may not be possible, but the control of symptoms usually can be attained.

► Discuss nutrition, stress reduction, exercise, and cessation of risky behaviors.

► Prevent or delay complications and functional decline.

► Improve self-care capacity.

► Discuss the medical regimen with patients and their families, explain the symptoms of exacerbation, and inform them how to contact healthcare providers.

► Work in partnership with older patients to manage chronic illness.

► Promote quality of life by improving functional capacity, delivering skilled end-of-life care, or both.

PAIN IN OLDER ADULTS

Although pain is not a normal part of aging, it remains a frequent companion of older adults. Therefore, it is imperative that gerontological nurses have a thorough understanding of this phenomenon, so they can advocate more effectively for patients.

This section is divided into five topical areas: understanding pain, barriers to effective pain management, pain assessment, nursing care for older adults in pain, and cultural responses to pain.

Understanding Pain

The literature provides a variety of definitions for *pain*. According to Pasero and McCaffery (2011), pain is best defined as what the patient him- or herself says it is. Aronoff (2002) has a more specific definition: "a subjective, personal, unpleasant experience involving sensations and perceptions that may or may not relate to bodily or tissue damage" (p. 304). Depending on the discipline, the exact definition of pain will vary.

Much like the definition, the causes of pain can be multiple. Many older adults often have back or joint pain. A typical pain occurs when there is a thinning of the intervertebral disks. This process leads to osteoporosis, arthritis, and other joint abnormalities. This pain is often chronic and nonmalignant, which in and of itself can pose a problem for many healthcare providers. Chronic pain affects about 100 million American adults—more than the total affected by heart disease, cancer, and diabetes combined. Pain also costs the nation up to $635 billion each year in medical treatment and lost productivity (Institute of Medicine, 2011).

Pain is divided into two types: acute and chronic. According to Louis and Meiner (2006), *acute pain* is rapid in onset and of short duration. It can be a sign of a new health issue that has to be addressed. *Chronic pain,* sometimes referred to as *persistent pain,* continues after healing and cannot be cured. Chronic pain is associated with functional decline and psychological problems. This type of pain requires a multidisciplinary approach.

In 2002, the American Geriatric Society (AGS) Panel on Persistent Pain identified four categories of pain:

1. *Nociceptive:* Visceral or somatic; may arise from inflammation, mechanical deformity, ongoing injury, or destruction of tissue; responds well to analgesics and nonpharmacological interventions.

2. *Neuropathic:* Involves the peripheral or central nervous system; does not respond well to traditional analgesics; agents such as anticonvulsants and antidepressants should be added to the regimen.

3. *Mixed or unspecified:* Has mixed or unknown mechanism; treatment is unpredictable.

4. *Other:* Rare; may include conversion reactions or psychological disorders.

The panel's position statement on pain is that perception of pain does not change appreciably with age.

In spite of these advances, pain is still unrecognized and undertreated in people age 75 or older (Louis & Meiner, 2006). Unrecognized and undertreated pain can result in deleterious consequences (see Box 11–2).

BOX 11-2.
HARMFUL EFFECTS OF UNRELIEVED PAIN

▶ Increased heart rate, cardiac output, hypertension, hypercoagulation, deep vein thrombosis
▶ Reduced cognitive function and disorientation
▶ Increased release of stress hormones
▶ Potential for development of persistent debilitating chronic pain (postmastectomy, postthoracotomy, phantom limb, and postherpatic pain)
▶ Decreased gastric and bowel motility
▶ Decreased urinary output, urinary retention, fluid overload, hypokalemia
▶ Depressed immune function
▶ Sleep disorders
▶ Increased depression, apathy, potential for suicide

Adapted from *Pain Management: Evidence, Outcomes and Quality of Life*, p. 343, by Wittink & Carr, 2008, New York: Elsevier.

Chronic pain is now recognized to be a disease in its own right, with the understanding that changes in the nervous system occur and often worsen over time. These changes have a profound effect on the physical and psychological function of a person, often with harmful effects (Institute of Medicine, 2011).

Barriers to Effective Pain Management

Many individuals, healthcare providers included, believe that pain is a normal part of aging. This myth can result in underreporting of pain and inappropriate assessment and treatment of pain. This same scenario occurs when older adults underreport pain. According to Louis and Meiner (2006), other barriers exist and interfere with adequate pain management in older adults:

▶ Inadequate access to diagnostic services, especially for those in long-term care and for frail older adults living in the community

▶ Pain assessment tools not validated with older adults

▶ Nurses who may be overly dependent on assessment tools to determine pain; patients with dementia who may not be able to demonstrate any of the behaviors or cues required for the assessment tool

▶ Physicians and nurses underestimating patient pain

▶ Fear of addiction (e.g., among healthcare providers, families, patients themselves)

▶ Lack of acceptance of the use of opioids for chronic nonmalignant pain

In addition, experts believe that many healthcare providers do not have adequate pain education while in training to appropriately assess and treat pain in the clinical setting (Gloth, 2000; Wittink & Carr, 2008).

Pain Assessment

Adequate pain assessment begins with gerontological nurses asking patients to describe their pain. Patients' reports should be taken as accurate and not second-guessed or discounted by healthcare providers. A thorough history and physical should follow.

The American Geriatrics Society (2002) developed some general principles for assessing pain in older adults:

▶ Patient report is the most accurate evidence that pain exists.

▶ Older patients may underreport pain in spite of severe impairments.

▶ Older patients may use words such as *uncomfortable, ache,* or *hurt* instead of *pain.*

▶ Unrelieved pain can impair functional status and decrease quality of life.

▶ Nonverbal cues and change in function should be used for accurate assessment of patients with cognitive or language impairments.

Numerous pain assessment tools exist in the literature. Numeric pain scales, visual analog scales, descriptive pain intensity scales, pain diaries, and pain logs are commonly used for pain evaluation. According to Louis and Meiner (2006), a pain scale that relies on activity level may be more specific to older adults. The PQRST acronym is recommended for investigation of a pain complaint:

▶ **P**rovocative (aggravating) and **P**alliative (relieving) factors

▶ **Q**uality of the pain (burning, stabbing, dull, throbbing)

▶ **R**egion (part of the body affected)

▶ **S**everity (1–10 pain rating)

▶ **T**iming (24-hour pain pattern, frequency, duration; Reuben et al., 2011)

Patient ability to resume activities or functions can be used to help clinicians determine whether pain is being adequately managed.

The physical exam should focus on the musculoskeletal and neurological systems. Autonomic, sensory, and motor deficits should be noted. Other areas that are important to examine include:

▶ *Functional status:* Activities of daily living (ADLs) and ambulation

▶ *Quality of life:* Pain effects on a patient's life

▶ *Depression:* Overall patient mood

According to Wittink and Carr (2008), quality of life is greatly impaired in people with chronic pain, which can rob the personality, sap energy, cause anguish, and create an unending cycle of depression, leading to sleeplessness and eating disturbances. Healthcare providers should evaluate quality of life by noting changes in any of the following areas:

▶ Social relationships

▶ Spiritual elements

▶ Energy level

▶ Sexual health

▶ ADLs

▶ Independence

▶ Freedom from pain and depression

▶ Positive coping patterns

▶ Personal strength

▶ Freedom from fatigue, constipation, and nausea

Following assessment and exam, the healthcare team and the patient should devise a comprehensive strategy to relieve or reduce pain.

Care for Older Adults in Pain

Older adults can respond unpredictably to analgesics (Institute of Medicine, 2011). Age-related changes in absorption, distribution, metabolism, and elimination require that prescribers adjust dosages of analgesics in older adults. Baseline bloodwork is needed in patients taking chronic pain medications—complete blood count (CBC), stool for occult blood, blood urea nitrogen (BUN), creatinine, and potassium. To prevent untoward drug interactions, providers should be aware of all medications an older patient takes, not just analgesics.

Pain management should be individualized to each patient. Drugs that are used for analgesia can be divided into three groups: mild analgesics, strong opioid analgesics, and adjuvant drugs. Table 11–1 depicts important summary points that gerontological nurses should be aware of regarding pain relievers.

TABLE 11–1.
CLASSES OF PAIN RELIEVERS AND NURSING CONSIDERATIONS

MEDICATION CLASS	DESCRIPTION	INDICATIONS FOR USE	NURSING CONSIDERATIONS
Mild analgesics	Includes nonopioid and some weak opioids, such as codeine and oxycodone	▶ Used as first line in drug-naïve patients ▶ Includes ibuprofen (Motrin, Advil), naproxen (Naprosyn, Aleve), and acetaminophen (Tylenol) ▶ Tylenol is considered first line for moderate musculoskeletal pain (maximum dose, 3,000 mg/day); 2,000 mg/day or avoid in patients with a history of alcohol abuse ▶ Nonsteroidal anti-inflammatory drugs (NSAIDs) can be effective for mild to moderate arthritic pain and bone pain from metastatic tumors; in older adults, associated with indigestion, gastric ulcers, renal insufficiency, increased bleeding	▶ Monitor patient for gastrointestinal side effects if NSAIDs are used ▶ Weaker opioids can cause constipation, nausea, and vomiting; nurses should be proactive in educating patients and beginning a bowel regimen
Opioid analgesics	Most opioid-based products, including morphine	Used in patients with chronic pain that cannot be controlled with other analgesics or for any end-of-life pain	▶ Monitor patients for side effects: nausea, vomiting, constipation, urinary retention ▶ Older adults are more sensitive to respiratory depression and sedation; starting dose should be low
Adjuvant drugs	▶ Supplement the effects of opioids ▶ Have intrinsic analgesic effects	▶ Helpful in treating chronic pain ▶ Include anticonvulsants, antidepressants, corticosteroids, some sedatives	Often used for postherpetic neuralgia, diabetic neuropathies, phantom limb pain

Adapted from *Geriatrics at Your Fingertips* (13th ed.), by D. Reuben, K. Herr, J. Pacala, B. Pollock, J. Potter, & T. Semla, 2011, New York: American Geriatrics Society; and *Pain Management: Evidence, Outcomes, and Quality of Life* by H. Wittink, & D. Carr, 2008, New York: Elsevier.

Many of the side effects of these pain relievers—nausea, sedation, and respiratory depression—are temporary. Patients seem to adjust to these troublesome side effects within 3 to 5 days. During that time, the dose may have to be adjusted downward or another agent given to help patients tolerate side effects. After the initiation period, patients will become less susceptible to side effects.

Certain analgesics are known to have untoward effects in older adults and should be avoided. According to the AGS-BEERS Criteria (American Geriatrics Society, 2012), agents to avoid include meperidine (Demerol), pentazocine (Talwin), indomethacin (Indocin), and non-Cox-selective NSAIDs (aspirin, Advil, etc.). In addition, skeletal muscle relaxants are not recommended because they are poorly tolerated by older patients and have anticholinergic side effects, cause sedation, and increase the risk of falls and fracture.

As mentioned earlier, the pain management plan should be tailored to each patient. In addition to analgesics, other therapies can be of great benefit to older adults in pain. Approaches that are not drugs are called *alternative therapies* and include *physical therapies* and *cognitive–behavioral therapies* (Institute of Medicine, 2011). Common physical therapies include:

► Heat and cold

► Massage

► Exercise

► Acupuncture and acupressure

► Transcutaneous electrical nerve stimulation

► Percutaneous electrical nerve stimulation

Common cognitive–behavioral therapies include:

► Hypnosis

► Meditation

► Imagery

► Progressive relaxation

► Jaw relaxation

► Distractions

► Music therapy

► Aromatherapy

► Therapeutic and healing touch

► Education

Cultural Responses to Pain

Pain can mean different things to different people; this realization should broaden the concept of *pain* to include the fact that people have different pain thresholds. Individuality and culture should be considered when addressing pain. Past pain experiences and individual attributes also influence a person's response to pain. Nurses must work closely with patients of diverse cultures and ethnicities to identify and manage pain appropriately. A patient's culture may indicate that certain remedies and practices should be used or avoided as part of the therapeutic regimen.

According to experts at the City of Hope Supportive Care Committee (2004) of the City of Hope National Medical Center, patients from culturally diverse backgrounds often use alternative therapies in their pain management regimens. Some of the more common alternatives include:

▶ Meditation

▶ Herbal therapies

▶ Relaxation

▶ Yoga

▶ Acupuncture

▶ Acupressure

▶ Topical applications of heat, cold, or herbal packs

Culture also influences how an individual reports pain. Professionals may assume that patients will self-report their pain if they are not asked about it; however, culture may preclude such behavior. Box 11–3 addresses some common cultural pain responses.

BOX 11-3.
RESPONSES TO PAIN BASED ON CULTURE AND UNIQUE HUMAN RESPONSE

▶ Minimizes pain with significant others
▶ Uses pain to elicit sympathy and support from others
▶ Carefully controls the expression of pain (is calm and unemotional)
▶ Is vocal about pain (cries or moans, complains)
▶ Withdraws and wants to be alone when pain is severe
▶ Seeks attention and presence of others when in pain
▶ Willingly accepts pain relief measures
▶ Avoids pain relief measures in the belief that they indicate weakness
▶ Wants and expects quick pain relief
▶ Accepts pain for long periods before requesting help (accepts pain as spiritual—from a higher power)

Adapted from *Cultural Responses: Diversity in Pain Management* by J. Matanky, 2009, retrieved from http://diversityinpain. wordpress.com/cultural-responses/.

REFERENCES

American Geriatric Society. (2002). AGS Panel on Persistent Pain in Older Persons: Management of persistent pain in older persons. *Journal of the American Geriatric Society, 46,* 635–645.

American Geriatrics Society. (2012). *AGS Beers Criteria for potentially inappropriate medication use in older adults.* Retrieved from http://www.americangeriatrics.org/files/documents/beers/2012AGSBeersCriter iaCitations.pdf

Aronoff, G. (2002). Drawing the line between pain management and addiction. *Psychopharmacology Update, 12,* 300–310.

Gloth, F. M. (2000). Factors that limit pain relief and increase complications. *Geriatrics, 55*(10), 46–54.

Institute of Medicine. (2011). *Relieving pain in America: A blueprint for transforming prevention, care, education and research.* Retrieved from http://books.nap.edu/openbook.php?record_ id=13172&page=22

Louis, M., & Meiner, S. E. (2006). Pain. In S. E. Meiner & A. G. Lueckenotte (Eds.), *Gerontological nursing* (pp. 304–327). St. Louis, MO: Mosby/Elsevier.

Matanky, J. (2009). *Cultural responses: Diversity in pain management.* Retrieved from http://diversityinpain. wordpress.com/cultural-responses/

McCaffery, M., & Pasero, C. (1999). *Pain: Clinical manual* (2nd ed.). St. Louis, MO: Mosby.

Passero, C., & McCaffery, M. (2011). *Pain assessment and pharmacological management.* St. Louis, MO: Mosby Elsevier.

Reuben, D., Herr, K., Pacala, J., Pollock, B., Potter, J., & Semla, T. (2011). *Geriatrics at your fingertips* (13th ed.). New York: American Geriatrics Society.

Robert Wood Johnson Foundation. (2010). *Chronic care: Making the case for ongoing care.* Retrieved from http://www.rwjf.org/files/research/50968chronic.care.chartbook.pdf

Tylenol. (2012). *Acetaminophen and the liver: Get relief responsibly.* Retrieved from http://www.tylenol.com/ getreliefresponsibly/index.jhtml?id=tylenol/getreliefresponsibly/aceta_liver.inc

U.S. Department of Health and Human Services. (2010). *Multiple chronic conditions—A strategic framework: Optimum health and quality of life for individuals with multiple chronic conditions.* Washington, DC: Author.

Wittink, H., & Carr, D. (2008). *Pain management: Evidence, outcomes, and quality of life.* New York: Elsevier.

ADDITIONAL RESOURCES

Chronic and Disabling Conditions: www.agingsociety.org/

Healthy People 2020: www.healthypeople.gov/2020/

ASSESSMENT OF LABORATORY VALUES

ASSESSING LABORATORY VALUES

Health maintenance and the treatment of illness in older adults includes pertinent historical information, appropriate physical exams, and other diagnostic parameters as indicated. The most common diagnostic used with this population is laboratory testing. This section reviews basic laboratory parameters and the effects of aging on the normal values of these diagnostic labs.

Because laboratory testing is expensive and often can be traumatic for frail older adults, common sense should be used when selecting and using diagnostic tests. For example, the simple act of drawing blood from an older patient can be a challenge because of the increased fragility of veins and the likelihood of severe bruising and discomfort afterward. Before undertaking any diagnostic testing, the healthcare provider should ask him or herself: "When I obtain the results of this test, how will I use the information to change the care plan and positively affect the health and well-being of my patient?" If this question cannot be answered easily, the test should not be performed.

For the most part, laboratory tests remain unchanged with age (see Table 12–1).

TABLE 12-1.
LABORATORY VALUES THAT DO NOT CHANGE WITH AGE

CHEMISTRY	NORMAL VALUES	
Erythrocytes	4.05–5.64 million/unit	
Hemoglobin	12.5–17.0 g/100 mL	
Hematocrit	40.5%–52.5%	
White blood cells	5.1–10.8 thousand	
Neutrophils	50%–70% 50%–65% (segmented) 0%–8% (banded)	
Eosinophils	1%–6%	
Basophils	0%–2%	
Monocytes	4%–12%	
Lymphocytes	25%–40%	
Folate	3–16 mg/mL	
Total iron binding	250–450 mg/100 mL	
Prothrombin	10.9–13.4 seconds	
International normalized ratio	2.0–3.0 average pt	

Adapted from *Geriatrics at Your Fingertips* (13th Ed.), by D. Reuben, K. Herr, J. Pacala, B. Pollock, J. Potter, & T. Semla, 2011, New York: American Geriatrics Society.

However, some lab values, such as these that reflect renal function, do exhibit more change with normal aging (see Table 12–2). How much these values change depends on a variety of issues, such as comorbid health problems, patient weight, medications taken by the patient, and patient biological age.

TABLE 12-2.
LABORATORY VALUES THAT CHANGE WITH AGE

CHEMISTRY	NORMAL VALUES	
Sodium	136–145 mEq/L	
Potassium	3.5–5.1 mEq/L	
Calcium*	98–107 mEq/dL	
Phosphorous*	2.6–4.9 mg/DL	
Magnesium	1.6–2.4 mg/DL (increases 15%)	
Fasting glucose	70–120 mg/DL	
Amylase**	3.4–122 units/l	
Albumin*	3.5–5.5 g/100 mL	
Blood urea nitrogen (BUN)*	7–22 mg/100 mL	
Creatinine	0.5–1.2 mg/100 mL	
B$_{12}$	200–800 pg/mL	

CHEMISTRY	NORMAL VALUES
Total cholesterol ▸ High-density lipoprotein (HDL) ▸ Low-density lipoprotein (LDL)	120–200 mg/100 mL > 45/100 mL = low risk 60–180 mg/100 mL
Alkaline phosphatase	0.11–0.60 units/L
Gamma-glutamyl transpetidase (GGT)	8–42 units/L
Uric acid	3.5–8.5 mg/dL; varies for men and women
Serum glutamic oxaloacetic transaminase (SGOT)	14–59 IU/L; varies for men and women

Note: * = values slightly lower with age; ** = values slightly increase with age.

Adapted from *Geriatrics at Your Fingertips* (13th Ed.), by D. Reuben, K. Herr, J. Pacala, B. Pollock, J. Potter, & T. Semla, 2011, New York: American Geriatrics Society; and *Current Medical Diagnosis and Treatment* (50th ed.), by S. McPhee & M. Papadakis, 2011, New York: McGraw Hill Medical.

Because gerontological nurses are critically involved in the process of assessing the health status of older patients, a brief review of the common laboratory parameters is useful. It also helps to reinforce common causes of alterations in these parameters.

Blood

The *complete blood count (CBC)* consists of the red blood cells (RBCs), white blood cells (WBCs), and platelets. Specialized WBCs can reveal important factors about the patient's immune response.

RBCs are oval-shaped discs that carry the hemoglobin molecule. When the RBC is low, *anemia* can result. This important diagnostic finding is a symptom that something more serious is happening internally. A high RBC value suggests a low oxygen state. Excess numbers of RBCs result in *polycythemia* and can be seen in chronic obstructive pulmonary disease (COPD), living in high altitudes, or uncommon hematological problems.

Hemoglobin is the oxygen transport mechanism in the blood. Like the RBC, alterations from normal can suggest anemia or other aspects of low oxygen states. Some hereditary conditions, such as sickle cell trait or disease, also can cause chronically low hemoglobin.

The *hematocrit* is the percentage of whole blood that is made up by RBCs. This value is calculated by the laboratory, based on the ratio of RBCs to the amount of liquid in the sample. Alterations from normal can be explained by the same factors as those for RBCs and hemoglobin.

There are five different types of *WBCs,* the body's main defense against infection: (1) neutrophils, (2) eosinophils, (3) basophils, (4) monocytes, and (5) lymphocytes. The first three are produced in the bone marrow and have granules in the nuclei. Often referred to as *granulocytes,* these specialized cells are involved with phagocytosis. In addition, the *basophil's* granules contain histamine, bradykinin, and serotonin, which are important in the normal inflammatory response (Huether & McCance, 2012). The function of the *monocyte,* which is also produced in the marrow, is to destroy large bacteria and viral-infected cells.

Lymphocytes, the smallest of the WBCs, are divided into two types: B and T. Lymphocytes are made in the bone marrow and thymus; they are stored in the lymph nodes, spleen, and tonsils. These cells produce immunity by manufacturing the human antibody and other specialized immune mediators (McPhee & Papadakis, 2011). These cells are thought to be less active with aging, resulting in the suppressed immune response to certain infections that is seen in older adults.

In the older adult capable of mounting an immune response, WBCs increase with infection and inflammation. However, drugs can cause a decrease in these cells. Any of the following medications can cause *leucopenia,* including:

▶ Antibiotics

▶ Anticonvulsants

▶ Antihistamines

▶ Antimetabolites

▶ Cytotoxics

▶ Analgesics

▶ Phenothiazines

▶ Diuretics (Rightdiagnosis.com, 2012)

Platelets, the small cells essential for clotting, are produced in the bone marrow, lungs, and spleen. When a vessel is injured, the platelet forms a "sticky" plug and stimulates the body's other clotting factors. A platelet count of less than 100,000 per cubic millimeter of blood is called *thrombocytopenia;* this finding should alert the healthcare provider that further investigation is needed. Nurses should watch for excess bleeding after procedures if the platelet count is less than 40,000/mm^3. Spontaneous bleeding can occur with platelet counts of less than 20,000/mm^3.

Prothrombin time (PT) is a plasma protein that is converted to thrombin in the first step of the clotting cascade. It measures how effectively the vitamin K–dependent factors of the extrinsic and common paths of the clotting cascade are working (Huether & McCance, 2012). The PT will be elevated in liver disease, vitamin K deficiency, bile duct obstruction, and use of warfarin (Coumadin).

Partial prothrombin time (PTT) measures the common pathway in the clotting cascade. Heparin is known to make prothrombin inactive; therefore, measuring the serum PTT while a person is taking heparin will give information about the adequacy of anticoagulation.

Erythrocyte sedimentation rate (ESR) is the rate at which RBCs fall through plasma; the rate depends largely on concentration of fibrinogen. The test indicates inflammation and is used to monitor the course of conditions such as rheumatoid arthritis, temporal arteritis, and polymyalgia rheumatic. Because the ESR does vary somewhat with age, interpretation must be used with the complete clinical picture in older patients to accurately reflect the state of inflammation.

Electrolytes

Electrolytes are inorganic substances: acids, bases, and salts. These substances dissolve in solution to form *ions*. An ion carrying a positive electric charge is a *cation*. An ion carrying a negative charge is an *anion*. Testing the blood will reveal how much of each electrolyte is in the circulating blood (extracellular fluid [ECF]).

Older adults do not tolerate electrolyte disturbances as well as younger adults. Dehydration is the most serious electrolyte disturbance seen in geriatric care.

Sodium (Na^+) is one of the important electrolytes and the major cation of ECF. Testing blood sodium reflects the balance between the ingested sodium and the amount excreted by the kidneys (McPhee & Papadakis, 2011). Sodium is important in maintaining normal blood pressure, transmitting nerve impulses, and regulating intracellular fluids (ICFs and ECFs).

Low serum sodium, *hyponatremia,* increases with age. Hypovolemic hyponatremia results from renal or extrarenal volume loss and hypotonic fluid replacement. In short, losses of water and salt are replaced by water alone. *Hypernatremia,* which is an excess of serum sodium, can be caused by infusion of high-sodium fluids, dehydration, excess water loss, diarrhea, or laxative abuse. Orthostatic hypotension and oliguria are typical findings. Both of these sodium abnormalities can cause changes in mental status (McPhee & Papadakis, 2011).

Potassium (K^+) is a cation that is most abundant in the ICF; the serum level reflects the small amount that is in the ECFs. This electrolyte is important in cell osmolarity, muscle function, transmission of nerve impulses, and regulation of acid–base balance (Huether & McCance, 2012). Because the cardiac muscle is especially sensitive to imbalances in this electrolyte, gerontological nurses should be alert to any abnormal elevation or low level of this cation. Elevations of potassium, *hyperkalemia,* can be caused by salt substitutes, potassium-sparing diuretics, excess use of potassium supplements, taking antihypertensives such as ACEIs or ARBs, or use of nonsteroidal antiinflammatory drugs (NSAIDs). Low potassium levels, commonly referred to as *hypokalemia,* can be caused by vomiting or use of diuretics. Low potassium can predispose older individuals to tachyarrhythmias or potentiate digitalis toxicity (Reuben et al., 2011).

Chloride (Cl^-) is an ECF anion that is closely associated with sodium. It combines with sodium to form a salt: sodium chloride (NaCl). For the most part, abnormalities in this electrolyte are closely tied to changes in sodium.

Calcium (Ca^{++}) is a cation that is found mainly in the bones and teeth; only 1% of the body calcium is in the ECFs. Calcium is important in blood clotting, conduction of nerve impulses, enzyme activity, and muscle contraction and relaxation. Calcium balance is quite complicated. The serum level is maintained by "stealing" calcium from the bone, which can be a major factor in osteoporosis. This cation is inversely related to phosphorus (see below); when serum levels of calcium are high, phosphorus is low, and vice versa. *Parathyroid hormone* (PTH) is integral to this relationship and influences the reabsorption of calcium and phosphorus to keep the levels in harmony. Low serum calcium levels are most commonly seen in renal disease, whereas elevations signal excess bone degradation: cancers with bony metastasis, prolonged immobility, or Paget's disease.

Phosphorus (PO4$^-$), as mentioned above, is closely linked with calcium. Elevated phosphorus levels are most commonly seen in renal disease. The roles of this anion is maintenance of homeostasis; metabolism of fats, carbohydrates, and proteins; and transfer of the storage form of energy: adenosine triphosphate (ATP; McPhee & Papadakis, 2011).

Magnesium (Mg$^+$) is an ICF cation that is important in the function of muscles (especially cardiac) and nerves. Low levels can be seen in malnutrition, malabsorption, and use of certain medications (e.g., thiazide diuretics, imipenem [Primaxin]). Elevated magnesium can be seen in hypothyroidism and renal insufficiency (McPhee & Papadakis, 2011).

Glucose is the most common sugar in the body and is the body's main source of fuel. Normal glucose should be maintained between 70 and 110 mg/dL. Glucose levels below 70 mg/dL are considered low; however, older adults may not have symptoms until this level falls below 50–60 mg/dL. Low blood sugar can cause hypoglycemia and mental status changes. High blood sugar, on the other hand, is diabetes mellitus. A normal fasting glucose in the older adult should be less than 100 mg/dL and a reading between > 100 mg/dL and < 126 mg/dL is considered "prediabetes" and > 126 mg/dL is consistent with the diagnosis of diabetes (Reuben et al., 2011).

Protein

Total protein measures the amount of albumin and globulin within the body. *Albumin* constitutes 60% of the body's total protein, with the remainder being *globulin*. Globulins are important in antibody formation and maintenance of osmotic pressure (McPhee & Papadakis, 2011).

Albumin is a protein in the body that is a measure of nutritional status. In gerontology, this protein is important for proper wound healing. Low levels are known to be associated with prolonged hospital stays, nonhealing wounds, and increased mortality. Low albumin levels can be seen in:

► Malnutrition

► Infection

► Heart failure (HF)

► Fluid overload

► Hepatic insufficiency

BUN is the measure of the amount of urea in the blood. *Urea* is the major remnant of protein catabolism; it is the result of ammonia conversion in the liver and is excreted by the renal system. Abnormal BUN levels can be indicative of either liver or renal disease (Huether & McCance, 2011). In older adults, elevated BUN usually indicates renal insufficiency or dehydration.

Creatinine is another byproduct of protein metabolism. In normal aging, a patient's renal function declines approximately 1% per year, beginning at age 40. However, there is no obvious change in creatinine level with age, unless a patient has a comorbid renal disease. Normal aging per se does not alter blood creatinine level. Therefore, in gerontology, creatinine level alone is not an indicator of renal disease. Creatinine is best used to calculate creatinine clearance (CrCl).

CrCl is a measure of glomerular filtration rate (GFR). It is done with a 24-hour urine collection and a serum creatinine on completion of the urine collection. Because this test is difficult for many older patients to complete, primary care providers will estimate the CrCl with the *Crockcroft–Gault formula,* which uses serum creatinine, body weight, and age to calculate the CrCl:

$$\text{CrCl (cc/min)} = ([140 - \text{Age} \times \text{Weight (kg)}] \div [72 \times \text{Serum creatinine (mg/dL)}]) \times .85 \text{ for women}$$

CrCl is important in drug dose calculations for older adults. In this population, a CrCl of 55 cc/min or more is desirable.

Enzymes

Alkaline phosphatase is an enzyme present in many tissues, especially the liver and bones. Measuring this enzyme helps identify bone and liver abnormalities.

Alanine aminotransferase (ALT), previously known as SGPT, is present in high concentrations in liver. It is a direct reflection of the function of the hepatocyte.

Aspartate aminotransferase (AST), previously known as SGOT, is less specific for liver disease than is ALT, because AST is found in many areas of the body: heart and skeletal muscle, kidney, pancreas, and liver. It can be helpful in monitoring for drug toxicity. Both the ALT and AST concentrations are normally < 30–40 IU/L.

Gamma-glutamyl transpeptidase (GGT) is present in the serum of healthy people. Increases are found with diseases of the liver, biliary tract, and pancreas. It reflects the same spectrum of disease as an elevated alkaline phosphatase, except that it is specific to the liver.

The major value of the serum GGT is in confirming organ specificity (liver) for an elevation of alkaline phosphatase. Elevated GGT is seen in patients who take barbiturates and diphenylhydantoin (Dilantin) or who drink large amounts of alcohol. An isolated elevation of GGT or an increase in GGT out of proportion to other liver function tests (LFTs) indicates alcohol abuse.

B Vitamins

Folic acid, one of the eight B vitamins, is a water-soluble vitamin needed for the normal functioning of the RBCs and WBCs. Low folic acid can indicate protein calorie malnutrition, macrocytic anemia, liver disease, or renal disease. Alcohol and certain drugs are notorious for lowering folate levels. Methotrexate and the drugs used to treat malaria will decrease folic acid levels (McPhee & Papadakis, 2011). Most recently, folic acid deficiency has been linked to prothrombotic states.

Vitamin B_{12}, also known as cobalamin, is another water-soluble B vitamin and is needed for normal RBC maturation and synthesis of nucleic acids. The structure of deoxyribonucleic acid (DNA) depends on normal B_{12} concentrations (Huether & McCance, 2012). B_{12}-deficient states can cause degeneration of the posterior columns in the spinal cord, leading to profound peripheral neuropathy. In addition, low B_{12} can cause mental status changes, fatigue, and macrocytic anemia.

Factors that can inhibit the absorption of B_{12} include:

- ► Gastric achlorhydria
- ► Pernicious anemia (lack of intrinsic factor)
- ► Pancreatic insufficiency
- ► Diseases of the ileum
- ► Parietal cell antibodies
- ► Chronic use of antireflux medications (histamine 2 blockers, proton pump inhibitors [PPIs]; Heuther & McCance, 2012)

The prevalence of B_{12} deficiency is rising as the population is living longer. B_{12} is given along with B_6 and folic acid to maintain a normal homocysteine (a precursor to the B vitamins) and reduce the chance of thrombotic events.

Miscellaneous Laboratory Parameters

Uric acid, a byproduct of purine metabolism, is excreted by the kidneys. Elevated uric acid is seen in patients with renal insufficiency or gout. In the latter disease, the excess uric acid accumulates in the body fluids and tissues. In high concentrations, crystals form that accumulate in the synovial fluids. As a result of these deposits (deposition), the joints become swollen, warm, and extremely painful (Reuben et al., 2011). Certain drugs are commonly used in geriatric health care place patients at risk for elevated levels of uric acid:

- ► Thiazide diuretics
- ► Caffeine
- ► Low-dose aspirin
- ► Anti-Parkinson's drugs

Amylase is produced in the pancreas and salivary glands and is important in the breakdown of carbohydrates. Several conditions may cause an increase in amylase. Elevated amylase and patient symptoms of nausea, vomiting, and abdominal pain usually indicate pancreatitis.

Lipase is an enzyme that the body uses to break down fat so that it can be absorbed in the intestines. Most older people produce enough lipase, but people with cystic fibrosis, Crohn's disease, and celiac disease may be lipase-deficient (University of Maryland Medical Center, 2011).

C-reactive protein (CRP), an acute-phase reactant that appears immediately with inflammation in the body, is used to assess cardiovascular status and risk, organ transplant inflammatory reactions, flares of chronic diseases such as irritable bowel disease, and recovery from surgery. It is a useful marker of inflammation and has an immediate response to increases and decreases in inflammation, making it a useful indicator or response to and guide for treatment (Bayless & Hanauer, 2011).

Brain naturetic peptide (BNP) is a neurohormone secreted from the ventricles of the heart when they are overstretched by too much circulatory volume. This test is used in the diagnosis and treatment of heart failure (Reuben et al., 2011).

Troponin is a measure of the cardiac myofibrillar proteins into the blood. These levels are specific for cardiac muscle death, and they appear 2 to 8 hours after an episode of cardiac hypoxia, usually caused by vessel occlusion. Troponins may remain elevated for 5 to 7 days following a myocardial infarction and, therefore, are not useful for evaluating suspected early reinfarction (McPhee & Papadakis, 2011).

Creatinine kinase (CK) enzyme is present in various parts of the body and is used as a marker of inflammation. There are three isoenzymes of CK, and each reflects specific areas of inflammation:

▶ *CK-BB:* found in the lungs and brain

▶ *CK-MM:* found in circulating blood and reflects skeletal muscle damage

▶ *CK-MB:* found in the cardiac muscle.

CK-MB levels rise after a myocardial infarction, generally normalize within 24 hours, and, thus, can serve as an indicator of further cardiac events (McPhee & Papadakis, 2011).

Lactate dehydrogenase (LDH) is an isoenzyme that is produced in the liver, but it appears throughout the body. It is not specific to liver disease and can be used as a helpful marker of myocardial infarction or hemolysis.

Prealbumin is used to measure nutritional status of adults over a short period of time. It will change earlier than serum albumin when an individual becomes malnourished. It also is helpful for judging the response of patient's nutritional therapy.

Prostate-specific antigen (PSA) is a test used to diagnose prostate cancer. Along with the physical exam, changes in this antigen level will provide clues about occult malignancy. Currently, the PSA is recommended as a diagnostic aid for men with symptoms suggestive of prostate cancer (urgency, frequency, large residual volume), but there is insufficient evidence to support its use for general screening in men up to the age of 75. Thus, the PSA is not recommended for general screening in men over the age of 75 (U.S. Preventive Services Task Force, 2012).

Cholesterol

Total cholesterol is a steroid compound that is important in stabilizing the cell membranes. The liver metabolizes cholesterol and binds it to the *low-density lipoprotein* (LDL) and *high-density lipoprotein* (HDL) receptors for transport into the bloodstream (McPhee & Papadakis, 2011). Total cholesterol and the HDL/LDL ratio are markers of cardiovascular risk.

Triglycerides (TGs) are the principal fat in the circulating blood. They are bound to proteins, and they form the HDLs and LDLs. TGs are manufactured in the liver from glycerol and fatty acids. These levels are markedly affected by dietary intake. An excess of TG particles in the system is stored in fat and high levels increase the risk of cardiovascular disease.

HDLs also are known as "good cholesterol." These cholesterol particles carry a greater amount of protein and less lipid content than LDLs; thus, they are referred to as the high-density lipid component. Approximately 25% of the cholesterol in the body is bound as HDL; this cholesterol particle is known to be cardioprotective. Diet per se does not affect the HDL level; omega-3 fatty acids (fish oils) and exercise are thought to increase HDL cholesterol levels (McPhee & Papadakis, 2011).

LDLs constitute the remaining 75% of cholesterol and are known as "bad cholesterol," since their level correlates with cardiovascular risk. The more LDL cholesterol a patient has in the blood, the higher the risk for cardiovascular and cerebrovascular events. LDL cholesterol in women is known to rise after menopause.

Thyroid

Thyroid function tests (TFTs) are a reflection of the status of the thyroid gland's functioning status. Thyroid physiology, in and of itself, is quite complicated. Three main serum tests are important: *thyroxine* (T4), *triiodothyronine* (T3), and *thyroid-stimulating hormone* (TSH). TSH is manufactured in the anterior pituitary and stimulates the gland to produce and release T3 and T4. T3 is thought to be the active thyroid hormone. In the periphery, T4 is converted to this active form (T3). Serum proteins have a critical effect on the TFTs, as the majority of both T3 and T4 are bound to proteins, and it is their unbound fraction that is out in circulation (and affecting body tissues).

In clinical practice, low serum-free T4 levels and high TSH levels signify *hypothyroidism*. This is the most common thyroid abnormality seen in older adults. In *hyperthyroidism*, the TSH is low and the free T4 is high. It is important for gerontological nurses to remember that older adults present atypically with thyroid disease; therefore, any unexplained symptoms—fatigue, change in bowel or sleep habits, or cardiac arrythmias—should always make one think of thyroid disease.

Urine

Urine is one of the major waste products of body metabolism; it is composed of 95% water. Composition of the urine excreted from the body can be helpful in providing clues to underlying illness. Production and excretion of urine is critical in body hemostasis. Each *urine electrolyte* is discussed below.

Urine protein is considered an abnormal finding. In healthy adults, essentially no proteins are released into the urine. The presence of proteins indicates some sort of disruption in the kidney's basement membranes. Proteinuria warrants a work-up for uncontrolled blood pressure or diabetes, infection, or intrinsic renal disease.

Urine glucose suggests that the amount of sugars in the infiltrate presented to the kidneys exceeds what the system can transport; the excess is excreted in the urine. Ordinarily, glucosuria is thought to signal diabetes. However, in older adults, the resorption of glucose is diminished as part of normal aging. That being said, glucose in the urine of older adults may or may not indicate diabetes, so a clinical evaluation is needed.

Urine bacteria are present in the urine in small amounts in healthy adults. A bacterium that is more than 105 colony-forming units (CFUs) per milliliter of urine indicates infection. *Urine leukocytes* are also seen in small amounts in healthy adults. When there are more than 10 white cells per mm³ of urine, this finding is considered *pyuria* (pus in the urine) and is indicative of infection.

Gerontological nurses should remember that the usual signs and symptoms of urinary tract infections (UTIs) may not be present in older adults and, instead, may present as confusion, lethargy, nocturia, or new onset of incontinence.

Urine ketones are never seen in normal healthy adults. They are a sign of fatty acid breakdown. Urinary ketones can be seen when the patient is ingesting a high-protein diet, is fasting or starving, or has ingested isopropyl alcohol (McPhee & Papadakis, 2011).

Urine pH reflects the acidity or alkalinity of the urine; pH assessment is important in certain types of infection and in the formation of kidney stones.

Blood in the urine is never a normal finding. *Hematuria* can indicate the following:

► Kidney stones
► Kidney trauma
► Inflammation
► Infection
► Malignancy

Hematuria always warrants investigation. It may be grossly visible or occult (microscopic hematuria). Regardless of the amount, a work-up is required.

REFERENCES

Bayless, T., & Hanauer, S. (2011). *Advanced therapy of inflammatory bowel disease.* Shelton, CT: People's Medical Publishing House: USA.

Cockcroft, D. W., & Gault, M. H. (1976). Prediction of creatinine clearance from serum creatinine. *Nephron, 16*(1), 31–41.

Huether, S., & McCance, K. (2012). *Understanding pathophysiology* (5th ed.). St. Louis, MO: Mosby.

Levey, A. S., Bosch, J. P., Lewis, J. B., Greene, T., Rogers, N., & Roth, D. (1999). A more accurate method to estimate glomerular filtration rate from serum creatinine: A new prediction equation. *Modification of Diet in Renal Disease Study Group, 130,* 461–470.

McPhee, S., & Papadakis, M. (2011). *Current medical diagnosis and treatment* (50th ed.). New York: McGraw Hill Medical.

Reuben, D., Herr, K., Pacala, J., Pollock, B., Potter, J., & Semla, T. (2011). *Geriatrics at your fingertips* (13th ed.). New York: American Geriatrics Society.

University of Maryland Medical Center. (2011). *Lipase.* Retrieved from http://www.umm.edu/altmed/ articles/lipase-000311.htm

U.S. Preventive Services Task Force. (2012). *Screening for prostate cancer.* Retrieved from http://www. uspreventiveservicestaskforce.org/uspstf/uspsprca.htm

ADDITIONAL RESOURCES

Chronic and Disabling Conditions: www.agingsociety.org/

Healthy People 2020: www.healthypeople.gov/2020/

National Osteoporosis Foundation: www.nof.org

Osteoporosis Screening: www.ahcpr.gov/clinic/3rduspstf/osteoporosis

CARDIOVASCULAR DISEASE

Cardiovascular disease (CVD) has been America's top cause of death for the past 80 years, but in the last 10 years, the death rate from CVD has declined 30.6% (American Heart Association [AHA], 2012). Even so, in 2008, CVD caused one of every six deaths in the United States. An estimated 82.6 million Americans (one-third) have one or more forms of CVD. In 2008, 33% of deaths from CVD occurred before the age of 75 years, which is well below the average life expectancy. The estimated direct and indirect costs of CVD in the United States for 2008 were $448.5 billion (AHA, 2012). It is not surprising that heart disease and stroke are one of the focus areas for Healthy People 2020 (www.healthypeople.gov).

All types of CVD have similar risk factors. Many of the diseases are risk factors for other problems. The AHA (2012) divides these risk factors into two categories: those that can be modified and those that cannot. Additional risk factors for each individual disease are discussed in the respective sections. Nonmodifiable risk factors include:

- ▶ Increasing age
- ▶ Male gender
- ▶ Heredity (including race)

Modifiable risk factors include:

- ▶ Tobacco smoking
- ▶ High blood pressure
- ▶ High blood cholesterol
- ▶ Physical inactivity
- ▶ Overweight and obesity
- ▶ Diabetes mellitus

The most common diagnoses of CVD encountered in older adults are hypertension, heart failure, ischemic heart disease/coronary artery disease/myocardial infarction, dyslipidemia, peripheral arterial occlusive disease, peripheral venous disease, cardiac arrhythmias, and atrial fibrillation.

Hypertension

Hypertension (HTN) is defined as a persistent elevation of the systolic or diastolic arterial blood pressure (BP) of both. Table 13–1 outlines the classification of high BP as presented in the Joint National Committee on Prevention, Detection, Evaluation and Treatment of High Blood Pressure (JNC-7) guidelines (U.S. Department of Health and Human Services, 2003).

HTN is very prevalent in older adults of all races, affecting 60%–80% of the population by late life. The disease occurs earlier and progresses more rapidly in Blacks (AHA, 2012). HTN is largely asymptomatic, earning it the name of the "silent killer." Despite campaigns and national guidelines for early detection and treatment to prevent other cardiovascular complications, only 34% of people treated for HTN have adequate control (BP < 140/90; U.S. Department of Health and Human Services, 2003).

TABLE 13-1.
CLASSIFICATION OF HYPERTENSION

CLASSIFICATION	SYSTOLIC	DIASTOLIC
Normal	< 120 mm Hg	< 80 mm Hg
Prehypertension	120–139 mm Hg	80–89 mm Hg
Stage 1 hypertension	140–159 mm Hg	90–99 mm Hg
Stage 2 hypertension	≥ 160 mm Hg	≥ 100 mm Hg

Adapted from *The Seventh Report of the Joint National Committee on Prevention, Detection, Evaluation, and Treatment of High Blood Pressure*, by the U.S. Department of Health and Human Services, 2003, Washington, DC: Author.

Identifying pre-HTN allows for earlier intervention with lifestyle modifications to prevent development of HTN. This classification is based on the average of two or more readings taken at two or more times, both standing and sitting after 5 minutes of rest.

HTN can be subdivided into *systolic–diastolic* or *isolated systolic*. The latter is most common in older adults, accounting for 65%–75% of cases. Treating systolic pressure to normal levels without lowering diastolic pressure too much is often difficult. Elevated systolic BP raises the risk of stroke, myocardial infarction (MI), left ventricular hypertrophy, renal dysfunction, and cardiovascular mortality (Reuben et al., 2011).

HTN can be divided into two categories: *essential* or *secondary*. Essential HTN accounts for about 95% of cases and is seen more commonly in obese patients, those with family histories of HTN, and certain groups such as Blacks. Secondary HTN occurs because of another cause and is potentially correctable. Causes include:

- ▶ Medications (e.g., corticosteroids, NSAIDs, decongestants, stimulants, anabolic steroids, cyclosporine)
- ▶ Renal disease
- ▶ Renal vascular disease (e.g., renal artery stenosis)
- ▶ Substances (e.g., salt, ethanol, street drugs)
- ▶ Endocrine disease (e.g., hyperthyroidism, hyperaldosteronism)
- ▶ Obstructive sleep apnea

Initial therapy for HTN depends on the level of BP elevation and the patient's comorbid conditions. Any patient with BP over 120/80 should be educated on lifestyle modifications, including:

- ▶ DASH diet (salt restriction)
- ▶ Moderation of ethanol (< 2 drinks/day)
- ▶ Weight reduction
- ▶ Calcium and magnesium supplementation
- ▶ Smoking cessation
- ▶ Regular exercise
- ▶ Stress management

When lifestyle interventions do not bring BP into normal range, antihypertensive medications should be started. The following classes of medication may be chosen to assist in controlling comorbid conditions (for compelling indications):

- ▶ Diuretics
- ▶ Beta-adrenergic blockers
- ▶ Calcium channel blockers
  - » Dihydropyridines
  - » Non-dihydropyridines
- ▶ Angiotensin-converting enzyme inhibitors (ACEIs)
- ▶ Angiotensin receptor blockers (ARBs)
- ▶ Direct rennin inhibitors
- ▶ Alpha-blockers
- ▶ Vasodilators
- ▶ Centrally acting drugs

The most common antihypertensive medications and their side effects are outlined in Table 13–2. Treatment of BP to normal or desirable levels often requires combinations of two or more classes of medications. Combinations of two drugs in low doses often work better than high doses of a single drug to lower BP, and lower dosing regimens can also minimize side effects. These combination products usually improve patient adherence, because they reduce the number of medications that a person must purchase and take each day. Many drugs are available that combine the following classes of medication:

▶ Diuretic and beta-blocker

▶ Diuretic and ACEI

▶ Diuretic and ARB

▶ Alpha-blocker and beta-blocker

▶ Calcium channel blocker and ACEI

▶ Calcium channel blocker and ARB

▶ Calcium channel blocker, ARB, and diuretic

Generally, it is desirable to reduce BP to as close to "normal" levels as possible. However, in many older adults, this goal may not be realistic or desirable, since aggressively lowering blood pressure levels may raise the risk of postural hypotension. As mentioned above, diastolic BP often will fall too low in patients who initially have isolated systolic HTN. Postural decreases in BP also are more common in older adults and may be aggravated by overzealous treatment of BP. One must balance the benefits of treating BP against the risks of falls and fractures. For patients older than 80 years of age without coexisting heart disease, a reasonable BP goal is < 150/80 mm Hg (Reuben et al., 2011).

TABLE 13-2.
ANTIHYPERTENSIVE MEDICATIONS

CLASS	MEDICATIONS	SIDE EFFECTS	POSSIBLE CONTRAINDICATIONS	COMPELLING INDICATIONS
Diuretics	Hydrochlorothiazide Chlorthalidone Furosemide Sprionolactone	Hypokalemia Hyperkalemia Hyponatremia Hypercalcemia Hyperuricemia Orthostatic hypotension	Gout	HF Diabetes CAD risk Recurrent stroke prevention
Angiostensin-converting enzyme inhibitors	Captopril Enalapril Lisinopril Ramnipril Trandolapril Benazepril	Cough Angioedema Hyperkalemia Acute renal failure with renal artery stenosis	Renal artery stenosis Pregnancy	HF Diabetes CAD Post-MI CKD Recurrent stroke prevention
Angiostensin receptor blockers	Losartan Valsartan Ibersartan	Hyperkalemia Acute renal failure with renal artery stenosis	Renal artery stenosis Pregnancy	HF Diabetes CKD
Direct rennin inhibitors	Aliskiren (Tekturna)	Diarrhea Cough Angioedema	Pregnancy	Not defined
Beta blockers	Atenolol Metoprolol Carvedilol	Bradycardia HF Bronchospasm Dyslipidemia Depression Insomnia Fatigue	Asthma Second- or third-degree heart block Depression	HF Post MI CAD risk
Calcium channel blockers	Dihydropyridines Amlodipine Nisoldipine Nicardipine Non-dihydropyridines Diltiazem Verapamil	Edema Tachycardia Headache Heart block	Second- or third-degree heart block Venous insufficiency	Isolated systolic HTN Diastolic HF CAD risk
Alpha blockers	Terazosin Doxazosin	Postural BP Dry mouth Fatigue	Caution in older adults	BPH

CONTINUED ▶

◀ **TABLE 13-2 CONTINUED**

CLASS	MEDICATIONS	SIDE EFFECTS	POSSIBLE CONTRAINDICATIONS	COMPELLING INDICATIONS
Vasodilators	Hydralazine Minoxidil	Tachycardia Headache Abnormal hair growth	Lupus Severe CAD	HF, especially in Blacks
Centrally acting drugs	Methyldopa Clonidine	Postural BP Fatigue Bradycardia	Hepatitis Cirrhosis	Refractory HTN

Note: CKD = chronic kidney disease, HF = heart failure, CAD = coronary artery disease, MI = myocardial infarction, BP = blood pressure, BPH = benign prostatic hypertrophy.

Adapted from *The Seventh Report of the Joint National Committee on Prevention, Detection, Evaluation, and Treatment of High Blood Pressure*, by the U.S. Department of Health and Human Services, 2003, Washington, DC: Author.

Patient education should focus on lifestyle modifications to control elevated BP, as well as potential medication side effects. Medication adherence and the need for routine follow-up with a provider also must be emphasized. For most patients, monitoring BP at home can be useful to assess the adequacy of control.

Heart Failure

Heart failure (HF) describes a syndrome in which the cardiac output is insufficient to meet the metabolic demands of the tissues. Nearly 5 million Americans have HF, with 75% of existing and new cases occurring in those over 65 years of age. It is estimated that treating heart failure and its complications accounts for approximately 17% of healthcare costs in the United States (McPhee & Papadakis, 2011).

In HF, reduced renal blood flow leads to activation of the rennin–angiotensin–aldosterone system (RAAS). Angiotensinogen is made in the liver and is converted by rennin in the kidney to angiotensin I. Angiotensin I is then converted to angiotensin II by angiotensin-converting enzyme (ACE). Angiotensin II is a potent vasoconstrictor and binds to the angiotensin II receptor type 1 (AT1), producing harmful cardiac effects, and also to the angiotensin II receptory type 2 (AT2), which has beneficial cardiac effects. Angiotensin II also stimulates the release of aldosterone, which leads to sodium and water retention in the kidneys (JNC-7, 2003).

In addition to RAAS activation, the sympathetic nervous system is stimulated through baroreceptor activation in the left ventricle, aortic arch, and carotid sinus, leading to catecholamine release, resulting in increased heart rate and vasoconstriction. Initially, these compensatory mechanisms improve cardiac output, but ultimately they lead to a more dysfunctional myocardial state. Heart failure is classified by functional status, using the New York Heart Association's classification (see Table 13–3; Morris & Alexander, 1999).

The American Heart Association and American College of Cardiology have also developed a heart failure classification system. The system is based on progression of the disease and allows healthcare providers to identify older persons at high risk for heart failure who do not yet have signs or symptoms of disease. Table 13–4 illustrates the AHA/ACC classification system.

TABLE 13-3.
NEW YORK HEART ASSOCIATION FUNCTIONAL CLASSIFICATION OF HEART FAILURE

CLASS	DEFINITION
I	No symptoms with regular activity
II	Mild symptoms with ordinary daily activity
III	Comfortable only at rest; symptoms with mild activity
IV	Symptoms at rest

Adapted from "The use of the New York Heart Association's Classification of Cardiovascular Disease as Part of the Patient's Complete Problem List," by J. W. Hurst, D. C. Morris, & R. W. Alexander, 1999, *Clinical Cardiology, 22*(6), 385–390; available at http://www.abouthf.org/questions_stages.htm.

TABLE 13-4.
AHA/ACC HEART FAILURE STAGES

STAGE	DESCRIPTION
A	People at high risk for developing heart failure but who do not have heart failure or damage to the heart
B	People with damage to the heart but who have never had symptoms of heart failure; for example, those who have had a heart attack
C	People with heart failure symptoms caused by damage to the heart, including shortness of breath, tiredness, inability to exercise
D	People who have advanced heart failure and severe symptoms difficult to manage with standard treatment

Adapted from *ACC/AHA 2005 Guideline Update for the Diagnosis and Management of Chronic Heart Failure in the Adult* by S. A. Hunt and colleagues, 2005, *Circulation, 112*, e154–e235.

Heart failure has multiple possible etiologies:

► Ischemic heart disease (IHD)

► HTN

► Cardiomyopathy

► Valvular heart disease

► Pulmonary HTN

IHD and MI are the primary causes of *systolic* HF, whereas HTN is the main cause of *diastolic* dysfunction.

Systolic HF results from damage to the cardiac muscle, leading to impaired contractility. In other words, the pump is broken. This type of HF is defined by a left ventricular ejection fraction (LVEF) of less than 40%. The example in Table 13–5 illustrates how, despite a dilated ventricle and large end diastolic volume (EDV), the cardiac output is very low because only a small amount of blood is propelled out of the ailing ventricle. Pure systolic dysfunction accounts for about one-third of cases.

Diastolic HF occurs when the ventricle is unable to fill with blood, most commonly because of a history of uncontrolled HTN that leads to left ventricular hypertrophy (LVH). The thickened ventricle becomes stiff and noncompliant, leading to inadequate filling volumes and high filling pressures. In this case, the LVEF will be normal or even high (> 60%), but cardiac output is reduced because of the small ventricular volume (see Table 13–5). Diastolic HF accounts for another one-third of cases but predominates in older adults, especially women. Normal aging results in increased stiffness of the ventricle, which, combined with longstanding HTN, makes diastolic dysfunction very common in people aged 60 or older.

The final one-third are a combined type, with those affected having both impaired pumping and impaired filling of the ventricle.

TABLE 13–5.
LEFT VENTRICULAR EJECTION FRACTION

NORMAL LVEF	HIGH LVEF	LOW LVEF
EDV = 100 ml	EDV = 60 ml	EDV = 120 ml
SV = 60 ml	SV = 50 ml	SV = 25 ml
EF = 60%	EF = 85%	EF = 20%
HR = 70	HR = 70	HR = 70
CO = 4.2 L/min	CO = 3.5 L/min	CO = 1.7 L/min

Note. EDV = end diastolic volume (amount of blood filling ventricle at end diastole), SV = stroke volume (amount of blood ejected with each ventricular contraction), EF = ejection fraction (percentage of blood ejected with each contraction), HR = heart rate, CO = cardiac output (amount of blood pumped in 1 minute; HR x SV).

Once present, HF can be exacerbated by several factors:

► Nonadherence to medications

► Excessive sodium ingestion

► Infection

► Arrhythmias (especially with rapid rate)

► Thyroid disease

► Anemia

► Digitalis toxicity

► New medications (particularly NSAIDs)

► Obstructive sleep apnea

Signs and symptoms of HF may include any or all of the following:

▶ Shortness of breath

▶ Orthopnea (inability to lie flat)

▶ Paroxysmal nocturnal dyspnea

▶ Edema

▶ Weight gain

▶ Tachycardia

▶ Jugular venous distention

▶ Wheezing

▶ Crackles on lung exam

▶ S3 or S4 gallop

▶ Altered mental status

▶ Cyanosis/pallor

The diagnosis of HF is primarily a clinical diagnosis based on history, physical exam findings, and diagnostic tests. An echocardiogram is useful for classifying the HF as systolic or diastolic, because the treatment approach will vary according to the primary problem. The following diagnostic tests may be ordered:

▶ Chest x-ray

▶ 12-lead EKG

▶ Electrolytes

▶ Renal function tests

▶ LFTs

▶ Urinalysis

▶ CBC

▶ Thyroid function tests

▶ Brain natriuretic peptide (BNP)

▶ Echocardiogram

▶ Cardiac stress test

The treatment of HF will depend on the type (systolic vs. diastolic), but both types require multiple medications to maintain optimum cardiac function. The medications used to treat HF are outlined in Table 13–6.

TABLE 13-6.
PHARMACOTHERAPY FOR HEART FAILURE

MEDICATION	ACTION/ INDICATION	BENEFIT	NURSING CONSIDERATIONS
Diuretics (usually loop)	Reduce volume overload	▸ Improve vascular congestion by reducing volume overload ▸ Provide most immediate symptom relief	Overuse can lead to volume depletion, further activation of the RAAS, and worsening renal function **Monitor for:** ▸ Electrolyte imbalance ▸ Hypotension
ACEIs	▸ Decrease activity of the RAAS ▸ First-line therapy ▸ Reduce ventricular preload and afterload by causing vasodilation	▸ Improve symptoms ▸ Improve LVEF ▸ Decrease LVH ▸ Reduce risk of death and hospitalization	**Monitor for:** ▸ Hyperkalemia ▸ Hypotension ▸ Cough ▸ Renal function ▸ Allergic reaction (e.g., rash, angioedema)
Angiotensin receptor blockers	▸ Block AT2 receptors ▸ Used in patients intolerant of ACEIs ▸ Similar effects to ACEIs ▸ May be combined with ACEIs in patients intolerant of beta-blockers	▸ Reduce hospitalizations (limited data, CHARM trial) ▸ Reduce mortality (limited data, CHARM trial)	8% chance of angioedema in patients with reaction to ACE inhibitors ("ACE Inhibitors vs. ARBs," 2007) **Monitor for:** ▸ Hyperkalemia ▸ Renal function
Beta-blockers	Block the effects of circulating catecholamines (norepinephrine)	▸ Reduce morbidity and mortality ▸ Improve LVEF	**Monitor for:** ▸ Bronchospasm ▸ Bradycardia ▸ Heart block ▸ Worsening HF symptoms ▸ Erectile dysfunction
Digoxin	For patients with systolic HF who continue with symptoms despite ACEIs, diuretics, and beta blockers (standard) therapy	▸ Increases exercise capacity ▸ Improves exercise tolerance ▸ Decreases hospitalizations	Narrow therapeutic index Target serum levels 0.5–0.8 mg/dL. May be ineffective and even harmful in women (Reuben et al., 2011) **Monitor for:** ▸ S/S toxicity (nausea, vomiting, diarrhea, halos around lights) ▸ Serum potassium

MEDICATION	ACTION/ INDICATION	BENEFIT	NURSING CONSIDERATIONS
Spironolactone	▸ Blocks aldosterone ▸ Indicated or Class III or IV failure despite ACEI, diuretic, beta blocker, and digoxin	▸ Decreases mortality ▸ Reduces hospitalizations	Avoid concomitant potassium Avoid artificial salt **Monitor for:** ▸ Hyperkalemia ▸ Gynecomastia
Hydralazine/isosorbide dinitrate	▸ Used in people intolerant of ACEIs ▸ Survival benefit in Blacks when added to standard therapy	▸ Decreases mortality ▸ Reduces hospitalizations (in Blacks)	Advise patients to report fever, malaise, or joint pain Avoid concomitant Viagra or similar medication **Monitor for:** ▸ Hypotension ▸ Dizziness ▸ Headache
Verapamil/diltiazem	▸ Contraindicated in systolic or combined HF ▸ Beneficial in pure diastolic HF ▸ Decrease myocardial contractility	Theoretical benefit in diastolic HF	**Monitor for:** ▸ Constipation ▸ Headache ▸ Edema

Note: RAAS = renin–angiotensin–aldosterone system, ACEIs = angiotensin-converting enzyme inhibitors, LVEF = left ventricular ejection fraction, LVH = left ventricular hypertrophy, HF = heart failure.

Adapted from *The Seventh Report of the Joint National Committee on Prevention, Detection, Evaluation, and Treatment of High Blood Pressure,* by the U.S. Department of Health and Human Services, 2003. Washington, DC: Author.

Patient involvement in the plan of care is vital to achieve optimal outcomes. Patients must be educated on the following:

▸ Limit sodium intake.

▸ Weigh themselves daily and record weight.

▸ Report 2–3 lb weight gain in 24–48 hours.

▸ Exercise regularly.

▸ Stop smoking.

▸ Limit alcohol ingestion (maximum: 1–2 drinks/day).

▸ Lose weight (if overweight or obese).

▸ Moderate fluid intake (restrictions only as indicated/ordered).

▸ Know importance of medication adherence.

▸ Avoid exacerbating factors (e.g., NSAIDs).

▶ Know signs and symptoms of exacerbation or worsening HF:

　　» Increased shortness of breath at rest or on exertion

　　» Chest pain

　　» Wheezing

　　» Inability to lie flat

　　» Waking at night because of gasping for breath or coughing

　　» Increased abdominal girth

　　» Nausea or anorexia

　　» Swelling in ankles or other locations

　　» Increased fatigue

　　» Altered mental status

▶ Manage end-of-life planning, and develop advance directives (because of increased risk of sudden cardiac death).

Left ventricular assist devices, cardiac resynchronization, implantable cardioverter defibrillators, and heart transplantation are sometimes considered in highly functional older people without comorbidities.

Ischemic Heart Disease, Coronary Heart Disease, and Myocardial Infarction

Ischemic heart disease (IHD), or *coronary artery disease* (CAD), is caused by atherosclerosis of the coronary arteries, which decreases blood flow to the myocardium. When myocardial oxygen demands exceed the available supply (during times of increased activity), myocardial ischemia occurs, resulting in *angina*. Angina presents as chest pain in the majority of people, but it may have an atypical presentation in older adults, those with diabetes, and women. Rather than crushing substernal chest pain, these people may experience shortness of breath, abdominal or back pain, profound fatigue, or confusion—or may have no symptoms at all. These unusual symptoms led to delays in seeking care, which may lead to sudden cardiac death, extensive cardiac damage, or pulmonary edema.

An acute coronary syndrome is caused by rupture of an atherosclerotic plaque that leads to either sub-total occlusion (unstable angina) or completed occlusion (MI) of a coronary artery. Clinically, the patient usually presents with an angina pattern that is different from usual; for example, severe chest pain that is not relieved by rest or nitroglycerine.

According to the AHA (2012), 16 million Americans have CAD. Just over 9 million have had an MI. Incidence increases with age. Before age 80, incidence is higher in men, but in the eighth decade, incidence equalizes between men and women.

In addition to the risk factors listed in the introduction to CVD, the following also influence risk:

► History of stroke

► History of peripheral vascular disease (PAD)

► Renal insufficiency

IHD is often suspected in individuals with one or more risk factors who present with symptoms of angina. Diagnosis is more difficult in those without typical chest pain. One common diagnostic test is the 12-lead electrocardiogram (ECG), which may be normal in up to 50% of people with active ischemia, but also may suggest a prior MI (presence of Q waves) or active ischemia or injury (ST segment depression or elevation). However, it is important to know that a normal ECG does not exclude severe CAD.

Traditional exercise testing is difficult in older adults because of deconditioning, gait and balance problems, and overall limited physical activities. When exercise testing is not possible, pharmacological stress testing with nuclear scans or echocardiography is used.

Other diagnostic tests include:

► *Serum creatinine phosphokinase:* Elevation occurs shortly after a MI and peaks at 24 hours, then returns to normal at 72 hours.

► *Cardiac troponin:* Specific to the cardiac cells; rises within a few hours of an MI. Various subtypes return to normal within 1–3 weeks of an event.

► *CBC:* Used to assess for infection or anemia.

► *Serum electrolytes:* Abnormally high or low levels can lead to fluid imbalances and cardiac rhythm disturbances.

► *Renal function tests:* Renal disease may worsen states of fluid imbalance and hasten development of pulmonary edema.

► *Lipid panel:* To detect hyperlipidemia, which is a significant risk factor for IHD. Determination of lipid levels is important in risk assessment and monitoring of ongoing lipid-lowering therapy.

► *Chest x-ray:* To determine overall size of the heart and detect vascular congestion or pleural effusion, which could indicate volume overload.

► *Cardiac catheterization:* The "gold standard" for detecting hemodynamically significant lesions in the coronary arteries.

► *Electron-beam computed tomography or ultrafast CT:* This computerized tomography test detects calcium deposits found in atherosclerotic plaques. A "calcium score" is assigned, which is helpful for risk stratification, as calcium deposits are one of the earliest signs of atherosclerosis. Although this test may be useful in younger people, it has little to no application in older adults, most of whom have significant calcium scores.

As with HF, lifestyle modifications are an important aspect of management of CAD and include the following:

▶ Smoking cessation

▶ Body-weight reduction (if overweight or obese)

▶ Regular exercise (gradual, steady increase in intensity and duration)

▶ Dietary modifications, including low-fat/low-cholesterol or the Mediterranean diet

▶ Control of comorbid conditions, such as HTN and diabetes

The following mnemonic has been suggested to guide initial treatment of CAD in older patients (Helmy, Patel, & Wenger, 2006):

▶ *A*—Aspirin and anti-anginal therapy

▶ *B*—Beta-blockers and blood pressure

▶ *C*—Cigarette smoking and cholesterol

▶ *D*—Diet and diabetes

▶ *E*—Education and exercise

TABLE 13-7.
MEDICATIONS FOR ISCHEMIC HEART DISEASE, CORONARY ARTERY, AND MYOCARDIAL INFARCTION

MEDICATION	ACTION/ INDICATION	BENEFIT	NURSING CONSIDERATIONS
Aspirin, Plavix, Effient	Inhibits platelet aggregation	▶ Decreases mortality rate of acute MI ▶ Lowers risk of MI in people with CAD	Not indicated in people at risk for GI or other bleeding No data showing benefit in primary prevention in women **Monitor for:** ▶ Dyspepsia ▶ S/S bleeding
ACEIs	Blocks conversion of angiotensin I to angiotensin II	▶ Prevents ventricular remodeling post-MI ▶ Reduces mortality in secondary prevention of CAD (Ramnipril, HOPE trial)	**Monitor for:** ▶ Hyperkalemia ▶ Hypotension ▶ Cough ▶ Renal function ▶ Allergic reaction (e.g., rash, angioedema)

MEDICATION	ACTION/ INDICATION	BENEFIT	NURSING CONSIDERATIONS
Statins	► Inhibit HMG-CoA reductase—enzyme that promotes cholesterol synthesis in liver ► First-line therapy in cholesterol reduction	► Reduce CAD mortality ► Reduce size and make plaques less prone to rupture	Drugs with shorter half-life will work better if dosed at bedtime (except atorvastatin and rouvastatin) **Monitor for:** ► Muscle pain ► Brown urine ► LFTs ► Lipid levels
Beta-blockers	Slow heart rate and decrease contractility, thereby reducing myocardial oxygen demand	► Improve survival after first MI ► Relieve angina	Use cautiously in patients with depression, asthma, PVD Contraindicated in severe bradycardia, sinus node disease, and high-grade AV block Abrupt discontinuation can precipitate angina **Monitor for:** ► Bronchospasm ► Bradycardia ► Heart block ► HF symptoms ► Erectile dysfunction
Calcium channel blockers	► Dilate coronary arteries ► Decrease contractility ► Usually second line for patients unable to tolerate beta-blockers	► Relieve angina ► Reduce myocardial oxygen demand	Verapamil and diltiazem contraindicated in overt HF (systolic) Dihydropyridines (amlodipine) should be used with bradycardia **Monitor for:** ► Constipation ► Headache ► Edema
Nitrates	► Dilate coronary arteries ► Reduces myocardial oxygen demand by decreasing preload and afterload	► Relieve or prevent angina ► No survival benefit	Contraindicated with severe aortic stenosis or hypertrophic cardiomyopathy Nitrate-free period necessary to avoid tolerance (usually 12 hours) **Monitor for:** ► Headache ► Flushing ► Dizziness ► Syncope ► Hypotension

Note: MI = myocardial infarction, CAD = coronary artery disease, GI = gastrointestinal, ACEI = angiotensin-converting enzyme inhibitors, HF = heart failure, LFTs = liver function tests, PAD = peripheral arterial disease, AV = atrioventricular.

Adapted from *The Seventh Report of the Joint National Committee on Prevention, Detection, Evaluation, and Treatment of High Blood Pressure,* by the U.S. Department of Health and Human Services, 2003. Washington, DC: Author.

Treatment for acute MI includes:

▶ Morphine sulfate for pain relief

▶ Oxygen at 2 LPM

▶ Nitroglycerine

▶ Aspirin (160–325 mg chewed) or Plavix

▶ Beta-blockers

▶ Heparin

Options for invasive treatment include percutaneous transluminal coronary intervention and angioplasty. Because of the multiple comorbid factors present in older patients, risk of complications does increase with age; however, age alone is not a contraindication to invasive therapy. Data from younger patients support improving quality of life and functional ability with invasive treatment, but no similar data exist for older patients. The following therapies should be considered, carefully weighing the risks and benefits of intervention:

▶ *Percutaneous transluminal coronary angioplasty* (PTCA): A balloon-tipped catheter is inserted into the coronary artery, under fluoroscopic guidance, to the level of blockage. The balloon is then inflated to compress the plaque and increase the lumen size of the coronary artery.

▶ *Coronary stent:* A stainless steel support is placed in the artery during PTCA to maintain patency of the artery.

▶ *CABG:* Blood flow is rerouted around sites of arterial obstruction by the use of grafts (either saphenous vein or internal mammary artery).

Patient education in CHD centers on prevention of disease progression and relief of symptoms. Lifestyle modifications discussed previously are paramount in the plan of care. As with HF, patients require multiple chronic medications, including daily aspirin, a beta-blocker, and an ACEI to treat CHD and improve outcomes. To achieve patient adherence to the plan of care, patients must understand the action and importance of each medication, as well as the need for regular medical follow-up.

Dyslipidemia

Abnormal lipid levels are a risk factor for all CVDs. Such abnormalities may include one or more of the following:

▶ Elevated LDL

▶ Elevated TGs

▶ Low HDL

Tables 13–8A–D outline the classification of lipid abnormalities according to the National Cholesterol Education Program (NCEP) guidelines.

TABLE 13-8A.
TOTAL CHOLESTEROL CLASSIFICATION

< 200	Desirable
200–239	Borderline high
> 240	High

TABLE 13-8B.
LDL CLASSIFICATION

< 100	Optimal
100–129	Near optimal
130–159	Borderline high
160–189	High
≥ 190	Very high

TABLE 13-8C.
HDL CLASSIFICATION

< 40	Low
>40	Optimal
≥ 60	High

TABLE 13-8D.
TG CLASSIFICATION

< 150	Optimal
> 150	High

Note: LDL = low-density lipoprotein, HDL = high-density lipoprotein, TG = triglyceride.

Adapted from the *Third Report on Detection, Evaluation, and Treatment of High Blood Cholesterol in Adults* by the National Cholesterol Education Program, 2011, Bethesda, MD: National Heart, Lung, and Blood Institute.

Target cholesterol levels for a given patient are determined according to the number of major risk factors for CVD that the patient has. Risk factors (excluding LDL) to be considered are:

► Cigarette smoking

► HTN (BP > 140/90 or on medication)

► Low HDL (< 40)

► Minus 1 risk factor if HDL ≥ 60

► Family history of premature CVD (first-degree male < 55 years; female < 65)

► Age (men ≥ 45; women ≥ 55).

Other forms of atherosclerosis, such as peripheral arterial occlusive disease (PAOD), symptomatic carotid disease, or history of stroke, are considered risk equivalents. Diabetes mellitus is also considered a risk equivalent, because having this diagnosis confers as much risk of having a heart attack in the next 10 years (20%) as already having had one. The percentage risk of having an event is determined based on Framingham scores. This risk can be quickly calculated by plugging in data from the following link: http://hp2010.nhlbihin.net/atpiii/calculator.asp?usertype=prof.

Tables 13–9 and 13–10 identify target levels for lifestyle and drug treatment according to NCEP guidelines. The term *therapeutic lifestyle choices* (TLC) describes the standard lifestyle changes of weight loss, exercise, and low fat–low cholesterol diet.

TABLE 13-9.
NATIONAL CHOLESTEROL EDUCATION PROGRAM GUIDELINES FOR RISK

RISK CATEGORY	LDL GOAL	INITIATE TLC	CONSIDER MEDICATION
Very high risk	< 70	> 70	≥ 70
CVD or risk equivalent	< 100	> 100	≥ 130 (100–129 drug optional)
2 or more risk factors; 10-year risk, 10%–20%	< 130	≥ 130	≥ 130
2 or more risk factors; 10-year risk, <10%	< 130	≥ 130	≥ 160
0–1 risk factors	< 160	≥ 160	≥ 190 (160–189 drug optional)

Note: LDL = low-density lipoprotein, TLC = therapeutic lifestyle choices, CVD = cardiovascular disease.

Adapted from the *Third Report on Detection, Evaluation, and Treatment of High Blood Cholesterol in Adults* by the National Cholesterol Education Program, 2011, Bethesda, MD: National Heart, Lung, and Blood Institute.

TABLE 13-10.
NATIONAL CHOLESTEROL EDUCATION PROGRAM GUIDELINES FOR MEDICATION

DRUG CLASS	MEDICATIONS	PRIMARY EFFECTS	NURSING CONSIDERATIONS
Statins	Lovastatin Fluvastatin Pravastatin Simvastatin Atorvastatin Rouvastatin Livalo	Lowers LDL Raises HDL Lowers TGs	**Monitor for:** ▸ Myalgias ▸ Dark urine ▸ LFTs
Fibrates	Gemfibrozil Fenofibrate Omega-3-acid ethyl esters	Lowers TGs Raises HDL	Contraindicated in severe hepatic and renal disease **Monitor for:** ▸ Gallstones ▸ GI upset ▸ Myopathy
Nicotinic acid	Niacin Niaspan	Raises HDL Lowers TGs Lowers LDL	Initial few doses cause severe flushing; aspirin taken 30 min before diminishes flushing **Monitor for:** ▸ Myopathy ▸ GI upset ▸ GI bleeding ▸ Liver function ▸ Hyperglycemia ▸ Hyperuricemia/gout symptoms
Cholesterol absorption inhibitor	Zetia	Lowers LDL Lowers TGs	**Monitor for:** ▸ Diarrhea ▸ Other GI symptoms
Bile acid resins	Colestipol Welchol	Lowers LDL	**Monitor for:** ▸ Constipation ▸ Elevated TGs
Fish oil	Lovaza	Lowers TGs Raises HDL	**Monitor for:** ▸ Eructation ▸ Taste perversion ▸ GI upset

Note: LDL = low-density lipoprotein, HDL = high-density lipoprotein, TG = triglycerides, GI = gastrointestinal, LFTs = liver function tests.

Adapted from the *Third Report on Detection, Evaluation, and Treatment of High Blood Cholesterol in Adults* by the National Cholesterol Education Program, 2011, Bethesda, MD: National Heart, Lung, and Blood Institute.

Nonprescription therapy includes:

- ▶ *Soluble dietary fiber:* Pectin from citrus fruits, psyllium seeds
- ▶ *Weight reduction:* Decreases cholesterol independent of dietary fat intake
- ▶ *Stress reduction:* Stress increases levels via effect of epinephrine or may decrease excretion
- ▶ *Smoking cessation:* Raises HDL and lowers TGs
- ▶ *Exercise:* Increases HDL and decreases TGs; also improves insulin sensitivity, lowers BP, and aids in weight loss
- ▶ *Plant sterols and stanols:* Substances found in plants; commercially available in various margarines and in tablet form
- ▶ *Soy protein:* Lowers LDL and TGs
- ▶ *Fish oil:* Lowers TGs
- ▶ *Red rice yeast:* Works like a statin drug by inhibiting HMG-CoA reductase

Peripheral Arterial Occlusive Disease

The major etiology of *peripheral arterial occlusive disease* (PAOD) is atherosclerosis affecting the lower extremities. Claudication, or pain with ambulation, often is the initial warning sign of this disease process and may be the first indicator of atherosclerosis. PAOD usually progresses slowly; therefore, symptoms are gradual in onset. However, as with MI, it is possible to have acute ischemia develop from plaque rupture, causing acute arterial occlusion.

Men are affected slightly more than women, but the numbers are converging. The presence of PAOD is a marker for widespread atherosclerosis, so it is associated with a significant increase in mortality, with most people dying from a coronary event. Amputation is the most feared consequence for most patients, but only 5% of those with claudication will need a major amputation (Brewster, 2009). Pain with ambulation can greatly limit functional status, and patients usually limit their activity to reduce their pain, creating the illusion that the disease is not progressing when in fact it is. See the interpretation of ankle-brachial index scoring in Table 13–13.

Subjective data include:

- ▶ Pain in extremity (e.g., location, severity, onset, duration)
- ▶ Aggravating and relieving factors (e.g., rest, activity)
- ▶ Walking distance before claudication
- ▶ Risk factor assessment (e.g., tobacco use, HTN, diabetes mellitus, dyslipidemia, obesity)
- ▶ Personal history of atherosclerosis (e.g., stroke, CAD)
- ▶ Family history of atherosclerosis
- ▶ Functional status and activity limitations
- ▶ Psychosocial status

Objective data include:

▶ Feet and legs (e.g., skin appearance/lesions, temperature, thickened nails, hair loss, sensation loss)

▶ Bruits (e.g., abdominal, femoral)

▶ Peripheral pulses (e.g., femoral, popliteal, dorsalis pedis [DP], posterior tibial [PT])

▶ Capillary refill

▶ Muscle tone and strength

▶ Elevation pallor and dependent rubor (patients with chronic ischemia will have blanching of skin on elevation of extremity, which will change to deep red color when foot is in the dependent position)

▶ Ankle–brachial index (see Box 13–1)

BOX 13-1.
MEASUREMENT OF THE ANKLE-BRACHIAL INDEX

Procedure
▶ Measure brachial BP in both arms, and record.
▶ Measure ankle BP in both legs, and record (see steps below).
▶ Divide the highest ankle pressure by the highest brachial pressure.
▶ Record ratio as ABI.

Measuring Ankle Pressure
▶ Place BP cuff just above ankle.
▶ Inflate and slowly deflate cuff with Doppler at the DP or PT site.
▶ Note pressure when signal is first heard.
▶ Record as ankle pressure.

Note: BP = blood pressure, ABI = Ankle brachial index, DP = dorsalis pedis, PT = posterior tibial.

TABLE 13-11.
INTERPRETATION OF THE ANKLE-BRACHIAL INDEX

ANKLE-BRACHIAL INDEX	SIGNIFICANCE
> 0.9	Normal
< 0.7	Claudication
< 0.5	Ischemic rest pain
< 0.3	Severe, limb-threatening

Diagnostic tests for PAOD include:

▶ Lower-extremity arterial segmental leg pressure study (by an accredited vascular lab)

▶ CT angiogram

▶ Magnetic resonance angiogram

▶ Arteriography (gold standard)

▶ Toe pressures in diabetics

Medical management includes:

▶ Antiplatelet medications (e.g., aspirin, clopidogrel)

▶ Pentoxifylline (Trental)

- Increases RBC deformity and decreases blood viscosity

- Increases walking distance in some patients

- Has low risk of side effects

▶ Cilostazol (Pletal)

- Inhibits platelet aggregation and dilates artery walls

- Increases walking distance by 50%

- Contraindicated in patients with HF

- Side effects of dizziness, headache, palpitations, and diarrhea

▶ Invasive therapies

- Bypass surgery

- Angioplasty/stenting

Nursing management for PAOD includes the following:

▶ Teach about smoking cessation.

▶ Teach control of diabetes mellitus.

▶ Encourage BP control and lipid management (e.g., compliance with medications, lifestyle changes).

▶ Teach about prevention of foot ulcers (e.g., importance of regular foot exams, daily washing, clean socks and protective shoes).

▶ Teach patient about progressive walking to improve collateral circulation (see Box 13–2).

BOX 13-2.
PROGRESSIVE AMBULATION PROGRAM

1. Walk a minimum of 5 days/week.
2. Gradually increase the total amount of exercise time (begin at 5 min/day and increase to 30–45 min/day).
3. Walk to the point of pain, then stop and rest until pain resolves.
4. Repeat process until the total time has been achieved.

Peripheral Venous Disease

Peripheral venous disease (PVD) includes *venous insufficiency, varicose veins, venous ulceration, and deep vein thrombosis (DVT)*. Venous insufficiency and varicose veins often occur together, although a person can have poor venous return in the legs without visible evidence of varicosities. Venous ulceration is a common complication of venous insufficiency.

Venous insufficiency is the most common cause of lower-extremity swelling. Risk factors for venous insufficiency and varicose veins include:

▶ Obesity

▶ Prolonged sitting or standing

▶ Tight-fitting garments

▶ Estrogenic hormones

▶ Trauma

▶ Family history

Signs and symptoms include:

▶ Ankle and lower leg edema, reduced by leg elevation

▶ Aching or leg cramps

▶ Skin changes (e.g., itching, rash, ulceration, brawny discoloration)

Management of venous insufficiency is aimed at minimizing swelling and skin irritation and preventing ulceration. Diuretics are not helpful, as the problem is not one of volume overload but, rather, one of increased hydrostatic pressure in the veins because of gravity, vein damage, or incompetent valves. The most effective therapy is preventing swelling by using compression wraps or venous compression stockings, applied first thing in the morning before the patient gets out of bed and removed at bedtime. A minimum of 20 mm Hg compression is required to effectively prevent swelling. These stockings will be "tight" and often impossible for an older person to put on without assistance. Periods of leg elevation, interspersed with exercise and walking, are also helpful to reduce edema.

Management of skin irritation and itching, using emollient creams, is important to maintaining skin integrity. Scratching can lead to skin disruption and secondary infection or cellulitis. Occasionally, topical corticosteroid cream will be prescribed to relieve itching and rash. Avoidance of medications that are likely to increase edema (e.g., calcium channel blockers) is another key management strategy.

Cardiac Arrhythmias

The prevalence of cardiac rhythm disturbances increases with age, because of a higher incidence of atherosclerosis, as well as the presence of age-related fibrosis in the cardiac conduction tissue. It always is important to exclude coronary ischemia as the cause of any cardiac arrhythmia in an older adult. The most common and serious arrhythmias include:

▶ *Atrial fibrillation* (AF): Chaotic depolarization of the atria in excess of 400 betas/min, with an irregular, often rapid (100–150 beats/min) ventricular response.

▶ *Sick sinus syndrome* or *sinus node dysfunction*: Alternating periods of *bradycardia* (rate < 60/min) and *tachycardia* (rate > 100/min), often with sinus pauses where the sinoatrial node fails to fire for several seconds, leading to temporary absence of cardiac pumping.

▶ *Heart block*: Delayed or blocked impulses between the atria and ventricles; classified as first degree, second degree (Type 1 or 2), and third degree; higher-degree heart block carries the most risk of complications.

▶ *Ventricular tachycardia*: Irritability of ventricular tissue, leading to rapid impulse firing and poorly organized ventricular contraction and, thus, reduced cardiac output.

Signs and symptoms of cardiac arrhythmias vary according to the type and ventricular rate. Both typical (palpitations) and atypical (falls or confusion) symptoms should be considered. Some common signs and symptoms are:

▶ Fatigue and weakness

▶ Palpitations

▶ Dizziness

▶ Near-syncope

▶ Chest pain

▶ Shortness of breath

▶ Nausea

▶ Confusion or altered level of consciousness

▶ Unexplained falls

▶ Slow, rapid, or irregular pulse

Available tests for detecting cardiac arrhythmias include a 12-lead ECG, 24-hour Holter monitor, and event or loop recorder. Occasionally, advanced electrophysiological studies or signal-averaged ECG will be required by a cardiac specialist.

Treatment of various cardiac arrhythmias depends on their associated symptoms, severity, frequency, and potential consequences (see Table 13–12).

TABLE 13-12.
TREATMENTS FOR CARDIAC ARRHYTHMIAS

TYPE OF ARRHYTHMIA	POSSIBLE TREATMENTS
Sick sinus syndrome	▶ Pacemaker to relieve pauses and treat bradycardia ▶ Calcium channel or beta-blockers to control rapid rates (once pacemaker is in place)
Ventricular tachycardia	▶ Beta-blockers (e.g., atenolol, metoprolol) ▶ Amiodarone ▶ Implantable cardioverter defibrillator
Heart block	▶ Avoid AV nodal–blocking drugs and digitalis ▶ First-degree or second-degree Type I—no treatment ▶ Second-degree Type II—careful monitoring for progression or pacemaker insertion ▶ Third degree—pacemaker
Atrial fibrillation	See discussion below

Note: AV = atrioventricular.
Adapted from *Heart Disease and Stroke Statistics: 2012 Update* by American Heart Association, 2012, retrieved from http://circ.ahajournals.org/content/125/1/188.full.pdf.

Atrial Fibrillation

Because of its high prevalence and devastating consequences in older adults, *atrial fibrillation (AF)* deserves additional discussion. AF has been diagnosed in 2.2 million Americans, affecting 6% of people age 65 or older and accounts for one-third of hospitalizations for arrhythmia in older adults (AHA, 2012).

In AF, rapid firing of atrial cells does not produce an organized contraction of the atria. Loss of atrial contraction leads to reduced ventricular filling. In the average person, atrial contribution or "atrial kick" is responsible for about 30% of the end-diastolic filling volume in the ventricle. In older adults who have developed stiffened ventricles, atrial contribution may provide for up to half of the filling volume in the ventricle. This decrease in ventricular filling leads to a reduced stroke volume, even when ejection fraction is preserved. Reduction of stroke volume means a reduced cardiac output, which may result in fatigue or functional limitations.

AF has numerous possible causes and predisposing factors, which may include the following:

▶ MI

▶ Pulmonary embolism

▶ Myocarditis

▶ Pericarditis

▶ Surgery

▶ Hyperthyroidism

▶ Alcohol consumption

▶ Infection

▶ Valvular disease (especially mitral disorders)

▶ HTN, with left ventricular hypertrophy

▶ Cardiomyopathies

▶ Cor pulmonale

▶ Obstructive sleep apnea.

AF carries a significant risk for cerebrovascular accident (CVA) because of the dislodgement of an intracardiac clot that travels into the cerebral circulation. About 15% of strokes occur in people with AF (AHA, 2012).

The major risk of AF is CVA, but functional limitations can occur because of fatigue caused by the arrhythmia. Symptoms are worse in people with rapid ventricular rates. Furthermore, a prolonged, rapid ventricular rate can lead to ventricular dysfunction and decreased contractility (tachycardia-induced cardiomyopathy). Treatment is, therefore, aimed at:

▶ *Rhythm control (symptom management):* Direct current cardioversion, anti-arrhythmic medications (e.g., amiodarone, dofetilide, ibutilide)

▶ *Rate control (symptom management):* Calcium channel blockers (e.g., verapamil, diltiazem), beta-blockers (e.g., metoprolol, atenolol, esmolol), and digoxin

▶ *Anticoagulation (stroke prevention):* Warfarin (Coumadin), dabigatran etexilate mesylate (Pradaxa), and aspirin (if contraindication to warfarin)

Warfarin therapy can be extremely important in stroke prevention, but it can lead to devastating bleeding consequences when not appropriately monitored. Regular international normalized ratio (INR) monitoring is essential. A newer drug, Dabigatran etexilate mesylate (Pradaxa), can be used in patients with nonvalvular atrial fibrillation and does not need INR monitoring.

Patients should be counseled to take medication as directed and at the same time each day, usually in the evening. Patients should following dosing instructions carefully and realize that these will change from time to time as their INR changes. They must keep scheduled appointments for blood monitoring. They should be advised that dark-green vegetables contain large amounts of vitamin K and can interfere with the action of the blood thinner. These foods should not be avoided, but patients should keep their intake consistent from week to week. An excellent patient handout on warfarin therapy is available from the Cleveland Clinic (2009) at http://my.clevelandclinic.org/drugs/coumadin/hic_understanding_coumadin.aspx.

For some older patients, taking warfarin and other thrombin inhibitors may present too much risk. Patients in this category include frequent fallers (at risk of subdural hematoma and other trauma-related bleeding), those who routinely miss medical and laboratory appointments, and those with cognitive impairment who administer their own medications (heightened risk of medication error).

REFERENCES

American Heart Association. (2012). *Heart disease and stroke statistics: 2012 update.* Retrieved from http://circ.ahajournals.org/content/125/1/188.full.pdf

Brewster, D. (2009). Management of peripheral artery disease. In *Primary Care Medicine: Office Evaluation and Management.* Philadelphia: Lippincott Williams & Wilkins.

Cleveland Clinic. (2009). Patient information—What you need to know about your warfarin therapy. *Cleveland Clinic Journal of Medicine, 70,* 372–373. Available from http://my.clevelandclinic.org/drugs/coumadin/hic_understanding_coumadin.aspx

Helmy, T., Patel, A. D., & Wenger, N. K. (2006). Cardiac disease. In T. Rosenthal, B. Naughton, & M. Williams (Eds.), *Office care geriatrics* (pp. 335–362). Philadelphia: Lippincott Williams & Wilkins.

Huether, S., & McCance, K. (2012). *Understanding pathophysiology* (5th ed.). St. Louis, MO: Mosby.

Hunt, S. A., Abraham, W. T., Chin, M. H., et al. (2005). American College of Cardiology; American Heart Association Task Force on Practice Guidelines; American College of Chest Physicians; International Society for Heart and Lung Transplantation; Heart Rhythm Society: *ACC/AHA 2005 Guideline Update for the Diagnosis and Management of Chronic Heart Failure in the Adult: A report of the American College of Cardiology/American Heart Association Task Force on Practice Guidelines* (Writing Committee to Update the 2001 Guidelines for the Evaluation and Management of Heart Failure): Developed in collaboration with the American College of Chest Physicians and the International Society for Heart and Lung Transplantation: Endorsed by the Heart Rhythm Society. *Circulation, 112,* e154–e235.

Hurst, J. W., Morris, D. C., & Alexander, R. W. (1999). The use of the New York Heart Association's classification of cardiovascular disease as part of the patient's complete Problem List. *Clinical Cardiology, 22*(6), 385–390.

McCaffery, M., & Pasero, C. (1999). *Pain: Clinical manual* (2nd ed.). St. Louis, MO: Mosby.

McPhee, S., & Papadakis, M. (2011). *Current medical diagnosis and treatment* (50th ed.). New York: McGraw Hill Medical.

Reuben, D., Herr, K., Pacala, J., Pollock, B., Potter, J., & Semla, T. (2011). *Geriatrics at your fingertips* (13th ed.). New York: American Geriatrics Society.

U.S. Department of Health and Human Services. (2012). *The seventh report of the joint national commission on prevention, detection, and treatment of high blood pressure.* Retrieved from http://www.nhlbi.nih.gov/guidelines/hypertension/express.pdf

ADDITIONAL RESOURCES

American Heart Association: www.heart.org/

Chronic and Disabling Conditions: www.agingsociety.org/

Healthy People 2020: www.healthypeople.gov/2020/

National Institutes of Health—Heart, Lung and Blood Institute: www.nhlbi.nih.gov/

RESPIRATORY DISEASES

Common respiratory diseases in older adults include chronic obstructive pulmonary disease, asthma or reactive airways disease, pneumonia, allergic rhinitis, carcinoma, and tuberculosis.

Chronic Obstructive Pulmonary Disease

Chronic obstructive pulmonary disease (COPD) describes lung pathology that leads to chronic and irreversible airflow limitation. COPD encompasses two main diseases: chronic bronchitis and emphysema. In 2008, 13.1 million U.S. adults were estimated to have COPD. However, close to 24 million U.S. adults have evidence of impaired lung function, indicating an underdiagnosis of COPD (American Lung Association [ALA], 2012a).

COPD is the third leading cause of death, behind cardiac vascular disease and cancer (Centers for Disease Control, 2012a). While the death rate from COPD has been declining for men, the same does not hold true for women. For 8 consecutive years, women have exceeded men in the number of deaths attributable to COPD. In 2007, almost 64,000 females died from it, compared to almost 60,000 males (ALA, 2012a).

Chronic bronchitis is characterized by a productive cough for 3 months in each of 2 successive years (when other causes have been excluded). *Emphysema* is characterized by abnormal, permanent enlargement and destruction of the alveolar airspaces (ALA, 2012a). Both problems often occur to varying degrees in the same person.

The most significant cause of COPD is cigarette smoking, accounting for 80%–90% of all deaths (ALA, 2012). Other risk factors include genetic abnormalities such as α_1-antitrypsin deficiency, which leads to a premature, accelerated form of emphysema. Occupational exposure to organic dusts and vapors, and indoor pollution from burning of fossil fuels, can cause COPD. Early childhood respiratory infections also seem to increase risk.

Symptoms often are absent early in the disease, delaying diagnosis until the disease has reached a moderate stage. Signs and symptoms may include:

▶ Dyspnea on exertion (early) and at rest (advanced)

▶ Chronic cough

▶ Sputum production

▶ Wheezing

▶ Decreased breath sounds

▶ Increased anterioposterior diameter of the chest

▶ Muscle wasting/cachexia (late)

▶ Cor pulmonale (late)

Diagnosis of COPD is made by pulmonary function tests (PFTs) or spirometry testing, which will show an obstruction to airflow that is not completely reversible with bronchodilator use (see Box 14–1). Chest x-rays may suggest COPD (e.g., flattened diaphragms, heart elongation, decreased lung markings, evidence of pulmonary hypertension [HTN]), but many people will have a relatively normal chest x-ray, yet have airflow limitations, as shown by spirometry. The presence of post-bronchodilator $FEV_1/FVC < 0.70$ confirms the presence of persistent airflow limitation and, thus, COPD (Global Strategy for the Diagnosis, Management, and Prevention of COPD, 2011). The GOLD guidelines (2009) divide COPD into stages based on the FEV_1.

BOX 14–1.
SPIROMETRY MEASUREMENTS*

FVC = Total amount of air that can be forcefully exhaled after deep inhalation

FEV_1 = Amount of air that can be forcefully exhaled in 1 second

FEV_1 / FVC or FEV_1 % = Percentage of total air leaving the lung in 1 second

*Many other measurements can be obtained, but those listed are considered the most useful.

The GOLD guidelines (2009) divide COPD into four stages (mild, moderate, severe, and very severe) based on the FEV_1 values that range from 80% for mild to 30% for very severe. Please refer to http://www.goldcopd.org/uploads/users/files/GOLD_PocketGuide_2011_Jan18.pdf for further information.

As with most chronic illnesses, education is a key component in the management of COPD. The following elements of management are essential for the best outcomes:

► Smoking cessation (most important)

► Regular exercise

► Weight control

► Limiting occupational exposure to air pollution and other toxins

► Adequate nutrition

► Immunizations (pneumococcal and annual influenza)

► Pharmacological therapy (stepwise approach based on symptoms and disease severity)

Pharmacological therapy includes beta$_2$-agonists, which stimulate beta$_2$ receptors in the lung, causing bronchodilation. The short-acting beta$_2$-agonists are the most important "rescue" medications for acute shortness of breath in both COPD and asthma, and include albuterol (Proventil), levolbuterol (Xoeponex), and pirbuterol (Maxair). They are administered by metered-dose inhaler or by nebulizer. Beta$_2$-agonists also are available in sustained-release or long-acting forms such as salmeterol (Serevent) and formoterol (Foradil). However, older adults with ischemic heart disease (IHD) can develop angina from the tachycardia caused by these medications, so they should be used with extreme caution.

Education about proper use of inhaled medications is critical. Many people do not receive full benefit from inhaled medications because of improper technique. Patients should be required to demonstrate the use of both new delivery devices and those that they have been using. Use of a spacer device on the standard inhaler can improve the delivery of medication to the lungs.

Inhaled anticholinergics inhibit vagal stimulation and prevent contraction of smooth muscle in the airway, as well as decrease mucous production. Iptratorpium bromide (Atrovent) is a short-acting medication that requires dosing four times daily. Tiotropium bromide (Spiriva) may be dosed once daily.

Inhaled corticosteroids are indicated in patients who achieve improvement in FEV$_1$ after a 6-to 12-week trial or who have frequent exacerbations. Examples are budesonide (Pulmicort) and fluticasone (Flovent). Inhaled corticosteroids should be considered if older patients in the *severe* or *very severe* categories have sufferred more than three COPD exacerbations (severe dyspnea, respiratory rate > 25, or PCO$_2$ 45–60) within the last 3 years (Reuben et al., 2011). Oral corticosteroids improve symptoms during acute exacerbations and decrease hospital lengths of stay.

Theophylline may be added to other therapies during times of exacerbation or for people with severe disease. Theophylline has bronchodilating effects and also improves respiratory muscle function. Major drawbacks are the potential for toxicity from multiple drug interactions and reduced clearance in older adults.

Supplemental oxygen is useful in patients with resting oxygen saturation < 88% by pulse oximetry or PaO_2 < 55 mm Hg by ABG. It also is useful in patients with symptoms of right-sided HF, even with slightly higher saturation levels. In addition, people who desaturate during sleep or exercise qualify for and benefit from oxygen therapy.

Broad-spectrum antibiotics often are prescribed to treat acute exacerbations believed to be secondary to bacterial infection. Because presence of a bacterial pathogen is difficult to prove (by sputum culture) in patients who are not intubated, clinical therapy usually covers this possibility.

Neither lung volume reduction surgery nor lung transplantation is appropriate for most patients. In general, patients age 65 or older are not candidates for lung transplantation. Pulmonary rehabilitation programs offer the best chance for improved symptom reduction and quality of life. These programs can have a profound impact on patients, even those with severe disease.

Asthma and Reactive Airways Disease

Asthma is a chronic inflammatory disorder of the airways characterized by variable and recurring symptoms, including airflow limitation, bronchial hyperresponsiveness, and underlying inflammation (National Asthma Education and Prevention Program, 2007). Symptoms result from acute bronchospasm and require treatment with bronchodilator therapy. Long-term treatment with inhaled corticosteroids targets airway inflammation to prevent alterations in airway structure (remodeling).

More than 18.7 million people have been diagnosed with asthma, with rates being higher in those age 0–17. In adults, women are affected more than men. The primary diagnosis of asthma accounted for more than 17 million visits to physicians' offices, outpatient clinics, and emergency rooms in 2007. In 2009, asthma accounted for 3,388 deaths in the United States (Centers for Disease Control and Prevention [CDC], 2012b).

An asthma attack may be triggered by many factors (see Box 14–2), and triggers vary. It is important for patients with asthma to know and avoid their triggers.

> **BOX 14-2.**
> **COMMON ASTHMA TRIGGERS**
> ► Allergens
>   ▸ Dust mites
>   ▸ Pollen
>   ▸ Molds
>   ▸ Animal dander
> ► Environmental changes
>   ▸ Heat
>   ▸ Cold
> ► Smoke
>   ▸ Tobacco
>   ▸ Wood
> ► Strong odors or fumes
>   ▸ Perfumes
>   ▸ Paint
>   ▸ Hairspray
> ► Respiratory infections

Signs and symptoms of an asthma attack include:

► Dyspnea

► Wheezing

► Increased respiratory rate

► Palpitations or tachycardia

► Use of accessory muscles

► Diaphoresis

► Pulsus paradoxus

Medication management for asthma is administered in a stepwise approach based on severity of symptoms and amount of lung compromise, similar to the approach to COPD (National Asthma Education and Prevention Program, 2007). Most of the medications used to treat asthma are discussed in the COPD section, with the exception of leukotriene modifiers (see Box 14–3).

Step 1: Mild intermittent asthma (symptomatic < 2/week, otherwise asymptomatic)

► No daily medication

► $Beta_2$ agonists, 2–4 puffs as needed for symptoms

Step 2: Mild persistent asthma (symptomatic < 2/week, < 1 day/week)

► Low-dose inhaled corticosteroids

► Alternative treatments such as Cromolyn, leukotriene modifier, nedocromil, or sustained-release theophylline

► $Beta_2$-agonists, 2–4 puffs as needed for symptoms

Step 3: Moderate persistent asthma (daily symptoms, daily use of beta$_2$-agonist)

▶ Low to medium dose inhaled corticosteroids and long-acting inhaled beta$_2$-agonists

▶ Alternative treatments such as increased-dose inhaled corticosteroids, leukotriene modifier, or theophylline

▶ Beta$_2$-agonists, 2–4 puffs as needed for symptoms

Step 4: Severe persistent asthma (continually symptomatic, limited physical activity)

▶ High-dose inhaled corticosteroids and long-acting inhaled beta$_2$-agonists

▶ If needed, oral corticosteroids

▶ Beta$_2$-agonists, 2–4 puffs as needed for symptoms

Gerontological nurses should be aware that systemic corticosteroids can have several adverse effects in older adults, including HTN, elevated blood glucose, cataracts, osteoporosis, and— especially in patients with underlying cognitive impairment—confusion and agitation.

BOX 14-3.
LEUKOTRIENE MODIFIERS

▶ Montelukast (Singulair)
▶ Zafirlukast (Accolate)

Block the action of *leukotrienes* (inflammatory mediators that cause asthma symptoms)

Patient education should focus on self-management and following the designated treatment plan. The proper technique for using inhaled mediations should be validated. The lifestyle modifications listed in the COPD section also apply to patients with asthma. In addition, patients must identify and avoid triggers for their disease.

Pneumonia

Pneumonia is an inflammatory illness of the lung, resulting in alveolar fluid accumulation. The infection can be caused by bacteria, viruses, fungi, or parasites. Pneumonia is the leading cause of infectious death in the United States. *Pneumococcal pneumonia* is the most common type of bacterial pneumonia. There are more than 40,000 cases of invasive pneumococcal disease in the United States a year, and approximately one-third of these cases occur in people 65 and older. Over half of the more than 5,000 annual deaths from invasive pneumococcal disease occur in people 65 years of age and older (Centers for Medicare & Medicaid Services, 2012).

Most pneumonia is caused by microaspiration of bacteria and viruses that colonize the oropharynx. Older adults have an increased risk of aspiration (especially with altered cognition, neuromuscular diseases, or altered level of consciousness), reduced ability to clear the airway, and decreased immune function. Hygiene issues can increase oral colonization, and poor nutritional status can further impair immune function. Furthermore, the presentation of pneumonia in an older adult is often atypical, which delays diagnosis and proper treatment (see Table 14–1).

TABLE 14-1.
CLINICAL PRESENTATION OF PNEUMONIA IN OLDER ADULTS

TYPICAL PRESENTATION	PRESENTATION IN OLDER ADULTS
Fever	Confusion
Cough	Falls
Shortness of breath	Anorexia
Leukocytosis	Decreased functional ability
Tachycardia	Dehydration
	Tachypnea
	Exacerbation of other illness (diabetes mellitus, coronary artery disease)

Pneumonia is diagnosed by the presence of an infiltrate on a chest x-ray. Measurement of oxygen saturation by pulse oximetry is important for assessing disease severity. An ABG may be needed to check for hypercarbia in patients who are hypoventilating. For community-acquired pneumonia, the decision to hospitalize a patient is based on:

▶ Chest x-ray (unilobar, diffuse, or multilobar infiltrates)

▶ Oxygen saturation

▶ Vital signs

▶ Mental status

▶ Evidence of volume depletion

▶ Functional status of patient or level of supervision or assistance available

The CURB-65 is a simple scoring system to help the clinician decide if an older patient should be admitted to the hospital. Points are assigned for each of five factors, including presence of confusion, blood urea nitrogen levels, respiratory rate, systolic blood pressure, and age. A total score of 3, 4, or 5 suggests the patient should be admitted to the hospital (Lim et al., 2001, 2003). Refer to http://reference.medscape.com/calculator/curb-65-pneumonia-severity-score for an electronic version of the CURB-65.

Pneumonia is divided into two categories:

1. *Community-acquired pneumonia* (CAP): No history of hospitalization or long-term care (LTC) residence for ≥ 14 days before symptom onset

2. *Hospital-acquired pneumonia* (HAP; also known as nosocomial pneumonia): Occurs ≥ 48 hours following admission to hospital or LTC facility

CAP and HAP differ in their likely causative organisms and, thus, in treatment.

Table 14–2 lists common organisms in pneumonia (Niederman, 2003).

TABLE 14–2.
CAUSATIVE ORGANISM IN PNEUMONIA

COMMUNITY-ACQUIRED PNEUMONIA	HOSPITAL–/NURSING HOME-ACQUIRED PNEUMONIA
Strep pneumoniae	*S. pneumoniae* (drug-resistant)
Hemophilus influenzae	*S. aureus* (MRSA)
Legionella sp. or atypical pathogens	Gram-negative enterics
Influenza, other viruses	Anaerobes
S. aureus (following influenza)	Chlamydia pneumoniae
Gram-negative bacteria	Fungi

Adapted from "Recent Advances in Community-Acquired pneumonia," by M. S. Niederman, 2003, *Chest, 131,* 1205–1215; and *Geriatrics at Your Fingertips* (13th Ed.), by D. Reuben, K. Herr, J. Pacala, B. Pollock, J. Potter, & T. Semla, 2011, New York: American Geriatrics Society.

Older adults should receive vaccinations against influenza and *Strep pneumoniae*. The flu vaccine is given annually in the fall. The pneumococcal vaccine can be given at any time of the year. Medicare covers one pneumococcal vaccination for every Medicare beneficiary. One vaccine at age 65 generally provides coverage for a lifetime, but a booster vaccine is needed for some high-risk people. Medicare will also cover a booster vaccine for high-risk people if 5 years have passed since their last vaccination. The Centers for Disease Control and Prevention (CDC, 2012c) recommends a single vaccine for people age 65 or older. People vaccinated before age 65 should have a second vaccination 5 years later.

The following nursing interventions are appropriate for a patient with pneumonia:

▶ Position for ease of breathing and airway clearance (Semi-Fowlers).

▶ Encourage coughing and deep breathing to promote airway clearance.

▶ Maintain hydration, but monitor fluid status.

▶ Monitor vital signs and oxygenation.

▶ For patients who must lie down, position with the good lung down to promote perfusion to the good lung and drainage of secretions from the affected lung.

Pneumonia is treated with antibiotics; most community-residing older adults can be treated on an outpatient basis. Antibiotics are usually administered for 8 to 10 days. The frail older adult may require hospitalization for supportive nursing care and administration of IV antibiotics. Inpatients should be treated until they have reached the following clinical indicators:

▶ Temperature < 100°F (37.8°C)

▶ Heart rate < 100 bpm

▶ Respiratory rate < 25/min

▶ SBP > 90 mm HG

▶ O$_2$ saturation 90%

▶ Ability to maintain oral intake (Reuben et al., 2011)

Allergic Rhinitis

The term *atopy* refers to the genetic predisposition to develop IgE-mediated hypersensitivity and often is used synonymously with *allergy*. *Allergic rhinitis* (AR) is the most common atopic disease. AR affects between 10% and 30% of all adults in the United States—there were more than 13 million physician office visits because of AR in 2010 (American Academy of Allergy, Asthma & Immunology, 2012). Management of upper-airway symptoms is critical for asthma control in people who have both conditions.

The most common symptoms of AR are:

▶ Sneezing

▶ Nasal itching

▶ Nasal congestion

▶ Rhinorrhea

▶ Postnasal drip

▶ Ocular itching or redness

Many people have seasonal symptoms, which usually represent an allergy to pollens or grass. Indoor allergens (e.g., pet dander, dust mites, cockroaches) usually produce perennial symptoms. Tobacco smoke, fumes, and cold air are other possible triggers for symptoms.

The three strategies for management of AR are:

1. Avoiding allergens

2. Medication therapy

3. Immunotherapy

Determination of allergens requires radioallergosorbent (RAST) or skin testing. Once allergens have been identified, environmental control measures can be taken to reduce exposure and, thus, reduce symptoms.

Medication management involves the use of various prescription or over-the-counter drugs. One medication often will control symptoms in a given patient, but occasionally someone with severe AR will require a combination of several medications to fully alleviate the symptoms. Examples of medications include:

▶ Antihistamines (e.g., loratadine, certirizine, diphenhydramine)

   » Nonsedating antihistamines are preferred in older adults.

   » Considerable mental clouding, worsened cognition, and increased risk of falling are possible with first-generation medications such as diphenhydramine.

▶ Oral decongestants (e.g., phenylephrine, pseudoephedrine)

   » Sympathomimetic medications can cause elevated blood pressure (BP), palpitations, restlessness, insomnia, and anxiety in older adults.

▶ Intranasal anticholinergic (ipratropium bromide, 0.03% and 0.06%)

   » This reduces production of nasal secretions, but can cause nasal dryness and nosebleeds.

▶ Intranasal glucocorticoids (e.g., fluticasone, budesonide)

   » These effectively relieve nasal symptoms and may be used daily (most effective) or as needed.

   » Side effects may include nasal irritation or bleeding.

   » Patients should point the spray away from the nasal septum (with chronic use), because septal perforations have been reported.

▶ Intranasal cromolyn sodium (Nasalcrom)

   » This must be used frequently (up to 4 times/day).

▶ Leukotriene modifiers (discussed in asthma management above)

   » These also are approved to treat seasonal and perennial AR.

For patients who do not achieve control with environmental measures and medications, a referral to an allergy specialist is warranted for consideration of immunotherapy. Therapy is usually effective in 1 year and is continued for 3–5 years. Patients must be observed for 20–30 minutes after injections for possible anaphylaxis.

Carcinoma

Lung cancer is the most common type of cancer and is the leading cause of cancer deaths in both men and women. In 2006, approximately 365,000 Americans had lung cancer. The national incidence rate for lung cancer was 63.1 per 100,000 population. The incidence rate was 77.7 per 100,000 for men and 52.5 per 100,000 for women. Lung cancer incidence rates among men have decreased by 29% since 1980, while they have increased by 60% among women (ALA, 2010b). Peak incidence occurs between ages 70 and 74 in women and ages 75 and 79 for men. Risk factors include the following:

- ▶ Cigarette smoking (plays a part in 90% of all lung cancers)
- ▶ Marijuana use
- ▶ Chronic exposure to talc
- ▶ Exposure to arsenic, ether, or chromates
- ▶ Exposure to coal-oven fumes, nickel, or petroleum products
- ▶ Exposure to radon
- ▶ Exposure to asbestos
- ▶ Vitamin A deficiency
- ▶ Vitamin E use in a person who smokes tobacco cigarettes (markedly increases risk of developing this malignancy)

Cigarette smoking is, by far, the most important cause of lung cancer, and the risk from smoking increases with the number of cigarettes smoked and the length of time spent smoking. This risk persists for 15 years after the individual stops smoking; after that point, the risk is similar to that of a nonsmoker (ALA, 2010b).

Signs and symptoms include persistent cough, hemoptysis, or recurring pneumonia or bronchitis. Many times, the symptoms are vague and do not include these signs. Anorexia, weight loss, or fatigue may be the only presenting symptoms. Symptoms of local metastasis include:

- ▶ Hoarseness, if the laryngeal nerve is encroached on by tumor
- ▶ Shoulder pain, if the tumor resides in the upper lobes and presses on the brachial plexus
- ▶ Dyspnea or dysphagia, if the tumor constricts the esophagus
- ▶ Head or neck swelling, if the tumor compresses the superior vena cava and blocks the venous return (ALA, 2010b)

Diagnostics may include chest x-ray, CBC, CT of the chest, ABGs, PFTs, EKGs, and sputum cytology. Bronchoscopy is used to confirm the diagnosis. If metastatic disease is suspected, total body bone scan and magnetic resonance imaging (MRI) of the brain are done before developing a treatment plan.

Lung cancers can be divided into two cell types: small cell (also called *oat cell*) and non–small cell. The non–small cell cancers are further subdivided into squamous cell, adenocarcinoma (most common), and large cell (anaplastic).

Small-cell lung cancers constitute nearly one-fourth of all lung malignancies and are associated with cigarette smoking (ALA, 2010c). The tumors grow and metastasize quickly; a poor prognosis is the usual outcome. These tumors most often respond to chemotherapy and radiation, and remission sometimes occurs. These tumors are not treated with surgery, because they tend to recur.

Squamous-cell cancers are also linked to cigarette smoking; they tend to occur in the central airways and bronchi, making them difficult to detect until very late in the disease. Adenocarcinomas are tumors that usually appear in the peripheral lung fields and are often found incidentally on a chest x-ray. These tumors appear as small, round, well-demarcated lesions on the x-ray, often referred to as *coin lesions*. Both cell types are best treated surgically. Postoperative radiation may be needed for the latter.

In 1998, the National Cancer Institute (NCI) established a new staging system for lung cancer. This staging system identifies the tumor by type and location and helps to guide treatment options (see Table 14–3).

TABLE 14-3.
STAGING OF NON-SMALL CELL LUNG CANCERS

STAGE	CRITERIA	TREATMENT
I	Non–small cell lung cancer	Surgery
II	Non–small cell lung cancer with lymph node or chest wall invasion	► Surgery ► Curative radiation or radiation, then curative surgery plus adjuvant chemotherapy
III–A	Non–small cell lung cancer with lymph node and chest wall invasion that requires resection of the lung and ribs	► Surgery ► Chemotherapy ► Surgery plus post operative radiation
III–B	Non–small cell lung cancer with more invasion than in Stage III–A; requires a wider, more invasive excision	► Radiation ► Chemotherapy ► Chemotherapy plus radiation ► Radiation, then surgical resection
IV	Non–small cell lung cancer with distant metastasis	Palliation of symptoms; therapies used only to curtail the life-quality-compromising effects of tumor

Adapted from *Lung Cancer: Staging Criteria* by the National Cancer Institute, 2012, http://www.cancer.gov/cancertopics/pdq/treatment/non-small-cell-lung/healthprofessional/page3#Section_478.

Many older adults with resectable lung cancers may not be surgical candidates because of comorbid medical conditions. The overall survival rates for lung cancer are based on stage of tumor at the time of diagnosis. Factors that have correlated with adverse prognosis include:

▶ Presence of pulmonary symptoms

▶ Large tumor size (> 3 cm)

▶ Metastases to multiple lymph nodes

▶ Vascular invasion (NCI, 2012)

Nursing assessment begins with identification of risk factors; the gerontological nurse's major role will be in management. Patients with lung cancer should be kept free of pain and given emotional support. The nurse plays a pivotal role in counseling and providing information about diagnostics and prognosis. Encouraging a patient to discuss his or her fears and concerns is an important and vital part of the nursing process.

Tuberculosis

Tuberculosis (TB) is an infectious disease caused by *Mycobacterium tuberculosis*. Today's older adults were alive when TB accounted for close to 35% of all deaths, in the first quarter of the 20th century. TB, which most often is seen in areas where people live in close quarters with little or no health or preventive care, is transmitted by droplet particles aerolized from a cough or sneeze of an infected person. On average, it takes several hundred bacilli to infect an immunocompetent person, yet only a few bacilli to infect a person in an immune-compromised state. TB is divided into two types: primary and active.

Primary TB occurs when the person who is exposed develops local illness in the upper lobes of the lungs, but manifests an immune response that "walls off" the infection. This patient does not have symptoms and is not contagious. TB can remain inactive in the body for decades.

Active TB occurs when the person is exposed and develops the illness. The bacillus causes inflammation and necrosis of the lung parenchyma. Active TB can be present in any patient who presents to a healthcare provider or facility with:

▶ Chronic institutionalization

▶ Corticosteroid use

▶ HIV/AIDS

▶ Frailty

▶ Cancer

▶ Kidney failure

▶ Malnutrition (Reuben et al., 2011)

In the older adult, TB may be reactivation of a dormant bacillus. Normal changes of aging that suppress the immune system make the older adult (who was previously exposed) more susceptible to a reactivation process. Risk factors for resistant organisms include HIV/AIDS, homelessness, IV drug abuse, previous treatment for TB, AFB-positive sputum smears after 2 months of treatment, and positive cultures after 4 months of treatment (Reuben et al., 2011).

Gerontological nurses should suspect TB in any older adult who presents with night sweats, atypical pneumonia, chronic low-grade fever, nonproductive cough, hemoptysis, and anorexia or weight loss. TB incidence is highest among individuals age 65 and older, especially those who have preexisting lung problems.

Diagnostics may include tuberculin skin testing, chest x-ray, CBC, electrolyte panel, sedimentation rate, and sputum test for acid-fast bacillus. Because TB skin testing often is unreliable in older adults, a two-step process must be carried out to achieve accurate results.

Mantoux testing involves giving five units (0.1 mL) of purified protein derivative intradermally into the forearm. This first step "wakes up the immune system." The same test is repeated in 2 weeks and read after 48 to 72 hours. If the person has 10 mm or more (5 mm in the HIV-positive person or those in recent contact with TB-positive people) of induration, the test is considered positive. At that point, the individual should have a chest x-ray.

The positive chest x-ray usually reveals an infiltrate in the upper lobes (apices) of the lungs. However, TB can look atypical on the x-ray of an older adult, because there may be lower-lobe nodular areas or a persistent infiltrate. A person who is asymptomatic is treated with 6 months of isoniazid (INH) in select cases as a prophylaxis against active disease. A patient who is symptomatic is referred to an infectious-disease specialist.

Usual regimens include four drugs—INH, rifampin, pyrazinamide, and ethambutol—for 2 months, with the INH and rifampin are continued for another 4 months. Pyridoxine (vitamin B_6) also is given to prevent resulting peripheral neuropathy from the INH. Reduction in the amount of bacillus is seen within 2 weeks. If the drug is resistant to INH and rifampin, it is said to be multi-drug–resistant TB (MDR-TB). The course of treatment for these individuals is 18–24 months with four drugs to which the bacillus is sensitive. MDR-TB is approximately 50%–60%, curable, compared with a 95%–97% cure rate for people with drug-susceptible TB (CDC, 2009).

Many of the new cases (40%) of TB in the United States occur in foreign-born individuals. This incidence is thought to be related to the widespread use of the Bacillus Calmette–Guérin (BCG) vaccine in Europe and other countries. Initially thought to be a vaccine for TB, this injection proved to have little effect on *M. tuberculosis* and, in some cases, may have made the disease worse (CDC, 2009).

Patients on active therapy should have their LFTs monitored monthly, as older adults are more susceptible to INH hepatitis than their younger counterparts. Dose reduction or discontinuation of the drug may be necessary.

Nursing assessment begins with symptom analysis and assessment of the lung fields. The gerontological nurse's main role in the care of these patients is education about the disease process and how it is transmitted, and in informing patients and family members or caregivers about the importance of taking all of medications and of good nutrition. Psychological support is needed in older adults with TB, because they were raised during a time when TB was considered "taboo" and required placement in a sanatorium (CDC, 2009). Current treatments and opinions have changed, so patients need to be informed of the changes in the societal view of TB.

Because the antitubercular drugs have a fairly high incidence of untoward effects, patients should be well versed in alarm symptoms and what is usual with these drugs. Table 14–4 illustrates important information that older adults should be given about the medications.

TABLE 14–4.
UNTOWARD EFFECTS OF ANTI-TUBERCULAR DRUGS

DRUG	NURSING CONSIDERATIONS	ALARM SYMPTOMS
Isoniazid	No alcohol	► Hepatitis ► Psychosis ► Muscle twitching ► Memory changes ► Dizziness ► Peripheral neuritis ► Agranulo-cytosis
Rifampin	► May turn urine, salvia, and tears orange ► Makes the patient photosensitive ► Makes OCP less effective	Skin rash
Pyrazinamide	Thrombocytopenia and nausea common	Aching joints
Ethambutol		► Tingling around the mouth ► Blurred or change in vision
Streptomycin	► Not a first-line drug ► Next drug added if patient intolerant to pyrazinamide or ethambutol	► Tinnitus ► Loss of hearing

Adapted from *Nurse Practitioners' Prescribing Reference,* 2012, New York: Haymarket Media Publication.

REFERENCES

American Academy of Allergy, Asthma, and Immunology. (2012). *Allergy statistics.* Retrieved from http://www.aaaai.org/about-the-aaaai/newsroom/allergy-statistics.aspx

American Lung Association. (2012a). *Chronic obstructive pulmonary disease (COPD) fact sheet.* Retrieved from http://www.lung.org/lung-disease/copd/resources/facts-figures/COPD-Fact-Sheet.html

American Lung Association. (2012b). *Understanding lung cancer.* Retrieved from http://www.lung.org/lung-disease/lung-cancer/about-lung-cancer/understanding-lung-cancer.html

Centers for Disease Control and Prevention. (2009). *Plan to combat extensively drug-resistant tuberculosis recommendations of the federal tuberculosis task force.* Retrieved from http://www.cdc.gov/mmwr/preview/mmwrhtml/rr5803a1.htm

Centers for Disease Control and Prevention. (2012a). *FASTSTATS–Leading causes of death.* Retrieved from http://www.cdc.gov/nchs/fastats/lcod.htm

Centers for Disease Control and Prevention. (2012b). *FASTSTATS–Asthma.* Retrieved from http://www.cdc.gov/nchs/fastats/asthma.htm

Centers for Disease Control and Prevention. (2012c). *FASTSTATS–Kidney disease.* Retrieved from http://www.cdc.gov/nchs/fastats/kidbladd.htm

Global Strategy for the Diagnosis, Management, and Prevention of COPD. (2011). *A guide for health care professionals.* Retrieved from http://www.goldcopd.org/uploads/users/files/GOLD_PocketGuide_2011_Jan18.pdf

Huether, S., & McCance, K. (2012). *Understanding pathophysiology* (5th ed.). St. Louis, MO: Mosby.

Lim, W. S., Macfarlane, J. T., Boswell, T. C., Harrison, T. G., Rose, D., Leinonen, M., & Saikku, P. (2001). Study of community acquired pneumonia aetiology (SCAPA) in adults admitted to hospital: implications for management guidelines. *Thorax, 56*(4), 296–301.

McPhee, S., & Papadakis, M. (2011). *Current medical diagnosis and treatment* (50th ed.). New York: McGraw Hill Medical.

National Asthma Education and Prevention Program. (2007). *Expert Panel Report 3: Guidelines for the diagnosis and management of asthma* (NIH Pub. No. 19-4051). Bethesda, MD: National Institutes of Health.

National Cancer Institute. (2012). *Non-small cell lung cancer treatment.* Retrieved from http://www.cancer.gov/cancertopics/pdq/treatment/non-small-cell-lung/healthprofessional/page1#Section_48499

Niederman, M. S. (2003). Recent advances in community-acquired pneumonia. *Chest, 131,* 1205–1215.

Nurse Practitioners' Prescribing Reference. (2012). New York: Haymarket Media Publication.

Reuben, D., Herr, K., Pacala, J., Pollock, B., Potter, J., & Semla, T. (2011). *Geriatrics at your fingertips* (13th ed.). New York: American Geriatrics Society.

ADDITIONAL RESOURCES

Chronic and Disabling Conditions: www.agingsociety.org/

Healthy People 2020: www.healthypeople.gov/2020/

National Heart, Lung and Blood Institute: www.nihlb.nih.gov/

GASTROINTESTINAL DISEASES

The gastrointestinal (GI) tract includes all of the organs and accessory organs that are involved in digestion and absorption of food and nutrients. These organs include the mouth and teeth, esophagus, stomach, liver, pancreas, and small and large bowels. Common problems of the GI tract include gingivitis and periodontitis, dysphagia, gastroesophageal reflux disease, hiatal hernia, gastritis, peptic ulcer, diverticular disease, enteritis, constipation, diarrhea, fecal impaction, fecal incontinence, colon polyps, hemorrhoids, bowel obstruction, and carcinoma.

Gingivitis and Periodontitis

The mouth, along with its support structures, is the initial organ involved in the digestive process. A common change that nurses see in older adults is loss of some or all of a patient's teeth. This loss may be a function of normal wear and tear on the teeth themselves or may result from diseases such as osteoporosis or periodontal disease.

In osteoporosis, the bones become fragile, as do the teeth, since those are the two major storage areas for calcium. In periodontal disease, the teeth become loose and fall out because the support structures and the gums become diseased and unable to hold the teeth in place (McPhee & Papadakis, 2011).

Inflammation of the gums is called *gingivitis*. This disease may cause pain and bleeding, and may lead to *periodontitis*—the progressive loss of bone around the teeth. Gingivitis may result from poor oral hygiene or from overgrowth of the gingivae from medications such as phenytoin (Dilantin; *Nurse Practitioners' Prescribing Reference*, 2012).

Nursing interventions to prevent and treat gingivitis and periodontitis include promoting good oral hygiene, regular dental visits, and maintaining normal nutrition. With each of these processes, prevention is the most important intervention.

Dysphagia

Dysphagia is difficulty in swallowing and can be the result of many underlying diseases, such as stroke, Parkinson's disease, or local trauma or damage to the esophageal tissues. Symptoms of dysphagia can be mild, such as a feeling like a lump is in the throat, to quite severe, such as a the complete inability to swallow food or fluids.

In older adults, dysphagia is quite common, usually the result of chronic acid reflux leading to esophageal stricture. However, dysphagia can be the symptom of other, more severe esophageal problems such as cancer. Gerontological nurses should assess patients for signs and symptoms of aspiration and alert other healthcare providers of the presence of dysphagia and its accompanying symptoms.

Gastroesophageal Reflux Disease

Gastroesophageal reflux disease (GERD) is the movement of stomach contents, usually hydrochloric acid, back into the esophagus. In normal health, the lower esophageal sphincter pressure prevents reflux of gastric contents; an incompetent sphincter is thought to be the main cause of acid reflux (McPhee & Papadakis, 2011). Risk factors include obesity and use of estrogen, nitroglycerin, and tobacco (Reuben et al., 2011). Other causes of GERD include hiatal hernia, which is discussed in a later section; infections; and certain illnesses such as lupus.

In GERD, the hydrochloric acid from the stomach alters the pH of the esophagus and allows the mucosal proteins to break down. These protein changes can cause inflammation, stricture, and scarring so severe that swallowing becomes difficult.

Symptoms of reflux disease can include acid taste in the back of the throat, heartburn and, in severe cases, chest pain. With esophageal chest pain, it often is difficult to discern whether the symptoms are cardiac or esophageal in nature. An emergency room evaluation to rule out cardiac disease often is necessary.

With chronic reflux, esophageal strictures can occur. When strictures are present, dysphagia begins to occur. In this case, a patient should be referred for an evaluation of the esophagus.

Treatment of GERD includes avoiding large and high-fat meals. Other common interventions are avoiding lying down for 3 hours after eating, and sleeping in a bed with the head elevated approximately 8 inches. Medications can include histamine blockers such as ranitidine (Zantac) and famotidine (Pepcid), or PPIs such as omeprazole (Prilosec) and pantoprazole (Protonix). A common prescription intervention is Nexium.

Esophagitis

Esophagitis is an inflammation of the esophagus. The most common causes include gastroesophageal reflux and prolonged vomiting. The amount of esophageal damage correlates with the contact time between irritation of the esophageal mucosa and the acidic gastric reflux.

Hiatal Hernia

A *hiatal hernia* occurs where a part of the stomach protrudes through the esophageal gastric junction. Part or all of the stomach and, in some case the intestines, may herniate up into the esophagus. The condition may be intermittent or continuous.

Hiatal hernia is a major cause of GERD and esophagitis in the older adult (see above). For the most part, hiatal hernias are asymptomatic; however, when they do cause symptoms, common ones include dyspepsia, heartburn, indigestion, and dysphagia. In severe cases, severe retrosternal chest pain and gastric ulcer can occur (Reuben et al., 2011).

Small hiatal hernias can be detected in most older adults. These hernias are also referred to as *diaphragmatic hernias* or *hiatus hernias*. By age 60, at least 60% of older adults have this condition. Risk factors include genetics and age-related changes in the esophageal wall. Diagnostics used to detect hiatal hernias include chest x-ray, barium contrast studies, endoscopy, and 24-hour esophageal pH monitoring (McPhee & Papadakis, 2011).

Treatments include lifestyle changes, the most important of which are weight loss (if needed) and restricting foods that cause irritation. Eating smaller meals more frequently also is recommended. Medicinal treatments include antacids, histamine-2 receptors antagonists such as ranitidine (Zantac), and PPIs such as omeprazole (Prilosec).

Treatment of this condition requires careful monitoring of medications taken, particularly if the older patient has a pulmonary or cardiac condition. Treatment of symptoms and monitoring for aspiration are other important interventions.

Gastritis

Gastritis is inflammation of the gastric mucosa and comes in two forms: acute and chronic. Although stomach acid is present in gastritis, it is not excessive. The major symptom is stomach pain; other indicators may include indigestion, early satiety, nausea, and vomiting (Stamm & Levy, 2006).

Acute gastritis is temporary inflammation, hemorrhage, or erosion of the gastric lining. Common causes include:

- ▶ Alcoholism
- ▶ Aspirin use
- ▶ NSAID use
- ▶ Smoking
- ▶ Severely stressful conditions (e.g., trauma, chemotherapy, radiation)

Chronic gastritis is inflammation that recurs over weeks or months. Common causes include:

▶ Vitamin deficiencies

▶ Chronic alcohol use

▶ Gastric mucosal atrophy (common in advanced age)

▶ Achlorhydria (common with chronic use of acid suppressive medications)

▶ Hiatal hernias (McPhee & Papadakis, 2011)

Chronic gastritis causes the older adult to lose healthy gastric tissue, which will lead to decreased gastric secretions. Decreased secretions can eventually lead to deficiency of all B vitamins (including vitamin B_{12}), peptic ulcer disease (PUD), or gastric cancer.

Peptic Ulcer Disease

Peptic ulcer disease (PUD) is ulceration in the GI tract. Ulceration occurs because of an imbalance between the effects of gastric acid and pepsin on the gastric and duodenal mucosa. The most common sites of ulceration are in the stomach and duodenum. The exact mechanism of PUD is unknown, but common causes include:

▶ *Helicobacter pylori* infection

▶ Overproduction of hydrochloric acid in the stomach (most common with duodenal ulcers; thought to occur because of increased acid secretion by the parietal cells

▶ Decreased resistance of gastric mucosa (can occur with the use of NSAIDs and in chronic gastritis)

H. pylori is the major cause of PUD, and NSAID use is the second most common cause (Reuben et al., 2011). *H. pylori* can be treated with antibiotic regimens that include PPIs (PPI plus clarithromycin plus amoxicillin; Reuben et al., 2011).

In gastric ulcers, the amount of hydrochloric acid is usually normal or reduced. The problem is with the increased diffusion of this acid back into the tissues. Common symptoms of gastric ulcers include epigastric pain, some relief of pain with eating, nausea, vomiting, and weight loss (McPhee & Papadakis, 2011).

With gastric ulcers, healing and recurrence is common. A small percentage of these ulcers will have an underlying cancer, so endoscopic documentation of healing is necessary.

In duodenal ulcers, the level of gastric acid is increased, as is the rate of gastric acid release from the stomach into the duodenum. If acid is not buffered in the stomach before it is passed to the duodenum, the unbuffered acid will irritate the duodenum. Experts believe that *H. pylori* migrate from the stomach into the duodenum. Most duodenal ulcers occur in the first part of the duodenum, close to the pylorus. Symptoms can include variable epigastric pain, pain that is relieved with food and antacids, pain that is worse when the stomach is empty, and weight gain (McPhee & Papadakis, 2011).

Nursing interventions for older adults with PUD include education about lifestyle modifications, and medications that are used to treat and heal the ulcer. Lifestyle changes include:

► Smoking cessation

► Avoiding alcohol

► Avoiding aspirin

► Avoiding NSAIDs

► Reducing stress

Dietary changes also may be in order—avoiding foods that irritate the stomach such as caffeine and alcohol and avoiding foods that cause symptoms to get worse.

Diverticular Disease

Diverticula are sac-like projections of the intestinal mucosa that develop in the GI tract. These sacs result from high pressure within the intestinal lumen. Diverticula are most often in the descending and sigmoid colon.

The true etiology of diverticular disease is unknown. Most experts believe that a diet that is low in dietary fiber is the main contributor to the increase of intraluminal pressure. When there is little stool volume, the intestinal muscles have to exert more force to propel the fecal matter through the colon; the end result is increased pressure. An individual who eats a diet very high in fiber needs less muscle for transit, which results in lower intraintestinal pressure.

Diverticulosis is very common in older adults, with two-thirds of those age 85 or older having diverticular disease. For the most part, diverticulosis is asymptomatic (Reuben et al., 2011).

Diverticulitis is inflammation or infection in and around a diverticular sac. It is usually the result of trapped undigested food, stool, or bacteria in the sac. The retained particles form a hard mass, called a *fecalith*. Common symptoms include a change in bowel habits; lower left abdominal pain; constipation; and increased flatus, nausea, and vomiting. However, many older adults with diverticulitis may be afebrile and have minimal abdominal symptoms.

When older patients present with suspected diverticulitis, gerontological nurses should assess for risk factors such as insufficient dietary fiber and chronic constipation. Diagnostic studies include abdominal CT or ultrasound and laboratory studies. A common laboratory finding is leukocytosis. Treatment may include bowel rest, analgesics, antibiotics, and, in severe cases, surgical resection.

Nursing management for older adults with diverticular disease includes prevention and elimination of constipation. A high-fiber diet is necessary for the older patient with diverticulosis. Patients should be instructed on foods to avoid, including nuts, popcorn, corn, celery, and other fresh, uncooked vegetables. Adequate fluid intake also is imperative in prevention of acute illness.

Enteritis

Enteritis, an inflammation of the stomach or small intestine, may be caused by bacteria, viruses, medications, ingestion of irritating foods, or some type of allergic response. Enteritis is also referred to as *gastroenteritis.*

Bacterial enteritis most often is caused by eating contaminated food *(food poisoning).* Common pathogens include *Staphylococcus aureus, Salmonella,* and *Clostridium botulinum.* Other infectious causes are parasites, such as amebiasis and trichinosis. Amoebae are found in tropical parts of the world where sanitation is poor. Trichinoses are transmitted through improperly cooked pork and game animals.

Acute enteritis occurs when a bacterium or virus invades the GI tract and produces a toxin that causes inflammation. Usually, there is increased fluid in the intestinal lumen, along with increased intestinal motility. The result is massive loss of fluid and electrolytes. Other symptoms include abdominal cramping, diarrhea, and vomiting.

Older adults are especially at risk for dehydration when they experience enteritis. Common electrolyte disturbances are hyponatremia and hypokalemia.

Nursing assessment with suspected enteritis includes:

▶ Recent foods eaten

▶ Symptoms

▶ Recent travel

▶ Recent use of antibiotics

▶ Any new routine medication

The most important nursing intervention is assessment and monitoring hydration status. In severe cases, the older patient must be hospitalized for intravenous hydration.

Constipation

Constipation is a diminished stool evacuation or difficulty in passing hard or dry feces. Constipation can be acute or chronic and may be constant or intermittent.

Common causes of constipation include:

▶ Low-fiber diet

▶ Medications

▶ Diabetes

▶ Thyroid disease

▶ Decreased motility or inflammation of bowel

▶ Mechanical obstruction (e.g., fecal impaction, tumor)

▶ Depression

▶ Functional issues (e.g., cannot reach the toilet, lack of privacy)

▶ Overuse or improper use of laxatives

Table 15–1 depicts common medications that can cause constipation.

TABLE 15–1.
COMMON MEDICATIONS THAT CAUSE CONSTIPATION

Aluminum-based antacids	Opioids
Calcium-based antacids	Antidepressants
Iron preparations	Anxiolytics
Anticholinergics	Antipsychotics
Calcium channel blockers	Barium sulfate

Adapted from *Constipation: Causes* by Mayo Clinic, 2011, retrieved from http://www.mayoclinic.com/health/constipation/ds00063/dsection=causes.

Diagnostic evaluation includes reviews of history and medications taken, and a rectal exam to rule out a mass. Labs are done to rule out metabolic causes. A colonoscopy is the screening test of choice. Assuming that no mechanical obstruction is detected, treatment is aimed at dietary and fluid management. Patients should be encouraged to increase fiber and fluids in the diet and to eat a diet low in fat. Behavioral modification includes light exercise, development of a regular toileting schedule, and responding to the urge to defecate.

Laxatives are used to treat constipation and are classified as bulking agents, surfactants, emollients, stimulants, saline cathartics, and osmotic agents. Table 15–2 includes the common agents used, based on category.

TABLE 15–2.
COMMON AGENTS USED TO TREAT CONSTIPATION

CATEGORY	COMMON AGENTS
Bulking agents	Bran, psyllium
Surfactants	Stool softeners (e.g., Surfak, Colace, docusate)
Emollients	Mineral oil
Saline cathartics	Milk of magnesia, magnesium citrate, sodium or potassium phosphate
Stimulants	Cascara, castor oil, Bisacodyl
Osmotic agents	Lactulose, Sorbitol, MiraLax

Adapted from *Geriatrics at Your Fingertips* (13th ed.), by D. Reuben, K. Herr, J. Pacala, B. Pollock, J. Potter, & T. Semla, 2011, New York: American Geriatrics Society.

Other agents that can be used but are not preferable include enemas and rectal suppositories.

Diarrhea

Diarrhea is an increase in the frequency of stools from increased bowel motility or from a problem with normal absorption of fluids and nutrients. The subjective data that nurses receive from patients are important in identifying the cause. Gerontological nurses should determine the cause by assessing:

▶ Onset

▶ Precipitating events (e.g., travel outside of the country, eating in a restaurant)

▶ Timing

▶ Other symptoms (e.g., fever, weight loss, abdominal pain, vomiting, foul smell, presence of mucous or blood, incontinence of stool)

▶ Recent dietary or medicine changes

▶ Recent antibiotic use

▶ Nocturnal diarrhea (suggests an organic cause)

Diarrhea can be classified as *acute* (< 2 weeks' duration) or *chronic* (> 4 weeks). Multiple causes exist, including diet, drugs, infections, endocrine disorders, neoplasia, impaction, and malabsorption syndromes. In frail older adults in long-term care (LTC), outbreaks of *E. coli* have a higher morbidity and mortality rate than outbreaks in younger adults.

Diagnostics may include evaluation for thyroid disease, diabetes, malabsorption such as sprue, and fecal impaction. Nursing care involves adequate nutrition and hydration. Suspect antibiotic-associated diarrhea or *Clostridium difficile* (C-diff) in older patients who have recent oral or parenteral antibiotic use or any of several antineoplastic agents, including cyclophosphamide, doxorubicin, fluorouracil, and methotrexate. Collect two separate stool stamples for C-diff toxin testing. Place patient in isolation and wash hands with soap and water to remove spores—hand sanitizers do not kill or remove spores. Treatment includes metronidazole 500 mg q 8h for 10 to 14 days. Vancomycin may be needed for severe cases and repeated occurrences (Reuben et al., 2011).

Depending on the cause, antidiarrheal agents (e.g., Imodium, Lomotil) may be used. Patient education regarding diet and fluid intake is needed: Advise patients to eat a bland diet, and to avoid gas-producing foods, vegetables, dairy, and spicy foods. It is safe to suggest clear liquids and the BRAT diet (bananas, rice, applesauce, and toast).

Fecal Impaction

Fecal impaction is a mass of hard feces in the lower rectum or colon that cannot be passed. Impactions usually occur because of unrelieved constipation. The typical presentation is abdominal fullness and oozing of liquid or soft stool. The patient may have anorexia because of the abdominal fullness.

Gerontological nurses should be suspicious of an impaction in the older patient who complains of diarrhea (rectal oozing) or constipation, especially if it is accompanied by a distended abdomen or complaints of abdominal fullness. Assessment should include checking for bowel sounds and taking a digital rectal exam (DRE). The rectal exam will reveal the hardened stool mass, which may or may not be amenable to manual removal. If removal is not possible, retention enemas or radiographic enemas may be necessary.

Prevention is of utmost importance. The nurse should educate the patient and caregivers about fluid intake and increasing fiber in the diet.

Fecal Incontinence

Fecal incontinence refers to the loss of control and inappropriate loss of stool. Fecal incontinence always requires evaluation. This problem impairs socialization and activities, causes embarrassment and anxiety, and may lead to institutionalization.

Fecal incontinence may be caused by:

▶ Colorectal lesions (e.g., perianal disease, proctitis, tumors)

▶ Neurological diseases

▶ Laxative abuse

▶ Fecal impaction

▶ Chronic diarrhea

▶ Chronic constipation (causing injured pudendal nerves)

▶ Stress

▶ Medications

▶ Decline in muscle tone related to aging

Diagnostics include physical exam to determine integrity of the neuromusculature, anal manometry, sigmoidoscopy, or anal ultrasound. Treatments include preventing constipation, biofeedback, adding fiber to the diet to provide bulk to the stool and prevent oozing, drug therapy in some cases (antidiarrheals), and surgical intervention.

Colon Polyps

Polyps are growths that protrude from a mucous membrane in the GI tract. Most commonly, polyps occur in the rectosigmoid area and are multiple. Polyps increase with patient age and vary by size, appearance, and etiology.

There are two appearances of polyps:

▶ *Sessile polyps:* Flat and broad; directly attached to intestinal mucosa

▶ *Pedunculated polyps:* Balloon-shaped; attached to the intestinal mucosa by a thin stem (Huether & McCance, 2012)

The most common type of polyp is nonmalignant—*hyperplastic*—and results from inflammation or abnormal growth of the mucosa. It has no malignant potential. The *adenomatous polyp,* or *adenoma,* comes from epithelial proliferation and dysplasia. This latter polyp is closely related to adenocarcinoma of the colon and rectum. Size is the main determining factor in malignancy, with larger polyps having more potential for malignancy (Stamm & Levy, 2006).

For the most part, polyps have no symptoms and often are discovered during screening procedures such as colonoscopy. Occasionally, they will produce bright-red blood in the feces.

Assessment should include any changes in the bowel elimination patterns and any symptoms of blood in the feces or on toilet paper. Nursing management involves education and reinforcement of the importance of colorectal cancer screening guidelines.

Hemorrhoids

Hemorrhoids are dilated veins in the mucous membranes inside or outside of the anus. They are related to varicose veins and can be thought of as varicose veins of the rectum. Predisposing factors include:

▶ Constipation

▶ Low-fiber diet

▶ Multiple pregnancies

▶ Liver disease

▶ Prolonged straining

▶ Irregular bowel habits

▶ Increased intra-abdominal pressure (Huether & McCance, 2012)

Internal hemorrhoids may cause bleeding with defecation. Dilated veins protrude into the anal and rectal canals where they become exposed. This exposure can cause pain, thrombus, ulcers, and frank red bleeding.

External hemorrhoids can cause pain as well as itching and irritation. Sometimes a palpable mass may be seen or felt. Bleeding can occur if the external hemorrhoid is injured or ulcerated (Reuben et al., 2011).

Assessment includes checking for or asking about constipation, pain, or bleeding. A physical exam may be normal except for a painful rectal area. If the hemorrhoid is prolapsed, it should be checked for swelling, thrombosis, and ischemia.

Stools that are positive for fecal occult blood (FOB) are common in patients with hemorrhoids. Nursing management includes education about a high-fiber, high-roughage diet that includes whole grains, legumes, fresh fruits, and vegetables. Adequate fluids, light exercise, and a regular toileting regimen also are important.

Over-the-counter (OTC) topical remedies such as Anusol or Tucks pads may help reduce symptoms. Sitz baths also can be used. Patients should be instructed to avoid constipation and straining with defecation, because both can make hemorrhoids worse (Reuben et al., 2011). Hemorrhoids may be treated by rubber band ligation and surgical removal of the hemorrhoids (hemorrhoidectomy).

Bowel Obstruction

A *bowel obstruction* occurs when there is complete or partial blockage of the small or large intestine. Obstruction can occur via a mechanical or nonmechanical mechanism. *Mechanical bowel obstructions* are the most common and can be caused by tumor, adhesions, hernia, or volvulus. A *volvulus* is caused by part of the intestine twisting up on itself; although an uncommon cause of obstruction, when it does occur, it is more common in older adults because of weakening of the mesenteric ligaments (McPhee & Papadakis, 2011).

Nonmechanical bowel obstructions occur from decreased or absent peristalsis. The most common causes are neurological or vascular compromise. A paralytic ileus is an example of a neurological obstruction and can occur in either the small or large bowel. The process occurs when peristalsis decreases or stops because of a noxious stimulus, such as anesthesia, peritoneal injury, interruption of circulation, surgical manipulation, abdominal injury, or electrolyte imbalances. Paralytic ileus is a common postoperative problem (McPhee & Papadakis, 2011).

Regardless of the cause, in obstruction, the bowel becomes distended by gas and air above the level of the obstruction. If left unchecked, gastric, biliary, and pancreatic solutions, along with water, electrolytes, and proteins, accumulate in and around the area, leading to increased intraluminal pressure and possible bowel perforation.

Symptoms include acute abdominal pain with a cramping sensation. With mesenteric ischemia, the presenting symptoms often are mild and nonspecific, especially in older adults. Other symptoms include:

▶ Abdominal distention

▶ Hyperactive bowel sounds above the obstruction but no bowel sounds below the obstruction

▶ Borborygmi (loud, high-pitched sounds caused by the rate and force of peristalsis above the blockage as the body tries to clear the obstruction)

▶ Vomiting

▶ Diarrhea (if the obstruction is incomplete, watery contents can pass around it)

A bowel obstruction is a medical emergency. Complications can be severe: perforated bowel, peritonitis, hypovolemic shock, or septic shock. Gerontological nurses should assess the onset, type, and frequency of vomiting and the exact location and severity of pain. The physical exam should assess bowel sounds (present or absent), abdominal distention, vital signs, and urinary output (McPhee & Papadakis, 2011).

Nursing management of bowel obstruction in older adults focuses on hydration and comfort. Intravenous fluids and electrolytes should be given as ordered. Nurses should monitor intake and output, urine-specific gravity, and signs of volume overload or dehydration. In many cases, surgery is necessary to rectify the obstruction.

Carcinoma

Cancers of the GI tract account for 25% of cancer deaths in the United States. This section reviews three GI carcinomas: esophageal, gastric, and colorectal (American Cancer Society, 2012).

Esophageal cancers were diagnosed in approximately 17,460 people (13,950 in men and 3,510 in women) in the United States in 2011 and resulted in about 15,070 deaths (12,040 in men and 3,030 in women; American Cancer Society, 2012). The symptoms usually are vague and nonspecific. As a result, most esophageal cancers are not diagnosed until they are well advanced. Risk factors include cigarette smoking, heavy alcohol intake, and GERD (specifically, Barrett's esophagus). Most tumors are in the middle and lower one-third of the esophagus; the usual cell type is squamous.

Classically, patients present with progressive dysphagia and weight loss. Unfortunately, individuals with esophageal cancer have the worst prognosis of all of the GI malignancies.

Gastric cancer develops slowly and often is not diagnosed until late in the course of illness. Gastric cancers are usually adenocarcinomas that occur as polypoid, ulcerative, or infiltrative disease. The ulcerative form is most common and produces symptoms much like that of peptic ulcers. The tumor is usually in the antrum (the lower one-third of the stomach) and causes ulceration, obstruction, and bleeding. Symptoms usually present after the disease is advanced, and include weight loss, pain, vomiting, anorexia, dysphagia, and an abdominal mass (American Cancer Society, 2012). The prognosis is poor.

Colorectal cancer is the most common GI malignancy and is the third most common cause of death from cancer in both genders. Age is a risk factor, as is a low-fiber, high-fat, and high-carbohydrate diet. Most tumors are adenocarcinoma cell types. Signs and symptoms depend on the location of the tumor. Cancers in the sigmoid and descending colon cause obstruction; therefore, patients with this disease present with change in bowel habits.

If the tumor is in the right lower colon, the symptoms are minimal, as the stool is still liquid in this area of the colon. If present, the symptom is mild abdominal cramps. Anemia may be present.

Left-side lesions can cause melena, diarrhea, constipation, and a feeling of incomplete evacuation. Right-side lesions may cause malaise, weakness, and weight loss (American Cancer Society, 2012). In either scenario, the stools are positive for FOB. Colorectal cancer metastasizes to the liver and lymphatics. Prognosis depends on the stage of the tumor at the time of diagnosis.

Nursing management for GI malignancies depends on stage and type of tumor. For the most part, gerontological nurses should monitor patients for weight loss and malnutrition. Small, frequent meals that are high in protein and calories are most helpful. Use of supplements, such as Ensure or Boost, may be in order. In some cases, tube feedings may be needed to maintain adequate nutrition for adequate treatment and healing.

HEPATOBILIARY DISEASES

The *hepatobiliary system* consists of the accessory organs of digestion and absorption: the gallbladder, pancreas, liver, and biliary tree (bile ducts). Common illnesses of these organs are cholelithiasis and cholecystitis, pancreatitis, hepatitis, cirrhosis of the liver, and carcinoma.

Cholelithiasis and Cholecystitis

The gallbladder is the storage organ for bile, which is important in the digestion of proteins and other nutrients. When gallstones form in the gallbladder, patients are said to have *cholelithiasis*. The majority of gallstones are made of cholesterol, usually from an increased saturation of cholesterol (e.g., from obesity, use of estrogen, previous surgery on the ileum, increased serum cholesterol). This increased level may be accompanied by an increased bilirubin from processes such as hemolysis. These two processes, along with decreased emptying of the gallbladder, cause collection of cholesterol crystals in the gland that eventually form gallstones (McPhee & Papadakis, 2011).

In many individuals, gallstones are asymptomatic. Risk factors include obesity, female gender, multiple pregnancies (increased levels of estrogens), sedentary lifestyles, use of oral contraceptive pills, and advancing age.

Symptoms usually begin soon after a large, high-fat meal. Patients may have right-upper-quadrant abdominal pain that radiates up to the scapula. The pain may last several minutes to several hours.

Gallstones cause symptoms because they obstruct the common bile duct (CBD) or cystic (most common) duct. The obstruction causes pressure and distention of the gallbladder. When the CBD is obstructed, bile cannot get into the duodenum; as a result, a patient will become jaundiced and have clay-colored stools. In addition, obstruction of the CBD can cause biliary pain (colic), pancreatitis, and or cholangitis (inflammation of the biliary tree itself.)

Cholecystitis, inflammation of the gallbladder from stones, can be acute or chronic. Cholecystitis can occur for other reasons, such as obstruction from tumor or stricture, but gallstones are the most common etiology. Chronic cholecystitis usually occurs from many mild attacks of inflammation that cause thickening of the wall of the organ and ineffective emptying.

Nursing assessment of patients with gallbladder disease begins with a symptom analysis of the pain. Nurses should assess the location, quality, and duration of the pain. Other symptoms, such as nausea and vomiting, should be documented. Precipitating factors, such as a large meal, and relieving factors also should be determined. The physical exam should focus on the abdomen, and may reveal tenderness in the right upper quadrant with or without jaundiced skin.

Nursing management includes providing pain relief and educating patients about the disease process. Patients should be given information about avoiding high-fat meals. Clear-liquid diets may be in order until symptoms abate. Treatment options include surgery, medical therapy to dissolve the stones, and lithotripsy.

Pancreatitis

Pancreatitis is inflammation of the organ and can occur in acute and chronic forms. Most commonly, *acute disease* is related to alcohol or biliary tract disease (e.g., stone, stricture, tumor). Activation of the pancreatic enzymes autodigests the organ. After the acute event, the pancreatic function returns to normal. Many times, acute pancreatitis is fatal.

Chronic disease usually results from alcoholism. The etiology is not well understood, and the organ does not return to a normal functioning state. The normal tissue is eventually replaced with scarred, fibrosed tissue.

Symptoms of pancreatitis include severe epigastric pain and pain in the right upper quadrant of the abdomen; nausea, vomiting, and fever are common. Patients with chronic disease may be weak, anorectic, and jaundiced. Steatorrhea (bulky, foul, fatty stools) are common later in the disease.

Assessment includes obtaining a history of alcohol use or gallstone disease. Symptoms of the abdominal pain should be documented. Nursing management centers on pain relief, maintenance of fluid and electrolyte status, and prevention of complications. Prevention of recurrence is a priority. If the disease is related to alcohol use, appropriate referrals should be made for counseling and alcohol cessation treatment. Teaching centers on the effects of alcohol and, in patients with biliary tract disease, dietary counseling is in order to reduce the lipid levels. Persons with fasting triglyceride levels of greater than 400 mg/dL are at increased risk of acute pancreatitis.

Hepatitis

Hepatitis is a global term that means inflammation of the liver. Most commonly, healthcare providers think of viral hepatitis when they hear this term. The most common etiologies are viruses, drugs, and alcohol.

The liver of an older adult is more susceptible to drugs and other toxins; in addition, older adults have a diminished ability to compensate physiologically when infection occurs.

Six documented viral agents can cause hepatitis. The most common versions of the disease in the United States are hepatitis A, B, and C. Table 15–3 shows the properties of the viruses. Once the virus has entered a person's circulation, it seeks out the liver tissue and then enters the hepatocyte and uses the host's own DNA to reproduce itself.

TABLE 15–3.
SPECIFIC PROPERTIES OF VIRAL HEPATITIS

	HEPATITIS A	HEPATITIS B	HEPATITIS C
Viral properties	RNA virus	DNA virus	Small RNA virus
Mode of transmission	Fecal–oral route; usually from contaminated food or water	Blood and body fluids	Blood and body fluids
Clinical course	Mild disease with short duration	More severe; increased risk for cirrhosis and hepatocellular carcinoma	Mild disease (in terms of symptoms); increased risk of hepatocellular carcinoma
Chronic state	No	Yes; 5%–10% incidence	Yes; more than 50% incidence

Adapted from "Gatrointestinal Function," by L. A. Stamm & R. A. Levy, 2006, in *Gerontological Nursing,* edited by S. E. Meiner & A. G. Lueckenotte, pp. 561–595, St. Louis, MO: Mosby/Elsevier.

Whenever a person contacts hepatitis, the disease progresses through three phases (assuming a normal immune response): the prodromal phase, the icteric phase, and the convalescent phase. Table 15–4 reviews the manifestations of each phase.

TABLE 15–4.
MANIFESTATIONS OF THE STAGES OF HEPATITIS

PRODROMAL STAGE	ICTERIC STAGE	CONVALESCENT STAGE
▸ Malaise, fatigue, nausea, vomiting, anorexia, and low-grade fever ▸ Right-upper-quadrant pain ▸ Person believes he or she has the flu, or symptoms are so mild that they are not noticed	▸ Jaundice (in some cases, this does not occur) ▸ Dark urine ▸ Pruritus ▸ Clay-colored stools	▸ Jaundice and other symptoms begin to disappear ▸ Patient feels fully recovered

Adapted from "Gatrointestinal Function," by L. A. Stamm & R. A. Levy, 2006, in *Gerontological Nursing,* edited by S. E. Meiner & A. G. Lueckenotte, pp. 561–595, St. Louis, MO: Mosby/Elsevier.

Assessment of patients with hepatitis should begin with questions related to possible exposure. Nurses should inquire about recent travel, blood transfusions, and food intake. Physical assessment should include skin color and abdomen tenderness or organomegaly. Patients should be questioned about changes in energy level, appetite, and weight.

Nursing management includes education about the type and course of illness of hepatitis. Patients should be made aware that complete resolution for normal liver function takes 3 to 6 months. Nurses should stress the ways to prevent spread of the virus, including hygienic practices. Other important teaching points include:

▶ Rest is an important part of recovery.

▶ A high-calorie, low-fat diet is ideal.

▶ Fluid intake should be increased.

▶ Jaundice will gradually abate, and the urine and stools will return to normal color as the jaundice fades.

▶ If itching is severe, OTC lotions (Sarna, Aveeno) and tepid baths may be helpful; these symptoms will resolve once the jaundice has cleared.

Hepatitis is also caused by the effects of drugs. The liver plays a major role in metabolism and detoxification of drugs. Tylenol (acetaminophen) is an example of a drug that causes direct toxicity to liver cells in doses above 4,000 mg in 24 hours for the healthy older adult, and 3,000 mg in 24 hours for the frail older adult, or those who drink three or more alcoholic drinks every day (Tylenol, 2012). Current recommendations for acetaminophen dosing are < 3,000 gm/24 hours in the healthy older adult and < 2,000 gm/24 hours in the frail older adult or those who drink three alcoholic drinks daily. This toxicity is reproducible, which means that the same reaction will occur in every person who exceeds this maximum level of the drug every time the excess ingestion occurs.

Many chemical products used in industry can injure the liver by exposure or ingestion. Carbon tetrachloride and chloroform are examples of this mechanism. In this scenario, normal metabolic pathways cannot clear the drug, so alternative avenues are found to clear the agents. These alternative mechanisms produce toxic byproducts (Health Protection Agency, 2009).

A third way that drugs and chemicals can cause liver damage is an unpredictable response, almost as if a person has a certain "sensitivity" to a drug; it is not related to dose and occurs rarely and in a random fashion—an idiosyncratic response. This type of drug-induced liver damage can result in massive hepatocyte damage. Agents that can cause damage by means of this mechanism include:

▶ Isoniazid (INH)

▶ Halothane

▶ Methyldopa

▶ Poisonous mushrooms

Other mechanisms of injury that can be seen in idiosyncratic response are cholestasis (disruption of the normal bile flow out of the bile ducts), oral contraceptive pills, and anabolic steroids (Stamm & Levy, 2006). A fatty liver also can result from idiosyncratic responses to drugs or chemicals (Kumar, 2009).

The clinical presentation of drug-induced liver disease is similar to that of viral hepatitis. The onset of symptoms may be immediate or may occur weeks or even months after the exposure. In some cases, the presentation is abrupt, with a short clinical course. This scenario is called *fulminant hepatitis*, and patients succumb to the event unless liver transplantation occurs.

Assessment involves obtaining information about the ingested substance, how much was taken, and when the ingestion occurred. Nurses must monitor patients for symptoms of liver failure. Physical assessment involves that of the liver, skin, sclera, and neurological status. Nursing management will be similar to what is done for patients with cirrhosis of the liver (see below).

Cirrhosis of the Liver

Cirrhosis means permanent, irreversible damage to the liver tissues. Normal liver tissue is replaced with scarlike tissue that does not have the same working ability as normal liver tissue. In the United States, the two most common causes of cirrhosis of the liver are *nonalcoholic steatohepatitis* (NASH; fatty liver from an obese state) and *alcoholic hepatitis* (liver damage from alcohol use). Alcoholic cirrhosis is sometimes referred to as *Laennec's cirrhosis.*

As the liver tissues are damaged, patients begin to show signs and symptoms of liver failure, including weakness, fatigue, disturbed sleep, muscle cramps, and weight loss (McPhee & Papadakis, 2011).

As the disease progresses, patients can have bleeding, ascites, portal HTN, and encephalopathy. Bleeding occurs because of a lack of clotting factors. The liver plays a pivotal role in producing clotting factors V, VII, IX, and X, as well as fibrinogen and prothrombin. A diseased liver does not make these factors in normal amounts and, in severe disease, produces only minimal amounts of these agents.

Ascites occurs because serous fluid collects in the abdomen. The accumulation occurs as a result of insufficient amounts of albumin (major plasma protein). When protein is lacking, plasma fluid escapes into the abdominal cavity. Increased venous pressure, which also is a manifestation of liver disease, forces serous fluids out of the vessels into the abdomen and its periphery.

Portal hypertension (HTN) is an increased pressure in the portal vein and its collateral vessels because of congestion in the liver. Portal HTN essentially causes blood to "back up" into areas such as the hemorrhoidal vessels, spleen, and small vessels that line the esophagus. Upper gastrointestinal tract bleeding may occur from varices or gastroduodenal ulcers (McPhee & Papadakis, 2011).

Encephalopathy is a manifestation of the diseased liver's inefficient detoxification of waste products and toxins. One end-product of protein metabolism is ammonia. Patients with rising blood ammonia levels will have mental status changes such as agitation, combativeness, and confusion. Patients with encephalopathy also can have muscle tremors, or asterixis.

Assessment begins with obtaining information about onset and duration of signs and symptoms. Patients should be asked about color of stools, any rectal bleeding, or bleeding in emesis. The physical examination should include all systems and pay particular attention to nutritional status. Diagnostics might include ultrasound, liver biopsy, and serum liver enzymes. Serum cholesterol levels will be decreased in patients with liver disease. These patients are susceptible to osteoporosis and osteomalacia, secondary to malabsorption of electrolytes such as calcium and vitamin D. The liver plays a role in absorption of these products; without adequate calcium and vitamin D, patients can develop the aforementioned disease states.

Nursing management focuses on preventing complications; skin care is a priority. Patients should be encouraged to reposition frequently. Many are most comfortable in the Semi-Fowler's position, because this position maximizes chest expansion and helps maintain oxygenation. The number of venipunctures should be limited, to minimize the bleeding risk.

Patients' psychomotor function should be carefully assessed, and nurses should reorient patients as indicated. Mouth care and small bland feedings are most often indicated. Dietary proteins should be severely restricted. Nurses also should encourage patients to discuss their feelings and reinforce their positive traits and abilities.

In older adults, end-stage liver disease is a chronic illness that often can be managed well for years. Gerontological nurses have an enormous role in educating patients about the illness and the medications and dietary alterations that will be necessary to control the symptoms and progression of the disease.

Carcinoma

Malignancies of the hepatobiliary system are not common; when they do occur, the presentation often is vague and nonspecific. As a result, these cancers often are not diagnosed until late into the course of illness.

Pancreatic cancer affects individuals ages 60 to 70, with men being more commonly affected. The American Cancer Society's most recent estimates for pancreatic cancer in the United States in 2012 are:

▶ About 43,920 people (22,090 men and 21,830 women) will be diagnosed with pancreatic cancer.

▶ About 37,390 people (18,850 men and 18,540 women) will die of pancreatic cancer.

Since 2004, rates of pancreatic cancer have increased about 1.5% per year. The lifetime risk of developing pancreatic cancer is about 1 in 71 (1.41%; American Cancer Society, 2012).

The illness is linked to alcohol abuse, high-fat diets, tobacco use, and chronic pancreatitis. The tumor itself is usually adenocarcinoma and affects the head of the pancreas in 70% of cases. As the tumor grows, it presses on the common bile duct, which results in jaundice. If the tumor encroaches on the celiac plexus (which is common if the tumor is in the tail of the organ), patients will experience a deep, boring-in, unrelenting pain in the abdomen. This cancer grows rapidly; 90% of cases have metastasized by the time of diagnosis.

This tumor presents with vague symptoms that are insidious in onset: anorexia, weight loss, nausea, and pain. Jaundice occurs late in the illness. Fewer than 20% of affected individuals are living at 1 year after diagnosis.

Cholangiocarcinoma is a rare malignancy of the bile ducts, often occurring in older patients who have previously been diagnosed with ulcerative colitis. This malignancy, if detected early enough, is treated with radiation, chemotherapy, and liver resection to remove the tumor. New protocols under development combine chemotherapy and radiation with liver transplantation, improving the chance of removing the entire source of cancer during surgery. The chemotherapy and radiation treat and sterilize the tumor bed, but using these options alone may eventually cause liver failure and may result in the need for liver transplantation (Emery Healthcare, 2012).

Hepatocellular carcinoma, another rare biliary tract malignancy, is usually thought to be related to chronic hepatitis B or C (the most common risk factor) and can occur sporadically. Patients can present with symptoms suggestive of hepatitis or may have a mass in the right upper quadrant of the abdomen. Treatment is resection or organ transplantation if the tumor affects more than one lobe of the liver.

Metastatic liver disease, much more common than hepatocarcinoma, is a site of metastasis from lung, breast, kidney, and other GI cancers. This disease usually indicates a terminal prognosis. Nursing management of these older patients is the same as for those with cirrhosis of the liver.

REFERENCES

American Cancer Society. (2012). *Learn about cancer.* Retrieved from http://www.cancer.org/Cancer/index

Bayless, T., & Hanauer, S. (2011). *Advanced therapy of inflammatory bowel disease.* Shelton, CT: People's Medical Publishing House: USA.

Cleveland Clinic. (2009). Patient information—What you need to know about your warfarin therapy. *Cleveland Clinic Journal of Medicine, 70,* 372–373. Available from http://my.clevelandclinic.org/drugs/coumadin/hic_understanding_coumadin.aspx

Emery Healthcare. (2012). *Liver transplant Cholangiocarcinoma treatment.* Retrieved from http://www.emoryhealthcare.org/medicaladvances/transplant/cholangiocarcinoma-bile-duct-cancer.html

Health Protection Agency. (2009). *Carbon tetrachloride: toxicology review.* Retrieved from http://www.hpa.org.uk/webc/HPAwebFile/HPAweb_C/1235032869649

Huether, S., & McCance, K. (2012). *Understanding pathophysiology* (5th ed.). St. Louis, MO: Mosby.

Kumar, V. (2009). *Robbins and Cotran pathologic basis of disease.* Philadelphia: Saunders.

Mayo Clinic. (2011). *Constipation: Causes.* Retrieved from http://www.mayoclinic.com/health/constipation/ds00063/dsection=causes

McPhee, S., & Papadakis, M. (2011). *Current medical diagnosis and treatment* (50th ed.). New York: McGraw Hill Medical.

Meiner, S. E. (2001). Gastrointestinal problems. In A. S. Luggen & S. E. Meiner (Eds.), *NGNA Core curriculum for gerontological nursing* (pp. 73–161). St. Louis, MO: Mosby.

Nurse practitioners' prescribing reference. (2012). New York: Haymarket Media Publication.

Reuben, D., Herr, K., Pacala, J., Pollock, B., Potter, J., & Semla, T. (2011). *Geriatrics at your fingertips* (13th ed.). New York: American Geriatrics Society.

Stamm, L. A., & Levy, R. A. (2006). Gastrointestinal function. In S. E. Meiner & A. G. Lueckenotte (Eds.), *Gerontological nursing* (pp. 561–595). St. Louis, MO: Mosby/Elsevier.

Tylenol. (2012). *Acetaminophen and the liver: Get relief responsibly.* Retrieved from http://www.tylenol.com/getreliefresponsibly/index.jhtml?id=tylenol/getreliefresponsibly/aceta_liver.inc

ADDITIONAL RESOURCES

Chronic and Disabling Conditions: www.agingsociety.org/

Healthy People 2020: www.healthypeople.gov/2020/

National Institute of Diabetes and Digestive and Kidney Diseases – National Institutes of Health: http://www2.niddk.nih.gov/

URINARY AND REPRODUCTIVE DISEASES

Urinary and reproductive diseases common among older adults include benign prostatic hypertrophy, prostate cancer, bladder cancer, urinary incontinence, urinary tract infections, sexual dysfunction, and postmenopausal conditions.

Benign Prostatic Hypertrophy

Benign prostatic hypertrophy (BPH) is age-related enlargement of the prostate gland that constricts the urethra and prevents the outflow of urine. This enlargement can lead to bladder outlet obstruction, urinary retention, and a distended bladder. Early in the disease, patients may be asymptomatic; however, as the gland enlarges, patients will begin to have hesitancy in urinating, decrease in the force of the urine stream, dribbling, and the sensation of incomplete bladder emptying. In severe cases, urinary tract infections (UTIs) and hydronephrosis may occur.

Diagnostics may include urinalysis, digital rectal exam (DRE), abdominal ultrasound, and serum prostate-specific antigen (PSA) to rule out malignancy. Assessment should include medical and surgical history, current medications, and voiding habits and patterns. The physical examination usually focuses on assessment for bladder distention, suprapubic tenderness, and costovertebral angle tenderness.

Nursing management includes education about the disease process and, if the patient opts for medical therapy, the importance of a voiding schedule. Patients should be educated about the actions of alpha blockers, such as Flomax, Hytrin, and Cardura, which are used to reduce symptoms of BPH. Patients also need information about medications that can make the symptoms worse, such as decongestants (e.g., Sudafed) and anticholinergics (e.g., Benadryl, Tylenol PM). Many individuals will be treated with surgical intervention, such as ablative transurethral techniques, intraprostatic stents, or transurethral prostatectomy.

Prostate Cancer

Prostate cancer is the most common cancer in older American men. Prognosis is usually quite favorable—more than 2 million men in the United States are prostate cancer survivors. It is estimated that there will be more than 241,000 new cases diagnosed in 2012, with 28,170 deaths (American Cancer Society, 2012).

The cause of prostate cancer is unknown; most tumors are adenocarcinomas. If the tumor metastasizes, the bones and pelvic lymph nodes are the most common sites. Many men are asymptomatic. As the gland enlarges, patients will experience obstructive urinary symptoms. Bone pain and pathological fractures are indications of metastatic disease. Diagnostics may include screening with a DRE and prostate-specific antigen (PSA). A prostate biopsy is done for the definitive diagnosis. Several treatment options are available: watchful waiting, radical prostatectomy, cryosurgery, high-intensity focused ultrasound, radiation, or hormonal therapy (Reuben et al., 2011).

Assessment is the same as for the men with BPH. Nursing management includes education on diagnostics and treatment options. Referral for sexual counseling may be needed. Education on the importance of follow-up with a urologist or primary care provider to follow the PSA level is paramount.

Bladder Cancer

Bladder cancer, the most common genitourinary tract malignancy, occurs almost exclusively in older adults age 50 to 70, with a predominance in men. Most early stage bladder cancers are resectable; however, in a few cases, the tumor metastasizes to the bladder wall, liver, lungs, or bone (WebMD, 2012).

Most bladder cancers are sporadic; however, 20% of them occur in individuals with exposure to industrial dyes, rubber, chemicals, benzene, and paint. Cigarette smoking is thought to be a risk factor. Signs and symptoms include painless hematuria, dysuria, urgency, and frequency.

Assessment should include a review of patient urinary patterns. Nursing management centers on patient education, psychosocial support, and pain control. Cystectomy and urinary diversion may be needed to resect the tumor. In those instances, patient education becomes even more important.

Nurses will need to educate patients treated with Bacillus Calmette-Guerin (BCG) about the actions and precautions related to this chemotherapeutic agent. Follow-up cystoscopy is required for several years after successful cancer treatment.

Urinary Incontinence

Urinary incontinence (UI) is not a normal change of aging, but results from the cumulative effects of comorbid conditions and medications, functional impairment, age-related changes, and genitourinary pathology. UI affects more than 30% of older adults who live in the community, with rates being higher in women (Agency for Healthcare Research and Quality, 2012). UI is frequently a major reason for admission to a nursing home.

UI can be either acute or chronic. In *acute incontinence,* patients suddenly develop the symptoms as the result of some other medical or surgical condition. Medications can be the culprit. According to Reuben and colleagues (2011), any new-onset UI should be considered acute in nature; determining the cause will allow symptoms to be treated and, most often, cured. Causes can include:

► UTIs

► Immobility

► Fecal impaction

► Delirium

► Diabetes mellitus that is uncontrolled

► Alcohol use in excess

► Medications (e.g., anticholinergics, alpha-blockers, calcium channel blockers, diuretics, psychotropics, benzodiazepines, opioids)

Chronic incontinence is persistent over time and often becomes worse with time. Chronic incontinence can present in five ways: stress incontinence, urge incontinence, overflow incontinence, functional incontinence, and mixed incontinence.

Stress incontinence (SI), the loss of urine because of a sudden increase in intra-abdominal pressure, occurs because the pressure within the bladder exceeds the urethral resistance to the force (in the absence of bladder contraction). These symptoms occur because of loss of normal support for the bladder neck or proximal urethra, or because the proximal urethra muscle is no longer functioning properly (McPhee & Papadakis, 2011). These problems can occur because of multiple pregnancies, vaginal deliveries, trauma during a surgical procedure, obesity, or chronic coughing.

Individuals with SI leak urine when exerting themselves, with, for example, exercise, lifting, coughing, sneezing, or laughing. Usually a small to moderate amount of urine is lost. This type of incontinence is uncommon in men, except when they have had a surgery or procedure that could have injured the urethral sphincter, such as prostate surgery or radiation.

Urge incontinence (UI) is usually associated with abnormal bladder contractions and is sometimes referred to as *overactive bladder.* Common causes include cystitis, urethritis, tumors, stones, bladder diverticula, and central nervous system disorders such as stroke, dementia, or Parkinson's disease.

UI usually presents with a sudden urge to void; before individuals can get to the bathroom, they experience a moderate to large amount of incontinence. This scenario can be precipitated by the sound of running water, exposure to cold weather, or the sight of a toilet (Reuben et al., 2011). According to the Agency for Health Care Policy and Research (AHCPR; 2012), UI can be classified into four types: detrusor hyperreflexia, detrusor instability, detrusor sphincter dyssynergia, and detrusor hyperactivity with impaired bladder contractility (see Table 16–1).

TABLE 16-1.
TYPES OF URGE INCONTINENCE

TYPE	MANIFESTATIONS	CAUSE
Detrusor hyperreflexia	Uninhibited bladder contractions	Neurological problem such as a stroke
Detrusor instability	Uninhibited bladder contractions	No underlying neurological problem
Detrusor sphincter dyssynergia	Uninhibited bladder contractions accompanied by contraction of the external sphincter; this problem can cause urinary retention	Suprasacral spinal cord lesions Multiple sclerosis
Detrusor hyperactivity with impaired bladder contractility	Uninhibited bladder contractions accompanied by impaired contractility with normal voiding; patient must strain to fully or partially empty the bladder	Seen in frail older adults

Adapted from *Management of Urinary Incontinence in Adults*, by the Agency for Health Care Policy and Research, 2012, http://qualitymeasures.ahrq.gov/content.aspx?id=32402.

In *overflow incontinence* (OI), a chronically full bladder obtains a high-enough pressure to voluntarily empty itself. This type of incontinence is not common and is seen in those with atonic bladders (diabetics) and those taking anticholinergic medications; with spinal cord injuries; or with an obstruction to emptying the bladder, such as enlarged prostate or uterine prolapse (AHCPR, 2012). OI also can be seen in persons with multiple sclerosis who have loss of function in the detrusor sphincter.

Individuals with OI usually complain of frequent loss of small amounts of urine; they have accidents during waking and sleeping hours. They also may complain of the feeling of incomplete emptying, frequency, and hesitancy.

Functional incontinence (FI) is the involuntary loss of urine that occurs because of inability or unwillingness to get to a toilet. Patients with physical problems may not be able to ambulate to the bathroom in a timely fashion. Patients with cognitive issues may not recognize that they need to urinate, while those with severe depression may not be motivated to get up and use the toilet by themselves. An older adult who is confined to a chair or bed is dependent on a caregiver to assist with voiding; if that help is not readily available, the person may be incontinent.

Mixed incontinence (MI) is a combination of two or more types of incontinence. A combination of UI and SI is most common. In older adults with severe dementia, a combination of UI and FI is most common.

Assessment should focus on identifying the type of incontinence that a patient is experiencing. The nursing history should include patient incontinence symptoms, and bladder and bowel habits; general health and functional status; current medications; and past medical, surgical, and obstetrical history. Nurses should specifically inquire about diabetes, HF, bladder and kidney infections, stroke, Parkinson's disease, memory loss, mobility problems, and neurological problems, because all of these can affect bladder functioning. To assess BPH symptoms, men should be questioned about frequency of urination, nocturia, quality of the stream, and hesitancy.

A brief functional assessment should be done. Nurses should ask about the ability of patients to perform their activities of daily living (ADLs), such as bathing, dressing, and grooming. Environmental barriers that could interfere with patients' ability to get to the bathroom should be identified. Psychological information should be gathered, focusing on the effects of the incontinence on the patient's lifestyle and caregiver assistance, if applicable.

The physical examination should include gait and balance, a neurological exam, and assessment of abdomen, rectum, and pelvis. The patient should be asked to keep a bladder diary that addresses frequency of urination, incontinent episodes, volume of incontinence, and any associated symptoms.

Diagnostics may include urine analysis or urodynamic studies to assess the detrusor muscle competency.

For all types of incontinence, the nursing management involves determining patient and caregiver motivation and willingness to participate in the self-care practices that will be required to reduce (or eliminate) the incontinence. After that is determined, management centers on behavioral therapies. For patients who are cognitively intact, interventions include bladder retraining, pelvic-floor muscle exercises, and biofeedback.

In *bladder retraining,* patients initiate an expanding voiding schedule. A specific schedule is set for voiding; patients are asked not to void except as delineated in the schedule (avoid voiding based on urge). This procedure is helpful in urge and frequency problems.

Pelvic-floor muscle exercises, first described by Dr. Arnold Kegel in 1948, involve alternating contractions and relaxations of the levator ani and the pubococcygeal muscles. These muscles in women are those of the pelvic floor and those that surround the mid-part of the urethra, respectively (Reuben et al., 2011). These exercises strengthen the pelvic floor, increase urethral resistance, and help older women avoid accidents.

Most older women need help to learn these exercises. Patients must practice the exercises at home; they should be encouraged to do the exercises in 8 to 12 contractions for 3 or 4 sessions per day. Patients can be taught to contract the pelvic muscles before activities that cause urine loss. Those with UI can be taught to take a few deep breaths and relax, then contract the pelvic floor muscles to abort a bladder contraction (Mayo Clinic, 2012). Pelvic-floor electrical stimulation and biofeedback can be used to help male patients post-prostatectomy.

For older patients with cognitive impairments, scheduled toileting, habit training, and prompted voiding can be used. *Scheduled toileting* means that patients are taken to the bathroom on a preset schedule. With *habit training,* a patient's normal voiding patterns are identified, and the patient is then assisted in the act of voiding at specific times. *Prompted voiding* is best used in patients who still understand what the urge to void is. The goal is to help patients understand this urge and to increase their ability to use the toilet themselves with a verbal cue.

Other nursing interventions include educating patients about the effects of caffeine (increases abnormal bladder contractions) and the importance of restricting large amounts of fluids late in the day. Patients should be encouraged to drink most of their daily fluid intakes before dinner. For patients with peripheral edema, spending several hours late in the day with the legs elevated will decrease the amount of edema at bedtime and, thus, reduce the amount of nocturia that the patient experiences. Patients should be encouraged to prevent constipation, because this problem sometimes makes UI worse.

Incontinence pads may be needed to provide convenience and comfort. Men may be able to use external collection devices for their urinary symptoms.

Persons with OI should be referred to a urologist. If the problem is not correctable, these patients can use the Credé maneuver to help empty the bladder; in this maneuver, patients gently apply pressure to the suprapubic area while voiding. If this is ineffective, patients may need intermittent in-and-out catheterization. The nursing role in patient education is critical here.

Other types of incontinence may be amenable to use of a pessary (for patients with a prolapsed uterus or bladder) or to surgery.

Urinary Tract Infections

Urinary tract infections (UTIs) and asymptomatic bacteriuria are common in older adults. Risk factors, which are more relevant in patients in institutions, include:

▶ Indwelling urinary catheter

▶ Cognitive impairment

▶ Bladder catheterization

▶ Functional incapacity

▶ Antibiotic use

Common pathogens include *E. coli, Proteus, Klebsiella, Enterobacter, Serratia,* and *Pseudomonas* strains. Clinical presentation is usually complaints of dysuria or frequency with or without hematuria. A patient with a UTI in the upper part of the genitourinary tract may have fever, chills, flank pain, and mental status changes. Gerontological nurses should remember that older patients often present atypically when they have infections and may present with atypical symptoms such as anorexia, falls, and altered mental status.

Diagnostics include urine analysis and cultures. Assessment begins with noting patients' normal voiding patterns and how they have changed. Characteristics of the urine should be determined. A mental status exam may be needed for patients who have had changes in their levels of consciousness.

Treatment involves hydration and antibiotics. Nursing management should include education on hygiene measures to prevent recurrence: wiping from front to back, going to the toilet to urinate when one gets the urge to do so, and emptying the bladder before and after sexual intercourse.

Sexual Dysfunction

Older adults desire closeness to and bonding with others. This need begins at birth and continues until death, and means that sexuality and physical function are important quality-of-life issues for older women and men.

Sexual dysfunction can affect both genders. In men, it is referred to as *erectile dysfunction* (ED); in women, it is referred to as *female sexual dysfunction* (FSD). ED is the persistent inability to achieve or maintain an erection adequate for sexual penetration and intercourse (Reuben et al., 2011). The etiology is thought to be hormonal, because circulating levels of testosterone and its aggregates decrease with age.

Women with FSD often have decreased libido, diminished arousal, and decreased ability or inability to achieve an orgasm. FSD may occur, in some part, because of normal aging. Estrogen levels decline with menopause. The vaginal tissues become thin and friable. As a result, women may find it more difficult to become aroused. The female arousal cycle is a neuroendocrine-mediated vascular and muscle response. Current research is focused on androgen deficiency as a probable cause.

Patients may have other contributing factors. Possible causes of sexual arousal disorder include:

▶ Vaginitis

▶ Cystitis

▶ Endometriosis

▶ Hypothyroidism

▶ Diabetes mellitus

▶ Depression

▶ Drugs (e.g., opioids, hormone replacement therapy [HRT], antihypertensives, sedatives, antidepressants)

Sexual function often is influenced by culture, ethnicity, emotional state, age, sexual experiences, disease state, and drug use. These issues must be kept in mind as a treatment plan is generated. Assessments should include biopsychosocial parameters. Information about sexual identity, behaviors, and physical issues that prevent or occur during the sexual encounter should be explored. Other contributing factors, such as fear of sexually transmitted infections (STIs), stress, and alcohol or drug use in one or both partners, should be assessed.

Patients taking medications known to cause ED or FSD should stop taking them, if possible. Treatments for men include use of sildenafil, vardenafil, tadalafil, testosterone, constriction devices with or without vacuum, and surgical penile implants, as well as use of bupropion, or testosterone replacement. Sildenafil should not be taken with nitrates because of the potentiating effects on vasodilation and side effects, including changes in vision, back pain, muscle pain, and prolonged erections. Testosterone is contraindicated in breast or prostate cancer. For women, the options are more limited. They include estrogen vaginal cream (Estrace) to treat dryness, itching, and burning; and removal of offending medications, if applicable (Tabloski, 2010).

According to the Hartford Institute of Geriatric Nursing (2012), gerontological nurses should use the PLISSIT model to intervene with patients with sexual dysfunction:

▶ *Permission:* Create an atmosphere where patients feel comfortable with discussing their sexual concerns.

▶ *Limited information:* Provide some useful information to clients.

▶ *Specific suggestions:* Offer some specific information based on the client's particular situation and readiness for intervention.

▶ *Intensive therapy:* Refer patients to an appropriate healthcare provider (e.g., urologist, therapist, counselor).

Post-Menopausal Conditions

With normal aging, both men and women experience a decline in the levels of their dominant sex hormones. Menopause denotes the final cessation of menstruation as a normal part of aging or as the result of surgical removal of both ovaries.

The average age of female menopause in the United States is 51 years (McPhee & Papadakis, 2011). Many women suffer mood swings, hot flashes, and depression at the time of menopause, but some of these symptoms may be coincidental with other life changes, such as children leaving home or the retirement of husbands or partners. Physical changes after cessation of menstruation for 1 year include vaginal atrophy and osteoporosis.

Laboratory evaluation to confirm menopause includes follicle-stimulating hormone and estrogen levels. Hormone replacement therapy (HRT) consisting of estrogen and progestin replacement is known to be associated with increased risk of coronary heart events, strokes, thromboembolic disease, breast cancer, and gallstones. The decision to alleviate hot flashes and treat menopausal symptoms with the use of HRT should be made by a menopausal woman only after long and careful discussion and after her healthcare provider has given her complete information about the risks involved.

Nursing assessment and management focus on education and offering solutions to the symptoms of some of these issues. Nurses should have information about weight-bearing exercise and adequate calcium and vitamin D intake. Information related to changes in sexuality also should be discussed. Symptomatic therapies include vaginal lubricants for the atrophic tissues and OTC melatonin to help with sleep issues that cause fatigue (which ultimately affects functional status and sexual life).

REFERENCES

Agency for Health Care Policy and Research. (2012). *Urinary incontinence in adults: Measure summary.* Retrieved from http://qualitymeasures.ahrq.gov/content.aspx?id=32402

Hartford Institute for Geriatric Nursing. (2012). *Sexuality assessment for older adults. Try this: Best practices in nursing care to older adults.* Retrieved from http://consultgerirn.org/uploads/File/trythis/try_this_10.pdf

Huether, S., & McCance, K. (2012). *Understanding pathophysiology* (5th ed.). St. Louis, MO: Mosby.

Levey, A. S., Bosch, J. P., Lewis, J. B., Greene, T., Rogers, N., & Roth, D. (1999). A more accurate method to estimate glomerular filtration rate from serum creatinine: A new prediction equation. *Modification of Diet in Renal Disease Study Group, 130,* 461–470.

Mayo Clinic. (2012). *Kegel exercises: A how-to guide for women.* Retrieved from http://www.mayoclinic.com/health/kegel-exercises/WO00119

McPhee, S., & Papadakis, M. (2011). *Current medical diagnosis and treatment* (50th ed.). New York: McGraw Hill Medical.

Meiner, S. E. (2001). Gastrointestinal problems. In A. S. Luggen & S. E. Meiner (Eds.), *NGNA Core curriculum for gerontological nursing* (pp. 73–161). St. Louis, MO: Mosby.

National Kidney Foundation Kidney Disease Outcomes Quality Initiative. (2007). KDOQI clinical practice guidelines for chronic kidney disease: Evaluation, classification, and stratification. *American Journal of Kidney Disease, 49*(2 Suppl. 2).

Nurse practitioners' prescribing reference. (2012). New York: Haymarket Media Publication.

Reuben, D., Herr, K., Pacala, J., Pollock, B., Potter, J., & Semla, T. (2011). *Geriatrics at your fingertips* (13th ed.). New York: American Geriatrics Society.

Tabloski, P. (2010). *Gerontological nursing* (2nd ed.). Upper Fall River, NJ: Pearson Prentice Hall.

U.S. Department of Health and Human Services. (2002). *Women's health initiative.* Retrieved from http://www.nhlbi.nih.gov/whi/index.html

U.S. Preventive Services Task Force. (2012). *Screening for prostate cancer.* Retrieved from http://www.uspreventiveservicestaskforce.org/uspstf/uspsprca.htm

WebMD. (2012). *Transurethral resection (TUR) for bladder cancer.* Retrieved from http://www.webmd.com/cancer/bladder-cancer/transurethral-resection-tur-for-bladder-cancer

ADDITIONAL RESOURCES

Chronic and Disabling Conditions: www.agingsociety.org/

Healthy People 2020: www.healthypeople.gov/2020/

CHRONIC AND END-STAGE KIDNEY DISEASE

Chronic kidney disease (CKD) affects about 3.9 million people in the U.S. population (Centers for Disease Control and Prevention, 2012); it was the ninth leading cause of death in the United States in 2010. A large percentage of all end-stage renal disease is attributed to diabetes mellitus and hypertension (HTN) as the result of end-organ failure. Given the aging population, increased longevity, and increasing prevalence of diabetes mellitus, these numbers will increase significantly over the next two decades.

The Kidney Disease Outcome Quality Initiative (National Kidney Foundation, 2007) defined five stages of kidney disease on the basis of the *Glomerular Filtration Rate* (GFR) and presence of albuminuria, including microalbuminuria (see Table 17–1). The GFR is the flow rate of filtration through the kidney. In clinical practice, this number is most commonly estimated by the calculated CrCl (see Box 17–1). This estimation of CrCl is particularly important in older patients, because serum creatinine alone does not adequately reflect declines in renal function in patients with reduced creatinine production—primarily those with decreased muscle mass. Of the formulas listed, the MDRD is probably most accurate as an estimate of GFR, but it is more difficult to calculate. Calculators are available online at www.kidney.org/professionals/KDOQI/gfr_calculator.cfm and www.nephron.com/mdrd/default.html.

TABLE 17-1.
CLASSIFICATION OF CHRONIC KIDNEY DISEASE

STAGE	DESCRIPTION	GFR ML/MIN/1.73M²
1	Persistent albuminuria with normal or ↑ GFR	≥ 90
2	Persistent albuminuria with mildly ↓ GFR	60–89
3	Moderately ↓ GFR	30–59
4	Severely ↓ GFR	15–29
5	Renal failure/dialysis	< 15

Note: GFR = glomerular filtration rate.

Adapted from "KDOQI Clinical Practice Guidelines for Chronic Kidney Disease: Evaluation, Classification, and Stratification," by the National Kidney Foundation, KDOQI, 2007, *American Journal of Kidney Disease, 49*(2 Suppl. 2).

BOX 17-1.
CALCULATING CREATININE CLEARANCE

GFR = 186.3 x (SCR)$^{-1.154}$ x (Age in Years)$^{-0.203}$ x 1.212 (if patient is African American) x 0.742 (if patient is a woman)

CrCl = ([140 − Age] x IBW)/(SCR x 72) (x 0.85 for women)

Note: GFR = glomerular filtration rate, SCR = serum creatinine, CrCl = creatinine clearance, IBW = ideal body weight.

Risk factors include:

▶ Diabetes mellitus

▶ HTN

▶ Family history of renal disease

▶ Advancing age

▶ Race (Black)

▶ Other diseases (e.g., lupus, multiple myeloma, sickle cell disease)

▶ Atherosclerosis

▶ Chronic NSAID use

A decline in renal function remains asymptomatic until approximately 50% of nephrons are lost (Stage 3). The laboratory values and clinical manifestations will vary from person to person. Possible signs and symptoms are listed in Table 17–2.

TABLE 17-2.
SIGNS AND SYMPTOMS OF RENAL FAILURE

GFR ML/MIN	> 50	20–50	< 20	< 10
Signs and symptoms	None except underlying disease	Elevated BUN and creatinine Metabolic acidosis ↑ Potassium Polyuria Anemia Fatigue	↓ Calcium ↑ Phosphate Metabolic acidosis Fluid overload	Uremia Nausea and vomiting HF Pruritis Fatigue Insomnia

Note: GFR = glomerular filtration rate, BUN = blood urea nitrogen, HF = heart failure.

Patients with CKD must be educated about the importance of controlling comorbid disease processes. Control of hyperglycemia has been shown to prevent kidney disease, as well as slow the progression of established disease (National Kidney Foundation, 2007). Most agencies have set the goal for hemoglobin A1c at < 7.0%. Controlling BP also slows the progression of kidney disease. Target BP is less than 130/80 mm Hg and should be achieved with use of ACE inhibitors or ARBs as part of the regimen (National Kidney Foundation, 2007).

Hyperlipidemia is another target for treatment, given the increased risk of patients for CVD. Patients who reach Stage 3 kidney disease and also have diabetes mellitus are more likely to die of CVD than to progress to Stage 5 kidney disease (National Kidney Foundation, 2007). Therefore, the LDL-cholesterol goal for these patients is less than 100 mg/dL. In cases of patients who have cardiovascular events, the goal may be less than 70 mg/dL.

Lifestyle changes, including smoking cessation, exercise, and nutritional changes (sodium, protein, and potassium restrictions), also are important. Patients should be warned to avoid medications with potentially nephrotoxic effects, such as NSAIDs, and to avoid dehydration. Because of the complex management of patients with CKD, a multidisciplinary approach is usually most beneficial.

Acute Renal Failure

Acute renal failure is classified as pre-renal, intrinsic, or post-renal failure. These terms refer to the origin of the failure. *Pre-renal azotemia* occurs as a result of decreased renal perfusion. Stenosis of the renal arteries can lead to decreased blood flow to one or both kidneys. Any cause of hypovolemia (e.g., dehydration, hemorrhage) or any cause of reduced cardiac output (e.g., myocardial dysfunction) or shunting of blood away from the kidneys, such as shock, can cause pre-renal failure. In addition, drugs that lower the GFR, such as NSAIDs and ACEIs, can cause this problem. This type of failure is potentially reversible with restoration of renal blood flow in a timely manner. Failure to improve renal perfusion will result in acute tubular necrosis, which is a form of intrinsic renal failure.

The causes of *intrinsic renal failure* are numerous and can include

▶ Nephrotoxic drugs (e.g., aminoglycosides, NSAIDs)

▶ Contrast dye

▶ HTN

▶ Glomerulonephritis

▶ Interstitial nephritis (e.g., medications, lupus, infection)

▶ Cholesterol embolization (postprocedure)

Post-obstructive renal failure is caused by a blockage after the level of the kidney. The most common cause is BPH in men. Other causes, such as stones or retroperitoneal tumors, are much less common.

End-Stage Renal Disease/Stage 5 CKD

With treatment advances in CVD, many older patients are living long enough to develop Stage 5 CKD. Dialysis in patients age 65 or older is common and often is appropriate even in patients who are in their seventh or eighth decade. Dialysis is indicated when severe hyperkalemia, acidosis, or volume overload cannot be managed with other therapies. Comorbidities and quality of life must be carefully considered when deciding on dialysis, which can either be chronic ambulatory peritoneal dialysis or hemodialysis. Although older adults have shorter life expectancies, functional older patients should be considered for kidney transplantation because they will benefit in the same way as middle-age adults receiving kidney transplants.

IMMUNOLOGICAL DISEASES

Sexually transmitted infections and HIV/AIDS occur in older adults.

Sexually Transmitted Infections (STIs)

Safe sex is a delicate issue and must be presented sensitively. Older adults belong to a generation that may not have used condoms in their lifetimes, and many may be unaware of the problems that await them when struggling with the need for intimacy in the shadow of loss. All older adults who are sexually active should have their sexual histories assessed. This history becomes more important for the person who has more than one sexual partner. Most safe sex programs do not focus on older adults, so it is imperative that gerontological nurses identify the instances in which this teaching is needed.

Common STIs include herpes, human papilloma virus, gonorrhea, syphilis, *Chlamydia, Trichomonas,* and HIV/AIDS. Although thought to be diseases of young people, these do occur in older adults. The major risk factor is unprotected intercourse with multiple partners. Because healthcare providers often do not maintain a high degree of monitoring of this population's sexual habits, diagnosis often is delayed. Patients may have signs and symptoms of tertiary disease, such as neurosyphilis, before the provider even considers syphilis as the cause of persistent shooting pains in the older adult's lower extremities.

Gerontological nurses must be diligent in history taking and remember that some older adults are not forthright in giving details about sexual issues. Sometimes, the situation requires that nurses directly ask patients, "Could this be a sexually transmitted infection?" If the question is phrased this way, patients may feel more comfortable in starting the conversation and divulging details.

Urethritis in older men or women should alert nurses to a possible *Chlamydia* infection, as should an abnormal female Pap smear that suggests inflammation. About 50% of all nongonococcal urethritis and cervicitis can be attributed to *Chlamydia* (McPhee & Papadakis, 2011).

HIV/AIDS

HIV/AIDS is a profound immune deficiency that is caused by the human immunodeficiency virus. The virus attaches to specialized WBCs (CD4 cells) and weakens the body's immune response, increasing the risk for opportunistic infections. Because HIV is much more virulent in older adults, a higher percentage of them will progress to AIDS than will their younger counterparts (Services and Advocacy for GLTB Elders, 2012).

Practicing unsafe sex is the most common reason that older adults acquire the infection. According to Resnick (2003), some reasons that older adults do not practice safe-sex behaviors include:

▶ They envision STIs as something that happens to other people (this mentality also applies to gay and bisexual men in this population).

▶ Older women do not fear getting pregnant, so asking partners to wear condoms is not a priority.

▶ Older women outnumber older men, and men have many partners to select from, so women may agree to unprotected intercourse to keep a partner.

▶ Older adults grew up in a time when men made most of the decisions; therefore, if a man does not want to use a condom, it is not used.

Other risk factors include blood transfusion (less of a risk), IV drug use, and some of the normal changes of aging. For example, as female vaginal tissues become thinner and more friable because of lack of estrogen, ongoing vaginal mucosal disruption can result, creating portals of entry for HIV (Resnick, 2003). The normal age-related decline in the immune system puts older adults at a higher risk of HIV than younger adults.

Diagnostics include laboratory studies to confirm presence of antibodies to the virus, exact amount of virus in each cubic millimeter of blood (viral load), and the measure of the T-lymphocyte cells (CD4 cells). Some patients present with illnesses or problems that suggest immunodeficiency such as Kaposi's sarcoma or *Pneumocystis carinii* pneumonia. Such entities are AIDS-indicator conditions and should prompt a work-up for HIV infection.

Assessment begins with a sexual history and a review of constitutional symptoms, such as fatigue, anorexia, weight loss, or memory difficulties. Nursing management focuses on preventing the illness and encouraging low-risk behaviors such as monogamous relationships, partner reduction, and use of condoms. For patients who have already been diagnosed, education about medications and the importance of adherence is imperative.

Common treatments include aggressive highly active antiretroviral therapy, along with antibiotic prophylaxis as indicated. Nurses are important in psychosocial intervention, oral hygiene, dietary intervention (high-calorie, low-fat diets), and the importance of *not participating in alternative and complementary therapies without checking with the healthcare provider first*, because many herbals have been known to interfere with the expected actions of the retroviral agents.

As the disease progresses, palliative care measures are needed, because there is no vaccine or known cure at this time. In the advanced stages of the disease, end-of-life care is an important consideration.

HEMATOLOGICAL DISEASES

Hematological diseases in older adults include anemia, pernicious anemia, and leukemia.

Anemia

Anemia is decreased RBCs, hemoglobin, and hematocrit and is a symptom of an underlying problem. Because oxygen sits on the hemoglobin to travel to the tissues, decreased hemoglobin means a decrease in the oxygen-carrying capacity of the blood. A person's symptoms relate to how the body has compensated for the lowered oxygen levels. If the anemia comes on insidiously, even the older adult with chronic illnesses can be fairly asymptomatic. On the other hand, if the anemia occurs quickly (as in GI bleeding or hemorrhage after trauma), patients are symptomatic and may have unstable vital signs (even if they are otherwise healthy; Huether & McCance, 2012).

Fatigue, pallor, and dizziness are common symptoms of anemia in older adults. In severe cases, patients may present with mental status changes (e.g., confusion, agitation, apathy, depression).

Anemias are classified according to RBC size (mean corpuscular volume [MCV]). If the MCV is elevated, the RBC is large and is called a *macrocyte,* resulting in a *macrocytic anemia.* If the MCV is decreased, the RBC is small and is called a *microcyte,* resulting in a *microcytic anemia.* If the MCV is within the normal range, the anemia is considered a *normocytic anemia.*

Certain types of anemia affect the size of the RBC; this alteration in cell size is used to guide clinicians in their search for the underlying cause of the anemia. Table 17–2 further explains the etiology and presentation of types of common anemia.

TABLE 17–2.
CLASSIFICATION OF COMMON ANEMIA

	LABORATORY VALUES	CAUSES	THERAPIES
Normocytic anemia	▸ MCV normal ▸ Serum iron low, while other iron stores normal (no iron deficiency)	▸ Acute blood loss ▸ Anemia of chronic disease	▸ Correct underlying problem (source of hemorrhage) or stabilize the chronic illness (e.g., renal disease, connective tissue disease) ▸ With chronic illness, RBC life span is shortened, and there may be a deficiency of erythropoetin to stimulate the bone marrow to make the RBC precursors (mechanism for anemia in renal disease)
Microcytic anemia	▸ MCV decreased ▸ Low ferritin ▸ FOB may be positive	▸ Iron deficiency anemia	▸ Usually GI bleeding is the culprit; source must be identified, then iron therapy instituted
Macrocytic anemia	▸ MCV increased ▸ Low B_{12} or folate levels (some patients can be deficient in both nutrients)	▸ B_{12} or folate deficiency	▸ Inadequate intake or absorption of one or both of these nutrients ▸ Treatment aimed at replenishing the levels

Note: RBC = red blood count, MCV = mean corpuscular volume, FOB = fecal occult blood, GI = gastrointestinal.

Adapted from *Geriatrics at Your Fingertips* (13th ed.), by D. Reuben, K. Herr, J. Pacala, B. Pollock, J. Potter, & T. Semla, 2011, New York: American Geriatrics Society.

Diagnosis is made on laboratory findings and evaluation of iron and vitamin studies; in some cases (not commonly), a bone marrow biopsy is indicated. Before any treatment can begin, the underlying cause must be found.

Assessment includes focusing on the underlying cause of the anemia. Nursing management centers on dietary education and balancing rest with activities of daily living. Patients should be provided with a list of foods high in the nutrient in which they are deficient.

Pernicious Anemia

True *pernicious anemia* (PA), which is a complete lack of production of intrinsic factor, is rare in older adults. Most individuals with true PA have been diagnosed as young or middle-age adults. Vitamin B_{12} deficiency is common in older adults.

With normal aging, the parietal cells atrophy and make less hydrochloric acid and intrinsic factor. This combination interferes with B_{12} absorption. In addition, use of acid-suppressing medications, such as H_2 blockers and proton pump inhibitors, further suppresses acid production, which compromises the body's ability to absorb B_{12} and other nutrients (McPhee & Papadakis, 2011).

Older people who have low vitamin B_{12} levels and macrocytic anemia should be treated with parenteral or oral B_{12}. If B_{12} levels fail to rise after a trial of oral vitamin B_{12} replacement, the older person may lack intrinsic factor (pernicious anemia), and parenteral B_{12} injections may be needed (Reuben et al., 2011).

Leukemia

Leukemia is a malignant proliferation of WBC precursors, or blasts, in bone marrow. The most common leukemia in older adults is chronic *lymphocytic leukemia* (CLL). This phenomenon usually is found accidentally, when patients are having a CBC drawn for another reason.

CLL is a disease of older people, with 90% of cases occurring after age 50 and an average age of diagnosis of 70 (McPhee & Papadakis, 2011). Most older adults have a normal life span and do not succumb to this illness. The etiology remains unknown.

Patients with CLL have a WBC count of 5,000/mcL to > 20,000/mcL, and 75%–98% of circulating cells are lymphocytes. All patients are referred to a hematologist. Common symptoms are lymphadenopathy, weakness, fatigue, weight loss, splenomegaly, abdominal pain, or fever. Painless lymphadenopathy is the most common sign.

There is no cure for this illness; patients are treated for symptoms, if any occur. Radiation, chemotherapy, and splenectomy may be done. A small percentage of patients will convert to *acute lymphocytic leukemia* (ALL); they are treated as are their younger counterparts, if their general health allows (McPhee & Papadakis, 2011).

Acute myelogenous leukemia (AML) is sometimes seen in older adults. This illness requires prompt treatment with chemotherapy or bone marrow transplant, or patients will succumb to it. Drugs commonly used include vincristine, prednisone, anthracycline, asparaginase, and cytarabine. In most cases of AML, remission can be obtained, but many older adults will experience a relapse.

Risk factors for leukemia are thought to be advanced age and exposure to prolonged radiation. Diagnostics may include laboratory tests, bone marrow aspiration, and histochemical stains.

Nursing management involves control of pain, education about activity intolerance (balancing rest with planned activities), and prevention of infection.

REFERENCES

Agency for Health Care Policy and Research. (2012). *Urinary incontinence in adults: Measure summary.* Retrieved from http://qualitymeasures.ahrq.gov/content.aspx?id=32402

Centers for Disease Control and Prevention. (2012). *FASTSTATS–Kidney disease.* Retrieved from http://www.cdc.gov/nchs/fastats/kidbladd.htm

Cockcroft, D. W., & Gault, M. H. (1976). Prediction of creatinine clearance from serum creatinine. *Nephron, 16*(1), 31–41.

Huether, S., & McCance, K. (2012). *Understanding pathophysiology* (5th ed.). St. Louis, MO: Mosby.

Levey, A. S., Bosch, J. P., Lewis, J. B., Greene, T., Rogers, N., & Roth, D. (1999). A more accurate method to estimate glomerular filtration rate from serum creatinine: A new prediction equation. *Modification of Diet in Renal Disease Study Group, 130,* 461–470.

McPhee, S., & Papadakis, M. (2011). *Current medical diagnosis and treatment* (50th ed.). New York: McGraw Hill Medical.

National Kidney Foundation Kidney Disease Outcomes Quality Initiative. (2007). KDOQI clinical practice guidelines for chronic kidney disease: Evaluation, classification, and stratification. *American Journal of Kidney Disease, 49*(2 Suppl. 2).

Nurse practitioners' prescribing reference. (2012). New York: Haymarket Media Publication.

Reuben, D., Herr, K., Pacala, J., Pollock, B., Potter, J., & Semla, T. (2011). *Geriatrics at your fingertips* (13th ed.). New York: American Geriatrics Society.

Services and Advocacy for GLTB Elders and National Center for Transgender Equality. (2012). *The lives of transgender older adults.* Retrieved from http://transequality.org/Resources/TransAgingPolicyReportFull.pdf

ADDITIONAL RESOURCES

Chronic and Disabling Conditions: www.agingsociety.org/

Diabetes and the Older Adult: http://ohioline.osu.edu/ss-fact/0166.html

Healthy People 2020: www.healthypeople.gov/2020/

MUSCULOSKELETAL DISEASES

Common musculoskeletal diseases of older adults include osteoarthritis and osteoporosis.

Osteoarthritis

Osteoarthritis (OA), also known as *degenerative joint disease,* is caused by gradual loss of cartilage at a joint articulation, with resulting development of bony spurs and cysts at the joint margins. OA affects approximately 27 million people in the United States and is a major cause of disability (Centers for Disease Control and Prevention [CDC], 2012). Prevalence increases with age, but age is not the only causative factor, nor does everyone develop worn-out, painful joints as they age.

Risk factors include the following:

▶ Advancing age (strongest factor)

▶ Joint trauma

▶ Obesity (particularly for weight-bearing joints)

▶ Overuse

▶ Familial tendency

The joints most commonly affected by OA are:

▶ Hands (distal interphalangeal—Heberden nodes, proximal interphalangeal—Bouchard nodes, carpometacarpal of the thumb)

▶ Knees

▶ Hips

▶ Spine (cervical, lumbar, thoracic)

▶ Feet (metatarsophalangeal, especially first joint)

The ankles, wrists, elbows, and shoulders usually are spared (Sweet, 2012).

The most common symptom is stiffening of the joint after prolonged inactivity, often called the *gel phenomenon*. This stiffness quickly subsides with movement, usually within 5–30 minutes. As further joint deterioration occurs, pain and aching become the predominant symptoms. Initially, pain is reported with joint use, but it may progress to pain even at rest or during sleep. OA of the hip can cause pain in the groin, but not the buttocks.

Examination in early disease may be normal. As the disease progresses, *crepitus* (grating or creaking noise) can be noted with range of motion. In addition, palpation at the joint margins usually elicits tenderness, and bony enlargement of the joints is usually apparent, most notably in the hands and knees. Joint alignment deformities may occur. Laboratory tests are not done unless it is necessary to exclude other diagnoses such as rheumatoid arthritis, gouty arthritis, or connective tissue diseases. Diagnosis is made by clinical exam and x-ray findings.

The pain associated with OA causes tremendous functional limitations, especially when weight-bearing joints are affected. Patients must be educated about the importance of pain control to maintaining a steady activity level. Decreases in activity can lead to muscle atrophy and further loss of functional ability. In addition, patients who are deconditioned have a higher risk of falls, which lead to further pain and disability. Splinting or support devices for weight-bearing joints can be helpful. Referral to a physical therapist for proper fitting and for instruction on assistive walking devices can improve mobility. Many older adults take the nutritional supplements glucosamine and chondroitin sulfate, but recent clinical trials have shown that these provide little or no benefit (National Center for Complementary and Alternative Medicine, 2008).

Osteoporosis

Osteoporosis is a reduction in bone mass and strength. In normal health, new bone is made by osteoblasts, and old bone is resorbed by the osteoclast cells. This cycle of bone remodeling takes about 4 months. Adults reach peak bone mass by about age 30. The sex hormones are important in regulation of normal bone remodeling by keeping the activity of the osteoclasts in check.

When these hormone levels begin to wane (menopause in women and about age 80 in men), bone thinning begins. In this process, the amount of resorption by the osteoclasts exceeds the amount of bone production by the osteoblast cells. A low vitamin D level in older adults contributes to this process, because it stimulates the parathyroid hormone (PTH), which is instrumental in regulation of calcium in the body. When PTH is stimulated inappropriately, it causes accelerated thinning of the skeleton. Low bone mass can be caused by the aforementioned process or can result from failure to reach peak bone mass, increased bone resorption that is not age-related, or decreased bone formation (McPhee & Papadakis, 2011).

Regular x-rays are not used to detect osteoporosis, because much bone loss is not detectable by this method. Bone densitometry is done with duel-energy x-ray absorptiometry (DEXA). Measurement areas include the femurs and lumbar spine (the wrist can be used as an alternate site in patients with hardware in those regions). The score is then compared to that of normal young adults of comparable height, weight, and gender (Reuben et al., 2011).

Osteopenia, which precedes osteoporosis, is a bone mineral density (BMD) loss that is from 1 standard deviation (SD) up to 2.4 SDs below normal. A patient with a BMD that reveals > 2.5 SD below normal has osteoporosis.

Osteoporosis is divided into primary and secondary disease. Primary disease is most common and is related to factors involving the bone itself; in secondary disease, another medical entity is causing the osteoporosis.

Primary osteoporosis is divided into Type I (postmenopausal) and Type II (age-associated) disease. *Type I osteoporosis* is related to estrogen deficiency and is seen in women ages 51–75; in this type, the trabecular bone in the vertebra, hips, and wrists becomes weak (Meiner, 2006). *Type II osteoporosis* occurs in both genders age 70 or older, as total bone production begins to wane. Cortical bone, which provides strength to the skeleton, is lost. Hip fractures are the common manifestation of this process. Vitamin D deficiency is thought to play a large role in this type of osteoporosis.

Secondary osteoporosis, which is the cause of 15% of osteoporosis, is the result of another illness or process that affects bone integrity (Sweet et al., 2009). Common entities that can cause secondary osteoporosis are:

- ▶ Parathyroid disease
- ▶ Cushing's disease
- ▶ Hypogonadism
- ▶ Alcohol abuse
- ▶ Liver disease
- ▶ Early amenorrhea (surgical or metabolic)
- ▶ Hyperthyroidism
- ▶ Neoplasms
- ▶ Prolonged immobility
- ▶ Gastrointestinal (GI) disorders that interfere with the absorption of nutrients, specifically calcium (e.g., bariatric surgery, malabsorption syndromes)
- ▶ Neoplasms
- ▶ Long-term use of steroids, methotrexate, and phenytoin
- ▶ Long-term use of heparin and aluminum-containing antacids

Risk factors for osteoporosis include female gender, increased age, White race, thin body frame, alcohol use, cigarette smoking, excess caffeine, and a diet low in calcium. Signs and symptoms may be as subtle as back pain or fatigue or as severe as spontaneous fracture of vertebrae, femoral neck, or wrist with normal activities such as bending or lifting.

Bone mass density should be assessed at least once in all women after age 65 and in all men after age 70. How often to repeat testing is uncertain, but some suggest every 3 years for older people with osteopenia and every 5 years for those with normal bone density. The value of monitoring bone mass density in patients already receiving treatment is unproven (Reuben et al., 2011). Gerontological nurses should be aware of the signs and symptoms of osteoporosis and suggest that patients discuss a DEXA scan with their primary care providers if any of the following are present:

- History of a fracture in a patient ages 40 or older
- Family history of osteoporosis
- Cigarette smoker
- Low body mass index (BMI)
- Dorsal kyphosis (hump on back, "dowager's hump")
- Loss of height

The goal of treatment is to increase bone mass density to prevent hip fracture. For each SD decrement in bone mass density, hip fracture risk increases about twofold. For each SD increment in bone mass density, hip fracture risk is approximately halved (Reuben et al., 2011).

Management includes a diet rich in calcium and vitamin D. Men and women should get 1,200 mg of calcium and at least 800 IU of vitamin D_3 daily (Reuben et al., 2011). Older adults can obtain the calcium in their diet by eating foods such as cheese, yogurt, collards, broccoli, and tofu. Skim milk and blackstrap molasses are both extremely good sources of calcium. Older adults who do not eat a diet high in calcium can obtain an adequate amount in supplements. Calcium carbonate contains 40% elemental calcium and is inexpensive. Smoking cessation, prevention of falls, and moderate alcohol use are all recommended. Patients taking PPIs such as Protonix, Nexium, and Prilosec should take calcium citrate, which is more easily absorbed in the presence of these agents. Weight-bearing exercise, such as walking, low-impact aerobics, vigorous water exercises, and walking with and lifting light weights are all thought to stimulate bone growth.

Options for treatment include estrogen therapy, bisphosphonates, selective estrogen receptor modulators, calcitonin, and PTH. Table 18–1 provides more information on each of the treatment options.

TABLE 18-1.
OSTEOPOROSIS MEDICATIONS

AGENT	MECHANISM OF ACTION	BRAND NAMES	ADDITIONAL CONSIDERATIONS
Estrogen	Antiresorptive	Estrace, Ogen, Premarin, many generics	▸ Use has come under great scrutiny since the results of the Women's Health Initiative in 2002 ▸ Although they provide a positive effect on bone, risk of thromboembolic events and breast cancer is increased ▸ Use strictly for osteoporosis prevention ▸ Treatment should be an individual decision between a well-informed patient and the healthcare provider ▸ Contraindicated in patients with history of CAD, thromboembolic disease of any type, and breast cancer
Bisphosphonate	Antiresorptive	Fosamax, Actonel, Boniva, Reclast	▸ Work well and can be given to both men and women ▸ Consider stopping after 5 years ▸ Prolonged use associated with atypical femoral fracture ▸ Can be given daily, weekly, monthly (Actonel, Boniva), every 3 months (Boniva), or yearly (Reclast) ▸ Use with caution in patients with dental or GI problems ▸ Reclast contraindicated in patients with present or past history of AF
Selective estrogen receptor modulator	Antiresorptive	Evista	▸ Works on the estrogen receptor; can be used in patients with a history (or an increased risk) of breast cancer ▸ Contraindicated in patients with a history of thromboembolic disease
Calcitonin	Antiresorptive	Miacalcin	▸ Nasal spray that can be used for osteoporosis of the spine (clinical trials show no effect on the hip)
Denosumab injection	RANK-ligand inhibitor	Prolia	▸ Stimulates bone growth and decreases bone resorption. ▸ Prolonged use may be associated with spontaneous bone fracture and delayed bone healing. Not effective at preventing fractures in patients with multiple myeloma.

CONTINUED ▶

◄ TABLE 18-1 CONTINUED

AGENT	MECHANISM OF ACTION	BRAND NAMES	ADDITIONAL CONSIDERATIONS
Parathyroid hormone	Stimulates bone production	Forteo	► Stimulates bone growth in individuals (men and women) at high risk for fracture because of severe disease ► Daily SQ injection for 2 years, then followed with biphosphonate therapy (to maintain the new bone that is formed) ► Contraindicated in people with history of radiation to the skeleton
Hydrochlora-thiazide	Decreases urinary excretion of calcium, thus slowing bone loss	HCTZ, Dyazide, Maxide	► Can be used in patients with concomitant HTN

Note: CAD = coronary artery disease, GI = gastrointestinal, AF = atrial fibrillation, HCTZ = hydrochlorathiazide, HTN = hypertension.

Nursing assessment begins with the health history, family history of osteoporosis, and presence of risk factors such as level of exercise, alcohol and caffeine intake, and smoking. Women need to be queried about onset of previous fracture, menopause, date of last mammogram, and history of gynecological cancer. Physical examination involves the back and assessment for kyphosis, gait impairment, and muscle weakness.

Nursing management includes:

► Control of pain

► Relaxation and repositioning techniques if the patient is in pain

► Education about the disease process

► Prevention of falls, injuries, and other deformities

► Stressing the importance of smoking cessation and decreasing alcohol use (if in excess)

► Limiting caffeine intake

► Recommending exercise at least every other day for 25–30 minutes

Additional educational information can be provided for interested patients through the National Osteoporosis Foundation (www.nof.org). The World Health Organization has supported the development of an instrument called the FRAX to assess the 10-year probability of hip, spine, forearm, or shoulder fracture on the basis of bone density readings. An online calculator is used to identify older people who are at risk for injury from falls and would benefit from aggressive treatment of their osteopenia or osteoporosis. See http://www.shef.ac.uk/FRAX/index.jsp for further information. (Mobility and falls are covered in Chapter 9.)

Osteomalacia is a metabolic disease characterized by formation of spongy bone due to inadequate and delayed mineralization. Although rare in the United States, it is common in Great Britain, Ethiopia, Pakistan, Iran, and India. Many factors contribute to the development of osteomalacia, but the most important is vitamin D deficiency, followed by renal tubular diseases, certain tumors, and a side effect of anticonvulsant drug therapy. Treatment of osteomalacia depends on the cause, but may include administration of vitamin D supplements, administration of calcium carbonate to adjust calcium and phosphorus levels, administration of biphosponates to strengthen bones, and renal dialysis if indicated (Huether & McCance, 2011).

ENDOCRINE AND METABOLIC DISORDERS

Common endocrine and metabolic disorders in older adults include thyroid disease and diabetes mellitus.

Thyroid Disease

Thyroid disorders, particularly hypothyroidism, increase dramatically in older adults. With age, the thyroid undergoes moderate atrophy and also some histopathological changes, decreasing the production of thyroxine by about 30% (McPhee & Papadakis, 2011). A hypofunctioning gland is termed *hypothyroidism.*

Hypothyroidism may result from defects in hormone production, target tissues, or receptors (McPhee & Papadakis, 2011). When the problem occurs at the level of the gland itself, it is *primary hypothyroidism;* if the decrease in hormone function occurs because of a problem in the anterior pituitary, the problem is *secondary hypothyroidism;* and, if the problem area is the hypothalamus, the entity is *tertiary hypothyroidism.* The latter two problems are rare.

The most common cause of hypothyroidism in older adults is autoimmune thyroiditis. The aged thyroid gland is more susceptible to the effects of Hashimoto's disease. Thyroiditis can be brought on by a virus, stress, or treatment of certain illnesses, such as Hodgkin's disease. On occasion, hypothyroidism can be the result of ingesting:

► Lithium carbonate

► Amiodarone

► Iodine

► Kelp

In addition, previous radiation to the head and neck (for malignancy) can render the thyroid nonfunctional, as can ablation of the gland with radioactive iodine (I_{131}) or surgery for the treatment of previous hyperthyroidism. The prevalence of hypothyroidism is higher in women.

Primary hypothyroidism is characterized by an elevated thyroid-stimulating hormone (TSH) and a subnormal serum-free thyroxine (T4) level. In older adults, its insidious onset of symptoms are often attributed to "getting old." Common presenting signs and symptoms include:

▶ Anorexia

▶ Weight loss

▶ Unstable gait or balance

▶ Arthralgias

▶ Muscle aches

▶ Weakness

▶ Unexplained lipid abnormalities (elevated TGs, cholesterol)

▶ Constipation or fecal impaction

▶ Depressed affect

▶ Mild cognitive impairment

Older adults may manifest more serious signs and symptoms than younger adults, such as bradycardia, angina, cold intolerance, syncope, muscle cramps, and numbness. Diagnostics include serum assays of TSH, free T4 levels, and thyroid antibodies (if there is a suspicion of acute thyroiditis).

Treatment includes replacement of the hormone with levothyroxine. The average dose is 75–100 micrograms (mcg) per day for older adults. Depending on the elevation level of the TSH, the starting dose is usually 25–50 mcg/day. Then, on the basis of TSH levels, which are checked every 8 weeks, the dose is titrated up until the TSH is 0.3–3 mlU/L (American Association of Endocrinologists, 2006). The patient's clinical picture and laboratory values are reassessed every 6–12 months after he or she has obtained a euthyroid state.

Assessment begins with questions about energy level; onset and pattern of fatigue should be identified, and any aggravating and alleviating factors. Any history of weight or bowel changes should be noted. A depression scale, a mental status exam, or both may be indicated as part of the assessment.

Nursing management includes education about the disease process, symptoms, and diagnostic testing that may be needed. Gerontological nurses should stress the importance of lifelong therapy and monitoring by the primary healthcare provider.

Hyperthyroidism is excessive secretion of thyroid hormones. *Primary hyperthyroidism* is usually associated with an enlarged gland (goiter). In older patients, the most common cause is multinodular goiter, rather than Graves' disease (which is seen in younger adults). Iodine-induced hyperthyroidism can be seen with the use of Amiodarone, which is 70% iodine and deposits iodine in the peripheral tissues.

The patient with hyperthyroidism has a suppressed TSH and an elevated free T4 and T3. The suppressed TSH is enough, along with the clinical picture, to confirm the diagnosis of hyperthyroidism.

Signs and symptoms of hyperthyroidism include insomnia, increased tremor, bowel movements, weakness, hair loss, heat intolerance, tachycardia, weight loss, and fatigue. Goiters are present in 60% of older adults with hyperthyroidism. In this population, in spite of the aforementioned signs and symptoms, AF is the most common presentation of hyperthyroidism (McPhee & Papadakis, 2011).

Medical management includes radioactive iodine (I_{131}). This therapy is curative and easily tolerated. Patients may be given beta-adrenergic blockers, such as propranolol, to control the symptoms of palpitations, tachycardia, and heat intolerance. However, beta-blockers have no effect on the etiology of the disease itself. After the ablation, patients must be monitored closely for indications of worsened illness (for the first 90 days) and then for signs and symptoms of hypothyroidism, which often occurs with radioactive therapy.

Assessment begins with gathering information about weight loss, body mass index (BMI), fatigue, and cardiac symptoms. Other comorbid states and medications should be noted. Nursing management focuses on education about the illness, diagnostics, and treatment. Many patients will require antithyroid medications (propylthiouracil [PTU] or Tapazole) before radioactive therapy. Nurses must inform patients of the importance of taking these "pretreatment" oral agents and what to expect with the I_{131} therapy. Nurses should alert patients about potential manifestations of eye disease (exophthalmus) from the hyperthyroid state and whom to notify if this occurs.

Diabetes Mellitus

Diabetes mellitus is a common disease found in Americans of all ages. In many cases, patients with diabetes have had a metabolic syndrome for years before becoming diabetic. This "prediabetic state" (fasting blood glucose levels between 100 and 126 mg/dL) is common; it is estimated that approximately 79 million Americans have prediabetes (American Diabetes Association, 2012).

Metabolic syndrome is a cluster of signs that are known to be associated with the risk of developing diabetes mellitus and cardiac vascular disease (CVD); obesity, sedentary lifestyle, genetic predisposition, age, and poor dietary habits are contributing factors. In 2005, the American Heart Association refined the criteria for diagnosis of metabolic syndrome and identified a series of interrelated risk factors that appear to promote the development of atherosclerotic cardiovascular disease. Any three of the five factors listed below establish the diagnosis of metabolic syndrome:

► Elevated blood pressure, > 130 mm Hg systolic BP or > 85 mm Hg diastolic BP or drug treatment for hypertension

► Fasting FBG > 100 mg/dL or drug treatment for elevated glucose

► Low HDL levels, < 40 mg/dL in men, < 50 mg/dL in women or drug treatment for reduced HDL

► Elevated waist circumference > 40 inches in men and > 35 inches in women

► Elevated triglycerides > 150 mg/dL or drug treatment for elevated triglycerides (Grundy et al., 2005)

Management includes weight loss, exercise, and dietary modifications. Patients should be encouraged to start with 5%–10% loss of their initial weight by decreasing their daily caloric intake by 500 calories per day, and to begin or increase their physical activity by 10–15 minutes per day until they are exercising 300 minutes per week (American Diabetes Association, 2012).

Food logs can be helpful. Pharmaceutical therapy may be an option for some older adults. For patients with a BMI of > 27 kg/m^2, orlistat may be prescribed. Bariatric surgery may be a consideration in selected older adults with a BMI of > 40 kg/m^2.

Diabetes mellitus is a hyperglycemic state that results from the impairment of insulin secretion, insulin action, insulin transport, or a combination of the three. It is characterized by repeated fasting blood sugar levels of > 125 mg/dL or any postprandial level of > 200 mg/dL. In many cases with older adults, the issue is insulin resistance rather than insulin absence.

The cause of diabetes is unknown, but experts believe that genetics, rising obesity levels, and environmental factors all play a role. The sequelae of diabetes can be devastating; thus, it is of paramount importance that this disease entity be identified and properly treated.

In type 1 disease, the insulin-secreting ability of the pancreas is absent or near absent. Patients with type II disease may have problems with insulin secretion, but they can still produce insulin in normal or supranormal levels (American Diabetes Association, 2012). Patients with type 2 diabetes often are obese, a state that is associated with high levels of native insulin production, which in turn may alter the number or function of the insulin receptors on the cell wall. For some reason, glucose cannot enter the cell, and excess insulin is produced to compensate for this problem, rendering a patient hyperinsulinemic.

Some patients with type 2 disease have defects in their insulin receptors that cause insulin to transport glucose ineffectively into the cells; other patients may have decreased or inadequate insulin secretion. The pathophysiological changes can vary from patient to patient.

Signs and symptoms may include polydipsia, polyuria, or polyphagia. Older patients may present atypically with fatigue, blurred vision, infection, or change in weight. Often, older adults are diagnosed when they present to a healthcare provider with another problem. Symptoms common in older diabetics include:

- ► Infection of foot or cellulitis of the leg
- ► Vaginitis
- ► Urinary tract infections (UTIs)
- ► Impotence
- ► Numbness of fingers or toes

Diagnostics include fasting and postprandial glucose levels, glycosylated hemoglobin, and urine for microalbumin. Medical management includes sulfonylureas, biguanides, secretagogues, thiazolidinediones, alpha-glucosidase inhibitors, insulin, and combinations of these agents.

Assessment includes review of medical history, medications, and family history for diabetes. For patients already diagnosed with diabetes, gerontological nurses should determine current medications, glucose monitoring, history of high or low blood sugars, and any self-care restrictions or issues that could interfere with managing the diabetic state. Nutritional assessment should be done and includes changes in weight, dietary patterns, signs/symptoms of nausea, vomiting, polydipsia, or polyphagia.

Nurses should assess patient readiness and ability to learn when beginning diabetes education. Past and present blood glucose readings should be reviewed. Patients should be asked about neurological sequelae of diabetes:

- ▶ Numbness
- ▶ Tingling
- ▶ Blurred vision
- ▶ Headaches
- ▶ Inability to feel temperature

The physical examination should include the skin, specifically that of the legs and feet. Nurses should document skin turgor, dryness, peeling, lesions, pedal pulses, and presence or absence of hair growth on the lower extremities (Reuben et al., 2011).

Nursing management includes education; diet and medication counseling; emergency identification; and instructions for monitoring, exercise, lifestyle changes, sick day management, skin changes, and wound infections. Referral to a nurse who is a certified diabetes educator (CDE) should be considered.

General diabetes education includes pathophysiology of the disease, why it is important to monitor glucose and urine ketones, etiology and manifestations of hypo- and hyperglycemia, foot and eye care, complications, and products/supplies.

Diet counseling should be directed by a dietitian. The cornerstone of dietary intervention is weight normalization and good nutrition. The American Diabetes Association recommends these nutritional guidelines:

- ▶ Eat lots of fruits and vegetables.
- ▶ Avoid starchy vegetables such as potatoes, corn, and peas.
- ▶ Eat fish 2–3 times per week.
- ▶ Choose lean meats, and remove skin from chicken and turkey.
- ▶ Choose nonfat dairy items such as skim milk, nonfat yogurt, and nonfat cheese.
- ▶ Avoid sugary drinks such as sweetened ice tea and soda.
- ▶ Choose liquid oils for cooking instead of solid fats.
- ▶ Cut back on ice cream and calorie-laden desserts.
- ▶ Watch your portion sizes—even "healthy" foods can add weight if eaten in large enough quantities.

Medication counseling includes education about the medications that have been prescribed such as insulin, oral agents, or both. Table 18–2 describes oral agents commonly used for older adults with diabetes, and Table 18–3 describes insulin preparations.

TABLE 18–2.
COMMON DIABETES MEDICATIONS USED FOR OLDER ADULTS

CHEMICAL CLASS	MECHANISM OF ACTION	COMMON DRUG NAMES (NOT INCLUSIVE)	GERIATRIC CONSIDERATIONS
Biguanides	▶ Decrease hepatic glucose production ▶ Increase skeletal muscle uptake of glucose	Metformin Metformin XR Fortamet	▶ Must have adequate renal function to use ▶ Calculated GFR should be 55 cc/min or more to use ▶ Not FDA approved for individuals ages 80 or older
Enzyme inhibitors	Increases the amount of enzymes naturally occurring in the body to lower blood sugar	Januvia Onglyza	Can lower HbA1C by 0.5%–1%. May be monotherapy or in combination with metformin or a thiazolidinedione.
Thiazolidinediones	▶ Decrease hepatic glucose production ▶ Increase skeletal muscle uptake of glucose ▶ Increase the efficiency and number of glucose receptors on the cell membrane	Rosiglitazone	▶ Contraindicated in Stages III and IV HF ▶ Can cause fluid retention
Sulfonylureas	Increase insulin secretion	Glipizide Glimepiride	Can cause hypoglycemia and weight gain
Secretagogues	Increase insulin secretion, but only for a limited time after each dose ingested (which is taken with each meal eaten)	Nateglinide Repaglinide	Can cause hypoglycemia and weight gain
Alpha-glucosidase inhibitors		Acarbose Miglitol	Can cause abdominal bloating and increased flatus; must titrate up dose slowly
Meglitinides	Increase insulin secretion	Starlix Prandin	Take 30 minutes before meals

CHEMICAL CLASS	MECHANISM OF ACTION	COMMON DRUG NAMES (NOT INCLUSIVE)	GERIATRIC CONSIDERATIONS
Injectable agents	Incretin mimetic actions. Works by stimulating the pancreas to secrete more insulin.	Byetta Victoza	Less weight gain than insulin. Avoid if CrCl < 30 mL/min. Victoza associated with risk of acute pancreatitis and possibly medullary thyroid cancer.

Note: CrCl = creatinine clearance, GFR = glomerular filtration rate, FDA = U.S. Food and Drug Administration, HF = heart failure.

TABLE 18-3.
INSULIN PREPARATIONS USED TO TREAT DIABETES MELLITUS

PREPARATION	ONSET/PEAK	COMMON DRUG NAMES (NOT INCLUSIVE)	GERIATRIC CONSIDERATIONS
Rapid-acting	20 min/0.5–1.5 hrs 15 min/0.5–1.5 hrs 30 min/1–3 hrs	Apidra Humalog Novolog	Monitor for signs and symptoms of hypoglycemia. Rotate injection site at least every 48 hours. Dosage decrease may be needed with renal dysfunction.
Regular	1–3 hrs	Humulin Novolin	May be mixed with other insulin and stored for future use.
Intermediate or long-acting	1–12 hrs 6–8 hrs 2–24 hrs 30 min–12 hrs	NPH – Humulin, Novolin Insulin detemir – Levemir Insulin glargine – Lantus Isophane and regular insulin inj, premixed – Novolin 70/30	Caution with dosing. Monitor blood sugars frequently during initiation of treatment. Increase dose in stress, illness, infection, and trauma.

Adapted from *Geriatrics at Your Fingertips* (13th ed.), by D. Reuben, K. Herr, J. Pacala, B. Pollock, J. Potter, & T. Semla, 2011, New York: American Geriatrics Society; and *Nurse Practitioner's Prescribing Reference*, 2011, New York: Haymarket Media Publication.

Emergency identification is important for patients with all types of diabetes; these patients should wear medic alert bracelets or necklaces. Home glucose monitoring is critical in the management of this disease. Older patients should be taught and expected to monitor their blood sugars at home. Some are as capable as their younger counterparts, while others may be capable of only limited efforts. Nurses and primary healthcare providers should work together to devise a monitoring schedule that works for each patient.

Exercise helps reduce insulin resistance and hyperglycemia. Patients should be educated about an appropriate exercise regimen on the basis of their comorbid illnesses. Patients should know to check their blood sugar before exercising, carry a source of carbohydrates in the event of low blood sugar, and not exercise if their blood sugar is > 250 mg/dL. When glucoses are high, insulin is insufficient because of some mechanism. Exercise can worsen high blood sugar and cause the production of free fatty acids and ketones; in addition, insufficient insulin stimulates glucose release from the liver (Huether & McCance, 2012).

Lifestyle changes may include avoidance of drugs of abuse, such as alcohol, tobacco, and illicit agents, as applicable to each patient. Sick day management also is an important education point. A sick day would be taken when a patient has an infection, viral illness, or flulike symptoms. During these times, patients may have quite elevated blood sugars and should have some guidelines on when to call their primary healthcare providers and when and how to adjust their medications, if applicable.

Skin changes from diabetes can include dryness, cracking, and fissuring of the plantar aspect of the feet. Patients with diabetes also may lose the ability to sweat, which can accentuate any potential foot problems. Patients should be taught the importance of daily diabetic foot exams and how to properly cleanse and dry their feet.

Wound infections are among the most serious complications of diabetes. *Diabetic foot syndrome* is the term used to describe the vascular and neurological changes that can be seen in the lower extremities of patients with diabetes. Decreased arterial flow and nerve damage from hyperglycemia contribute to this condition and can lead to amputation. A patient who presents with a foot lesion should be inspected critically. If the foot is red and swollen, yet the lesion is small and without drainage, the real problem may be deeper in the tissues, such as an abscess below the fascia. Patients with foot ulcers may present with pain, swelling, redness, or no symptoms at all. The infections often are polymicrobial and include *Klebsiella, Enterobacter, Corynebacteria, Bacteroides fragilis,* and *Clostridia.*

NEUROLOGICAL DISEASES

During aging, the changes in the neurological system can range from pronounced to subtle and can lead to cerebrovascular disease—specifically stroke and movement disorders.

Stroke

Stroke or a *cerebrovascular accident* (CVA) occurs when impaired circulation to the brain disrupts the supply of oxygen. The signs occur suddenly and last more than 24 hours. A stroke is a medical emergency. A *transient ischemic attack* (TIA) consists of the same symptoms but lasts less than 24 hours. For patients with manifestations of a stroke or TIA, treatment is of upmost importance; however, the cause of the event must be identified to prevent future episodes.

Stroke is the fourth leading cause of death and the leading neurological disability in the United States. Strokes are divided into two types: ischemic and hemorrhagic. Ischemic stroke, which occurs when blood clots block the blood vessels to the brain, is the most common type of stroke, representing about 87% of all strokes (CDC, 2011).

When blood flow to an area of the brain is reduced, hypoxia occurs. This process can cause tissue ischemia and death. Short-term hypoxia causes the signs and symptoms of TIA, while prolonged hypoxia causes CVA. When an infarct occurs, the affected brain tissue is deprived of oxygen and becomes necrotic. The amount of brain damage depends on the location and size of the vessel affected and adequacy of collateral circulation.

Risk factors include inflammatory artery disease, sickle cell anemia, HTN, atherosclerosis, emboli, previous heart surgery, smoking, hyperlipidemia, family history of strokes, thrombosis, substance abuse, diabetes mellitus, AF, and head trauma.

Ischemic strokes can have one of three etiologies: thrombosis, cardioembolic, or small-vessel intracerebral occlusion (lacunar strokes). The most common causes of ischemic strokes, as mentioned above, are atherosclerosis, inflammatory disease, or a thrombus from a place outside the brain (such as the cardiovascular system).

Hemorrhagic strokes, on the other hand, are divided into two etiologies: *subarachnoid* and *intracerebral* (CDC, 2011). The most common cause is uncontrolled HTN. According to Huether and McCance (2001), other causes of hemorrhagic events include:

▶ Intercerebral aneurysm rupture

▶ Arteriovenous malformation (AVM)

▶ Bleeding from a tumor

▶ Hemorrhage from anticoagulation or blood dyscrasia

▶ Head trauma

▶ Illicit drug use, specifically cocaine

Risk factor identification and modification for TIAs and both types of strokes are important nursing responsibilities. Of course, some risk factors, such as age, are not modifiable, but those that are should be addressed:

▶ HTN

▶ Diabetes

▶ CVD

▶ AF

▶ Dyslipidemia

▶ Smoking

▶ Obesity

▶ Sedentary lifestyle

▶ High stress levels

▶ Heavy alcohol use

▶ Illicit drug use, especially cocaine

▶ Operable occlusion of an arterial vessel (carotid or vertebral)

▶ Patent foramen ovale

▶ Abrupt cessation of antihypertensive regimen that precipitates a hypertensive crisis (CDC, 2011)

Clinical symptoms depend on the area of the brain involved. If the anterior circulation (internal carotid arteries) is involved, patients may have blurred vision, temporary loss of central vision in one eye (amaurosis fugax), paresthesias, or weakness. If the posterior circulation is involved (vertebral/basilar arteries), patients may have ataxia, diplopia, facial weakness, circumoral numbness, bilateral sensory abnormalities, or bilateral motor abnormalities. Early warning signs of a TIA that is thrombotic in nature include transient paresis, dysarthria or loss of speech, abnormal sensory changes, and paresthesias of one side of the body.

Signs and symptoms that can precede a hemorrhage stroke may include occipital headache, fainting, paresthesias, epistaxis, dizziness, or retinal hemorrhage (Reuben et al., 2011). Diagnostic tests are important to the way an acute neurological event is treated. Any patient with an acute stroke is given a noncontrast CT or MRI of the brain to determine if the stroke is caused by a hemorrhage or a thrombus. An EKG is also done to assess for cardiac cause of the event (such as new onset of AF). Additional tests that may be ordered are chemistry and hematologic profiles, echocardiogram, transeophageal echocardiogram, or carotid artery Doppler studies.

The National Institute of Neurologic Disorders and Stroke (NINDS) revolutionalized the treatment of stroke when it completed its 1996 landmark study. This study proved that use of thrombolytic agents within a 3-hour window of onset of symptoms reduced morbidity and mortality from stroke. How patients are treated greatly depends on how soon they present to the emergency room or stroke center. Patients who present within 3 hours of when symptoms begin and have no exclusion criteria (noted below) are treated with recombinant tissue plasminogen activators (r-TPA). These agents dissolve the clot and restore circulation to the hypoxic tissues. According to NINDS (1997, 2012), exclusion criteria for use of r-TPA include:

▶ Current use of an anticoagulant

▶ Prothrombin time of > 15 seconds

▶ Use of heparin within the past 48 hours

▶ Platelet count of < 100,000 per mm^3

▶ History of recent heart attack

▶ Bleeding from the urinary tract within the past 3 weeks

- ► History of intracranial bleeding
- ► Major surgery within the past 2 weeks
- ► Rapidly improving neurologic signs
- ► History of stroke or head trauma within the past 3 months
- ► Presence of very mild, isolated (a single) neurological deficits, such as ataxia, sensory loss, dysarthria, and minimal weakness
- ► Elevated BP readings before the use of r-TPA that are > 185 systolic or > 110 diastolic

If the patient is not a candidate for r-TPA, other agents that are given include anticoagulants (e.g., Heparin, Lovenox) and antiplatelet therapy (aspirin or clopidogrel [Plavix]). These drugs are used to reduce the growth of the clot (Reuben et al., 2011).

The BP of patients who are acutely ill and hospitalized is monitored closely. Pressors are titrated to keep BP > 180/105 and hypotension (which can worsen the neurological insult) is avoided. Common agents used to decrease blood pressure are labetalol or nitroprusside. If the stroke was caused by a subarachnoid hemorrhage, calcium channel blockers such as nimodipine are used to decrease or prevent vasospasm of the vessels (NINDS, 2012).

In some cases, the treatment of choice for stroke or TIA is surgical intervention, most commonly an internal carotid endarterectomy. Other surgical management used in specific stroke cases includes:

- ► Extracranial to intracranial bypass
- ► Vertebral artery endarterectomy
- ► Repair of AVM
- ► Repair of cerebral aneurysm
- ► Evacuation of intracranial bleeding

Acute nursing management includes positioning to prevent an increase in intracranial pressure by elevating the head of the bed 30–45 degrees. Vital signs must be monitored closely. Other nursing interventions include:

- ► Range-of-motion exercises
- ► Reposition patient every 2 hours
- ► Monitor lower extremities for signs of DVT
- ► Resume and monitor dietary intake (after a swallowing evaluation has been done)
- ► Teach alternate methods of communication for patients with dysarthria
- ► Teach patients with visual field defects how to turn the head to enlarge the visual field
- ► Collaborate with physical and occupational therapists throughout the course of rehabilitation (NINDS, 2012)

Education of patients about the etiology of stroke and preventative strategies also is in order. Patients will slowly improve in varying degrees over time, and the gerontological nurse's role in this process is critical. Nurses should evaluate stroke patients using these criteria:

► Cerebral perfusion status

► Respiratory status

► Signs and symptoms of aspiration

► Prevention of contractures

► Skin breakdown

► Pain

► Fecal and urinary status (e.g., incontinence)

► Dependent edema on the affected side

► Functional status (e.g., mobility; compensation for sensory, motor, visual, and speech deficits)

► Ability to discuss feelings about the stroke

► Involvement of family and or significant others

Stroke can leave older patients with significant functional disability after the acute phase of the illness. Rehabilitation is extensive, with family counseling and education as priorities.

Movement Disorders

Older adults often experience common movement disorders, such as essential tremor, Parkinson's disease, and various forms of dizziness.

Essential tremor (ET) is usually a mild tremor of the head and upper extremities. The upper-extremity manifestations involve purposeful movements, such as holding a coffee cup or signing a check. These symptoms are relieved with rest and ingestion of small amounts of alcohol. For the most part, individuals with ET first develop signs and symptoms in their mid- to late 40s, and the symptoms progress mildly over time. This entity, although common, is benign in nature and responds well to low doses of beta-blockers, such as propranolol, nadolol, and mysoline. For the most part, patients with ET remain active and can complete all of their own ADLs (NINDS, 2012).

Parkinson's disease (PD) is a slowly progressive deterioration of the basal ganglia that destroys the dopamine pathways. It presents in patients as progressive slowness of movement, resting tremor, muscular rigidity, and loss of postural reflexes. Additional diagnostic criteria include muscle rigidity (cogwheeling), slowness of movement, and impaired righting reflex after a sternal nudge (Reuben et al., 2011). Parkinson's disease occurs in approximately 1% of persons age 60 years and in about 4% of those age 80 years. Because overall life expectancy is rising, the number of individuals with Parkinson's disease will increase in the future (MedicineNet.com, 2012).

The *basal ganglia* is a neuronal area located deep in the cerebellum. These cells control muscle tone and smooth voluntary movements. These normal movements are controlled by the secretion of acetylcholine (ACh), which is an excitatory neurotransmitter, and dopamine, which is an inhibitory substance. Dopamine itself is produced in the substantia nigra, and it is transported for its actions to the basal ganglia. Without dopamine, there is no way to control fine motor and voluntary movements (Huether & McCance, 2012).

In PD, the deterioration in the dopamine pathways causes a lack of dopamine in the basal ganglia; therefore, there is an imbalance between ACh and dopamine. This imbalance causes the classic symptoms of hypertonia such as tremor, rigidity (dyskinesia), slowness of movement (bradykinesia), or lack of movement (akinesia).

Risk factors include:

► Drug-induced Parkinsonism

► Toxin-induced Parkinsonism

► Exposure to certain herbicides and pesticides

► Trauma to the midbrain

► Stroke

Despite the aforementioned risk factors, most cases are idiopathic. In most individuals, the symptoms begin insidiously.

Resting tremor is probably the most common sign. Most patients with PD have difficulty with balance and feel as if their muscles are "weak." Patients will experience difficulty getting up out of a chair, walking backward, or turning around in a small area. During the trajectory of the disease, these individuals also develop the following:

► *Festination:* Patients can take only small steps.

► *Freezing:* Patients suddenly stop, as if frozen in place.

► *Propulsive gait:* Patients walk flexed forward, taking small steps, and their gait gets progressively faster (as if they are running); they may not be able to stop themselves unless they fall or run into an object.

► *Retropulsion:* Patients walk and then have a tendency to fall backward.

Patients also experience rigidity of the muscles around the face and head. As a result of this rigidity, patients develop a staring gaze.

The autonomic nervous system is markedly affected by PD. Patients experience postural hypotension, excess perspiration of the face and neck (yet none on the trunk or extremities), constipation, seborrhea on the face and neck, and heat intolerance. As the disease becomes more progressive, patients become more disabled, having mood disturbances, sleep disturbances, dysphagia, and frequent falls (usually backward).

PD is a clinical diagnosis, which means that no specific tests can be done to "prove the diagnosis." Diagnosis is made based on the patient's signs and symptoms. Drug screens or MRI of the brain might be in order if there is a question about an endogenous cause. For the most part, the diagnosis is made in the healthcare provider's office, and it is confirmed when the patient responds to anti-Parkinson medications.

Management is centered on relieving symptoms, improving functional status, and decreasing injury. PD is one of the few diseases in which patients will improve with more medications. Patients will have to take more and more medications throughout the duration of illness to continue to be mobile. Table 18–4 describes some medications commonly used to treat PD.

TABLE 18–4.
COMMON MEDICATIONS USED IN PARKINSON'S DISEASE

DRUG CLASS	DRUG NAMES	MECHANISM OF ACTION
Monoamine oxidase inhibitors	Selegiline (Eldepryl) Rasagline (Azilect)	Inhibit monoamine oxidase Type B from converting chemical byproducts into neurotoxins that can cause cell death in the substantia nigra
Dopamine agonists	Ropinirole (Requip) Pramipexole (Mirapex)	Stimulate the dopamine-producing cells to work more effectively, thus increasing endogenous dopamine levels
Dopaminergics	Amantadine (Symmetrel) Carbidopa-levidopa (Sinemet, Sinemet CR)	Supply exogenous dopamine in an attempt to replace what is deficient
Catechol O-methyltransferase (COMT) inhibitors	Tolcapone (Tasmar) Entacapone (Comtan)	Prevent the peripheral degradation of dopamine before it enters the central nervous system, therefore increasing the amount of usable dopamine supplied to the brain (from the oral dopaminergics being given to the patient)
Anticholinergics	Cogentin Artane	Monitor for delirium and other anticholinergic side effects

Adapted from "Cognitive and Neurological Function," by K. Imperio & E. Pusey-Reid, 2006, in S. E. Meiner & A. G. Lueckenotte (Eds.), *Gerontological Nursing* (pp. 653–591), St. Louis, MO: Mosby/Elsevier; and *Geriatrics at Your Fingertips* (13th ed.), by D. Reuben, K. Herr, J. Pacala, B. Pollock, J. Potter, & T. Semla, 2011, New York: American Geriatrics Society.

Although most of the aforementioned agents work well initially, the effects seem to wane with duration of use. When this happens, patients will develop an "on-and-off" response, as if the drugs suddenly have worn off, and patients become unable to move.

As the population has aged, more and more research has been done on treatments for PD. Currently, three categories of surgical therapies can be used in certain patients:

▶ *Ablation:* Certain neuronal tissues are destroyed, decreasing the amount of tissue that can produce the excitable neurotransmitter ACh.

▶ *Deep brain stimulation:* This works in the same fashion as ablation.

▶ *Transplantation with fetal neural tissues:* The idea is to give patients normal dopamine-producing brain cells; this procedure is still in the experimental phase.

In addition to medication, maintenance of function status is critical. Patients will require the help of physical therapy, occupational therapy, and speech therapy. Patients also will need structured exercise programs.

Nursing interventions include teaching patients the importance of exercise, the use of assistive devices, and strategies to prevent injuries. Gerontological nurses should assess patient speech pattern and nutritional parameters. Patients and their family members should be referred to community resources such as the American Parkinson's Disease Association (www.apdaparkinson.org) and the National Parkinson's Foundation (www.parkinson.org). Education should include the fact that PD is progressive and will require many medications over the duration of illness. Involvement of the family is of utmost importance in the care of patients with PD.

Dizziness is the most common complaint of older adults and often has multiple causes in the same individual:

▶ Vertigo

▶ Pre-syncope

▶ Imbalance or disequilibrium

▶ Nonspecific lightheadedness

▶ "Mixed" dizziness

There are numerous causes for each type of dizziness, making the complaint one of the most perplexing to diagnose (Table 18–5).

TABLE 18-5.
TYPES OF DIZZINESS

VERTIGO	PRE-SYNCOPE	DISEQUILIBRIUM	LIGHT-HEADEDNESS
Acute ▸ Infection ▸ Seizure ▸ Drug toxicity ▸ Trauma ▸ Tumor ▸ Vascular event **Recurrent** ▸ Hypothyroidism ▸ Ménière's disease ▸ Migraine ▸ Multiple sclerosis ▸ Seizure ▸ Syphilis ▸ Transient ischemic attack **Positional** ▸ Benign positional ▸ Cervical spine disease ▸ Postinfectious ▸ Posttrauma	**Orthostatic hypotension** ▸ Increased vagal tone ▸ Acute stress ▸ Pain ▸ Urination ▸ Vasovagal reaction ▸ Hyperventilation	**Cervical spine disease** **Medication toxicity** **Multiple sensory impairments** **Muscle weakness** **Unstable joints** **Neurologic disease** ▸ Cerebellar degeneration ▸ Myelopathy ▸ Parkinson's disease ▸ Peripheral neuropathy ▸ Stroke	▸ Carbon monoxide intoxication ▸ Hyperventilation ▸ Medications ▸ Psychiatric disorders ▸ Stroke ▸ Visual disorders

Adapted from *Geriatrics at Your Fingertips* (13th ed.), by D. Reuben, K. Herr, J. Pacala, B. Pollock, J. Potter, & T. Semla, 2011, New York: American Geriatrics Society; *Understanding Pathophysiology* (5th ed.) by S. Huether & K. McCance, 2012, St. Louis, MO: Mosby; and *Current Medical Diagnosis and Treatment* (50th ed.) by S. McPhee & M. Papadakis, 2011, New York: McGraw Hill Medical.

Vertigo and orthostatic hypotension are the most common etiologies of dizziness in older adults. *Vertigo* can be divided into two broad classes: peripheral or central. *Peripheral vertigo* originates in the vestibular system of the inner ear. *Central vertigo* results from a disruption of blood flow to the cerebellum, which is the brain's balance center.

The most common causes of peripheral vertigo in older adults are acute labyrinthitis, recurrent vestibular syndromes, and benign paroxysmal positional vertigo (BPPV). *Labyrinthitis* is caused by a viral infection or vascular injury to the labyrinth. This condition presents with sudden onset nausea, vomiting, and vertigo. If the auditory portion of the labyrinth is affected, tinnitus and hearing loss also may occur.

Recurrent vestibular syndromes encompass Ménière's disease and recurrent vestibulopathy. Ménière's disease causes recurrent attacks of vertigo accompanied by tinnitus and hearing loss. Usually there is associated ear pain or fullness. Ménière's is treated with salt restriction, diuretics, and discontinuation of caffeine and nicotine. *Recurrent vestibulopathy* is a syndrome that often follows an acute cause of vertigo but usually resolves with time. It also can be migraine-related.

BPPV causes short episodes of vertigo (less than 1 minute) that are brought on by changes in head or body position. BPPV is caused by calcium particles (otoliths) that break off from the sacule or uticle, then migrate into the semicircular canal. Attacks of BPPV usually last 1 to 2 weeks, but often recur months or years later. Symptomatic treatment with meclizine is sometimes prescribed. Vestibular retraining exercises are useful to diminish symptoms.

Many age-related changes in the cardiovascular system favor the development of *orthostatic hypotension* in older adults (see Box 18–1). Other factors may aggravate this tendency, such as:

▶ Anemia

▶ Deconditioning

▶ Dehydration

▶ Hypokalemia

▶ Medications—Sinemet, nitroglycerine, anticholinergics, tricyclic antidepressants, diuretics, narcotics, benzodiazepines, and various antihypertensives

▶ Varicose veins

▶ Aortic stenosis

▶ Hypertrophic obstructive cardiomyopathy

BOX 18–1.
AGE-RELATED CHANGES IN THE CARDIOVASCULAR SYSTEM
▸ Changes in arterial compliance
▸ Impaired diastolic filling
▸ Impaired renal sodium conservation
▸ Lower rennin, angiotensin, and aldosterone levels
▸ Increased levels of atrial naturetic peptide
▸ Lower maximum heart rate

The textbook definition of orthostatic hypotension requires a 20 mm Hg drop in systolic BP or 10 mm Hg drop in diastolic pressure on standing. Many older adults do not meet this standard definition, yet still have significant symptoms. Often, a drop in BP will not occur for several minutes after standing, and dizziness may affect older adults once they begin to walk. Another high-risk time is after eating, when circulation is shunted to the stomach and intestines to aid in the digestion of food. Orthostatic hypotension can result in increased risk of falls and fractures, stroke, and MI (Reuben et al., 2011).

Treatment involves eliminating aggravating factors or reversible causes, increasing fluid and salt intake, and elevating the head of bed. Education must include information about standing up slowly and using support until dizziness passes. This is particularly important after meals. In addition, wearing compression stockings during the day is helpful for most patients.

When symptoms persist despite these measures, it may be necessary for patients to take a medication to raise BP, such as Florinef (fludrocortisone acetate) or ProAmantine (midodrine).

REFERENCES

Centers for Disease Control and Prevention. (2012). *Osteoarthritis and you.* Retrieved from http://www.cdc. gov/Features/OsteoarthritisPlan/

Grundy, S., Cleeman, J., Daniels, S., Donato, K., Eckel, R., Franklin, B., Gordon, D., Kraus, R., Savage, P., Smith, S., Spertus, J., & Costa, F. (2005). Diagnosis and management of metabolic syndrome: An American Heart Association/National Heart, Lung, and Blood Institute Scientific Statement Executive Summary, *Circulation 112,* e285–e290.

Huether, S., & McCance, K. (2012). *Understanding pathophysiology* (5th ed.). St. Louis, MO: Mosby.

McPhee, S., & Papadakis, M. (2011). *Current medical diagnosis and treatment* (50th ed.). New York: McGraw Hill Medical.

Meiner, S. E. (2006). Musculoskeletal function. In S. E. Meiner & A. S. Luggen (Eds.), *Gerontological nursing* (3rd ed., pp. 596–629). St. Louis, MO: Mosby/Elsevier.

National Center for Complementary and Alternative Medicine. (2008). *Questions and answers: NIH Glucosamine/Chondroitin arthritis intervention trial primary study.* Retrieved from http://nccam.nih. gov/research/results/gait/qa.htm

Nurse practitioners' prescribing reference. (2012). New York: Haymarket Media Publication.

Reuben, D., Herr, K., Pacala, J., Pollock, B., Potter, J., & Semla, T. (2011). *Geriatrics at your fingertips* (13th ed.). New York: American Geriatrics Society.

Sweet, R. (2012). *Osteoarthritis.* Retrieved from https://www.louortho.com/documents/ OSTEOARTHRITISoverview_001.pdf

Sweet, M., Sweet, J., Jeremiah, M., & Galazka, S. (2009). Diagnosis and treatment of osteoporosis. *American Family Physician, 79* (3), 193–200.

U.S. Department of Health and Human Services. (2010). *Multiple chronic conditions—A strategic framework: Optimum health and quality of life for individuals with multiple chronic conditions.* Washington, DC: Author.

World Health Organization Collaborating Centre for Metabolic Bone Diseases, University of Sheffield, UK. (2012). *Frax. WHO Fracture Risk Assessment Tool.* Retrieved from http://www.shef.ac.uk/FRAX/index.jsp

ADDITIONAL RESOURCES

Chronic and Disabling Conditions: www.agingsociety.org/

Healthy People 2020: www.healthypeople.gov/2020/

National Osteoporosis Foundation: www.nof.org

Osteoporosis Screening: www.ahcpr.gov/clinic/3rduspstf/osteoporosis

DISORDERS OF THE INTEGUMENTARY SYSTEM

The skin is considered the largest organ of the human body and, like other systems, it changes with normal aging. Many skin manifestations seen later in life are the result of prior sun exposure and become common geriatric dermatoses: benign skin growths, inflammatory skin conditions, eczema, herpes zoster, scabies, carcinoma, and pressure ulcers.

Benign Skin Growths

Benign lesions have no malignant potential; however, they are very common in older adults, who often question nurses or primary healthcare providers about these "unsightly areas." It is important to be able to recognize these common dermatoses to reassure patients. The common benign skin growths of aging are cherry angiomas, seborrheic keratosis, and acrochordons (see Table 19–1).

TABLE 19-1.
COMMON BENIGN SKIN LESIONS OF OLDER ADULTS

LESION	DESCRIPTION	COMMON LOCATION	TREATMENT
Cherry angioma	▸ 1–5 mm red or deep-purple, dome-shaped lesions ▸ New growth resulting from increased vascularity in the dermis	Trunk	None
Seborrheic keratosis	▸ Scaly brownish-black lesions that have a "stuck-on" appearance ▸ Can be 2–4 mm in size ▸ Has a greasy brown appearance, but, because of the dark color, patients are concerned that they have a melanoma	Sun-exposed areas such as face, neck, and trunk	▸ Cryotherapy ▸ Removed for cosmetic purposes or if inflamed
Acrochordon	▸ "Skin tags" ▸ Small, stalk-like lesions, usually flesh-colored	Neck Axilla Breasts Groin	▸ Electrocautery Cryotherapy ▸ Cut off with scissors ▸ Removed for cosmetic reasons only

Inflammatory Skin Problems

The three most common inflammatory skin problems of older adults include seborrheic dermatitis, intertrigo, and psoriasis. Summary information, based on Friedman's (2006) synopsis of each of these lesions, is presented in Table 19–2.

TABLE 19–2.
COMMON INFLAMMATORY SKIN CONDITIONS OF OLDER ADULTS

LESION	DESCRIPTION	LOCATION	THERAPY	NURSING CONSIDERATIONS
Seborrheic dermatitis	▸ Inflammatory response with scaling ▸ Thought to be a reaction to the yeast, Pityrosporum ovale ▸ White or yellow scale with the appearance of a plaque on an erythematous base	▸ Begins in scalp and moves downward symmetrically to ear canals, eyebrows, eyelashes, nasolabial folds, axilla, breasts, chest, and groin	▸ Shampoo the affected areas with solutions that contain selenium, zinc, or ketoconazole ▸ Shampoo should be left on for 20 minutes twice weekly for 3 weeks ▸ Hot oil treatments with peanut oil will reduce the amount of scale in the scalp ▸ Low-to-moderate-potency hydrocortisone ointments for inflammation ▸ T-cell modulators, such as pimecrolimus (Elidel) can be used on face and in recalcitrant areas	▸ This condition requires repeated treatments, because it is chronic ▸ Patient should understand the recurrence of symptoms is common and, when symptoms recur, treatment regimens should be restarted
Intertrigo	▸ Form of seborrheic dermatitis that results from friction of skin surfaces ▸ Areas are erythematous and itchy	▸ Armpits ▸ Inner aspects of thighs ▸ Skin beneath the breasts ▸ Abdominal folds	▸ Weight loss ▸ Keeping the skin clean and dry ▸ Topical antifungals ▸ In rare cases, topical hydrocortisone may be indicated	▸ Lifestyle modifications are critical ▸ Keeping the areas dry and use of an antifungal powder after morning shower or bath may be needed to prevent frequent recurrences
Psoriasis	▸ Considered an autoimmune disease ▸ Well-demarcated pink plaques covered with silver-white scale; when the scale is removed, there is pinpoint bleeding ▸ Scales are the result of accelerated replication of the dermis and epidermis ▸ Patients may have constitutional symptoms such as fever, arthralgias, and leukocytosis	▸ Skin of the elbows, knees, scalp, lumbosacral, and intergluteal areas ▸ Affects the nails in 30% of patients (yellow-brown discoloration with thickening and onycholysis)	▸ Topical steroids or coal tar preparations ▸ Topical vitamin D_3 for moderate cases—Calcipotriene ointment (Dovonex) ▸ Topical retinoids (vitamin A analogues) such as tazarotene (Tazorac) with/without ultraviolet B light therapy for more severe cases ▸ Therapy of choice is ultraviolet A light therapy plus oral or topical psoralen (PUVA therapy)	▸ Avoid triggers such as smoking and excess stress ▸ Teach the etiology and ≠chronicity of this illness; patients should understand that treatment may be lifelong

Adapted from "Integumentary Function," by S. Friedman, 2006, in S. E. Meiner & A. G. Lueckenotte (Eds.), *Gerontological Nursing* (pp. 693–729), St. Louis, MO: Mosby/Elsevier; and *Geriatrics at Your Fingertips* (13th ed.), by D. Reuben, K. Herr, J. Pacala, B. Pollock, J. Potter, & T. Semla, 2011, New York: American Geriatrics Society.

Eczema

Eczema is a chronic inflammatory dermatitis. Affected individuals often will have a history of atopy. This entity is characterized by dry, pruritic skin. Dermatologists often refer to eczema as the "itch that rashes." Because of the intense pruritus, patients develop 4–5-cm coin-shaped plaques on the dorsum of the hands, antecubital fossas, and anterior parts of the lower legs.

Classically, patients are men with a history of dry skin. Patients develop grouped papules on an erythematous base. With persistent scratching, these papules coalesce and become well demarcated and thickened (lichenified). As a result, patients will have easy-to-identify coin-shaped (nummular) lesions.

Treatment for this chronic condition includes avoidance of irritants and use of emollients and low- to medium-potency topical steroids. Gerontological nurses should be alert for bacterial and fungal suprainfection in these individuals. Nursing interventions include education about the chronicity of this disease and the importance of preventing excess dryness of the skin.

Herpes Zoster

Herpes zoster, or *shingles*, is an eruption caused by reactivation of latent varicella virus in the dorsal root ganglia. The virus remains in the dorsal root ganglia after an earlier episode of chickenpox. For the most part, the varicella virus recurs because of depression of immune response. A wide variety of causes of this immunosuppression can lead to shingles:

▶ Age (most common)

▶ Stress

▶ Fatigue

▶ Radiation

▶ HIV/AIDS

▶ Any malignancy

▶ Chemotherapy

▶ Steroids

Herpes zoster is not infectious except in individuals age 6 months or older who have not had chickenpox or the vaccine for chickenpox. Up until age 6 months, infants have maternal antibodies that protect them from the virus.

Shingles most commonly occurs on the thorax; however, it can be seen in the cervical and lumber areas (10%) or in the ophthalmic areas (15%). Herpes zoster in the ophthalmic branch of the trigeminal nerve is a true medical emergency; patients should be seen urgently by an ophthalmologist. These individuals can develop blindness from scarring of the cornea.

Usually, a patient with shingles will have a prodrome with no lesions but will have pain, burning, paresthesias, or itching along the affected dermatome. Three to 5 days later, patients will have eruption of the vesicles. The lesions appear as grouped vesicles on an erythematous base. These lesions will follow one to two dermatomes (sometimes three dermatomes are involved), and they will not cross the midline. Over the next 7 to 10 days, the vesicles will ulcerate and crust over. An average case of shingles lasts 3 weeks (Reuben et al., 2011).

Complications include bacterial suprainfection and *postherpetic neuralgia* (PHN), which consists of chronic, lancinating pain that persists after the lesions have cleared. In fact, some patients experience pain for the rest of their lives. PHN can be quite debilitating. The virus should be treated with antivirals within 72 hours of the rash's appearance in an attempt to decrease the incidence of PHN (Reuben et al., 2011).

Assessment includes documentation of patient symptoms and a history of pertinent risk factors, such as childhood chickenpox and recent chemotherapy or radiation. Nursing management includes education about the disease process and its sequelae. Pain management is of paramount importance in these individuals. One of the most effective topical agents for the pain of shingles is Domeboro soaks, which provide a cooling sensation to the painful areas and can be obtained without a prescription.

Gerontological nurses should discuss the shingles vaccine Zostavax. The new vaccine reduces the occurrence of both shingles and PHN, and should be administered to all older adults (except those who have a weakened immune system caused by treatments that they are taking, such as chemotherapy, radiation, a class of drugs called corticosteroids, or from conditions such as AIDS, cancer of the lymph, bone or blood), even if they have had shingles in the past (Food & Drug Administration, 2012).

Scabies

Scabies is caused by a mite, *Sarcoptes scabies,* that burrows under the skin and causes inflammation and severe itching. In older adults, the presentation often is muted; patients will experience a chronic mild itching of the hands, wrists, and genitalia. Nurses may not be able to detect any type of rash.

With close inspection using a magnifying glass, primary healthcare providers may be able to detect fine, wavy lines in the finger webs or blisters and eruptions with small, dark particles in the center (these dark particles are the mites themselves). This mite is spread by direct contact, and scabies is considered a communicable disease. The incubation period may range from 4 to 6 weeks. Diagnosis is confirmed by skin scrapings (Reuben et al., 2011).

This condition is treated with local application of 5% permethrin cream to the entire body at bedtime. The following morning, all bed linens and bed clothes must be washed in hot water to eradicate the mite.

Nursing interventions include education about transmission and telling the patient that one treatment is usually curative. Gerontological nurses must assess all older adults on admission to acute or long-term care (LTC) for infection with this mite.

Carcinoma

Many older adults have skin problems, which may range from irritated, reddened, itchy areas to a mass or nodule. Many of the lesions in aged skin are benign or premalignant. A common premalignant lesion is *actinic keratosis* (AK). Commonly seen in fair-complexioned people, these lesions occur because of exposure to sun. They begin in vascular areas as reddish macules or papules with a rough, yellowish-brown scale (Reuben et al., 2011). AKs may itch and become rough to the touch. AKs have an abundant blood supply, so any attempt to remove the rough areas can cause bleeding. On occasion, an AK will have a cutaneous horn on the top of the lesion, which results from excess keratin formation.

These lesions commonly are found on the dorsum of the hand, forearms, scalp, helix of the ear, and face. The concern with these premalignant lesions is that they may progress to *squamous cell cancer*. Gerontological nurses should be alert for these lesions in all older individuals. They may appear atypically in patients who use emollients on the skin, appearing as smooth, reddened macules or papules. Nurses should educate patients about wearing protective clothing outdoors and using sunscreen with a sun protection factor (SPF) of at least 15. AKs should be evaluated by primary care providers, because some may require dermatological removal.

True skin malignancy is common in older adults. The most common lesion is basal cell cancer. Other skin cancers that are prevalent are squamous cell carcinoma, as mentioned above, and malignant melanoma.

Basal cell cancer is a lesion most commonly seen in fair-skinned, blonde, or red-headed individuals who have had marked sun exposure. This cancer commonly occurs on the face and scalp and in areas of scarring or chronic irritation (e.g., on the nose where the eyeglasses rest). For the most part, these lesions do not metastasize and are slow growing. Lesions usually appear as pearly papules with depressed centers. These lesions have rolled edges with telangiectasia in and around the edges.

On occasion, a basal cell cancer can have a different appearance. The *pigmented basal cell carcinoma* is a blue-black, pearly nodule, and the *superficial spreading basal cell carcinoma* is a lesion, usually on the thorax, that appears as a red, scaly macule that has eczematous features.

As with AKs, assessment begins with identification of risk factors, such as sun exposure and previous skin lesions. A thorough skin assessment should be done, and these lesions should be identified. Patients should be referred to their primary healthcare providers so that dermatological intervention can take place.

Basal cell cancer lesions are removed with cryotherapy (if they are small) or incision. Patients should be educated on the importance of wearing sun-protective clothing and the use of sunscreen.

Squamous cell carcinoma is the second-most-common skin cancer in older adults. This cancer also arises from the epidermis. Lesions are most commonly found on the scalp, helix and pinna of the ears, dorsum of the hands, and lower lip.

This cancer can develop in chronic leg ulcers. Approximately 20% of squamous cell carcinoma will metastasize. The causative agent is chronic sun exposure; therefore, the closer to the equator a patient lives, the more likely he or she is to have this cancer.

Lesions from a squamous cell carcinoma appear as a thick scale with well-defined borders; this lesion usually has an ulcerated or crusted center (Reuben et al., 2011). On occasion, these lesions look like a common wart or skin tag; the base may be inflamed, reddened, or bleeding, or it may appear as totally benign growth. Patients may be able to remember when the lesion appeared. New skin lesions in older adults should always arouse suspicion about skin malignancy, especially because squamous cell carcinoma arises from benign AKs (see above).

As with patients who have basal cell carcinoma, nurses should assess such patients for risk factors and examine the lesion. Because all of these lesions must be removed, patients should be referred to their primary healthcare providers. Nursing intervention will vary, depending on the extent of the surgical removal.

Malignant melanoma originates from the pigment-forming cells—the melanocyte. These lesions, which are capable of metastasizing at an early stage, are becoming more common throughout the United States because of the increased use of tanning booths and recreational sun exposure. Early detection is critical. These lesions grow both laterally and vertically; the vertical growth causes the metastasis.

Malignant melanoma most often occurs in fair-skinned individuals who have a tendency to sunburn. In addition, people with red or blonde hair, who have multiple moles, and those with a tendency to freckle are thought to be at high risk. Malignant melanoma appears as an irregularly shaped mole, papule, or plaque that has recently appeared or changed in color or size. The American Cancer Society (2012) reminds nurses to use the ABCDs of skin assessment for all lesions concerning for melanoma:

- ► **A**symmetry
- ► **B**order irregularity
- ► **C**olor variation (red, white, blue, gray)
- ► **D**iameter > 6 mm

As the melanoma advances, it may begin to itch or bleed. Any lesion that meets these criteria should be examined by a dermatologist.

Melanoma prognosis is determined by how much vertical growth has occurred. Dermatopathologists use *Breslow's depth,* which refers to how deep into the tissues the melanoma has grown; this depth determines prognosis, not the lateral size of the wound. According to the American Cancer Society (2012), the sooner the melanoma is discovered and treated, the better the diagnosis.

All melanomas are treated with wide and deep excisions in hopes of getting skin margins that are free of tumor. Malignant melanoma can have one of four presentations (see Table 19–3).

TABLE 19–3.
TYPES OF MALIGNANT MELANOMA

TYPE	APPEARANCE	INCIDENCE	LOCATION
Superficial spreading melanoma	Flat, slightly elevated, pigmented papule with irregular borders and varied colors within the lesion	70% of all melanomas Slow growing	Back in men Extremities in women
Nodular melanoma	Hard, dark nodule occurring in a preexisting mole	▸ 15%–30% of all melanomas ▸ Worst prognosis as it grows vertically at an early stage	▸ Usually not seen on head, neck, or trunk ▸ More common in black and dark-skinned individuals
Lentigo maligna melanoma	Brownish-tan macule with variable pigment and irregular borders	5%–10% of all melanomas	Commonly seen on the face
Acral-lentiginous melanoma	Resembles lentigo maligna; flat, irregular-shaped macule with discoloration	10% of all melanomas	▸ More common in older adults ▸ Found on palms, fingers, soles, and toes

Adapted from *Clinical Dermatology* (4th ed.), by T. P. Habif, St. Louis, MO: Mosby; American Cancer Society, 2012.

Nursing assessment and intervention is the same for patients with malignant melanoma as it is for those with other skin cancers. The key for successful therapy and cure is early detection.

Pressure Ulcers

Pressure ulcers are caused by unrelieved pressure over a bony prominence denying the skin tissue of circulation and oxygen, thus, causing necrosis and damage. Each year, more than 2.5 million people in the United States develop pressure ulcers. These skin lesions bring pain, associated risk for serious infection, and increased healthcare use. About 60,000 patients die as a direct result of a pressure ulcer each year. In 2008, Medicare said it would no longer reimburse for hospital-acquired pressure ulcers but that pressure ulcers present on admission will qualify for a higher reimbursement rate. The presence of pressure ulcers on admission must be identified, coded, and noted in the chart, with documentation by the admitting physician. A full skin assessment is now part of the standard hospital admission (McPhee & Papadakis, 2011).

Epidemiology of pressure ulcers, which varies on the basis of the environment assessed, is measured in terms of incidence, number of new cases, and prevalence over a specific time period. According to the Agency for Healthcare Research and Quality (AHRQ, 2011), the following data details occurrence rates of pressure ulcers by location:

► Hospitals
  ► Incidence 12%
► Long-term care facilities
  ► Incidence 23%

Highest-risk patients

► Patients with quadriplegia
► Older patients with hip fractures
► Immobile patients, regardless of diagnosis
► Reduced sensory perception
► Urinary or fecal incontinence
► Poor nutritional status
► Friction and shear forces
► Patients in critical care units

The most common areas of occurrence are:

► Sacrum
► Ischial tuberosity (especially when patient is seated)
► Lateral malleolus
► Greater trochanter
► Heels

Increased pressure leads to capillary closure; this change is compounded by the length of pressure and tissue tolerance. The result is tissue anoxia, ischemia, and edema, which can cause tissue necrosis if not relieved.

Capillary pressure ensures movement of blood through the smallest arteries and veins in the body. This pressure maintains oxygenation and nutrition to the tissues. If these capillaries collapse from increased or prolonged pressure, the result will be tissue anoxia, ischemia, reactive erythema, leakage of plasma into the interstitial areas, and microvascular hemorrhage (manifested by nonblanchable erythema).

Shearing, which is the sliding of parallel surfaces, will cause stretching and occlusion of the arterial supply of fascia and muscle. When the head of the bed is elevated, the body slides down, which can cause shear pressure or movement of the skin away from its underlying support structure. *Friction,* which is the rubbing of the skin against another surface, can cause a superficial abrasion of the epidermis and dermis. Both friction and shearing are thought to be major contributors to pressure ulcer formation.

Protein deficiency lessens tissue tolerance, making the soft tissues more susceptible to damage from increased or prolonged pressure. Patients who have serum albumin of less than 3.5 g/dL are at increased risk of ulcer development and poor wound healing (Lyder & Ayello, 2011).

The aging skin also is an important consideration. A person age 70 or older has a thin epidermis with less elasticity. Age also causes vessel degeneration and reduced blood flow to the skin appendages (Lyder & Ayello, 2011). As a result, the early warning signs of pressure ulcer development, such as erythema, may be muted. Healing is slowed with normal aging, as is the immune response. All of these changes put older adults at high risk for ulcer development.

Low blood pressure and dehydration reduce microvascular circulation; these issues can be important in older and acutely ill patients in pressure ulcer development. Adequate oxygenation, whether in the form of pressure reduction or elevation of blood pressure, is the most important factor in wound healing and prevention.

Early identification of at-risk individuals is critical to preventing pressure ulcers. According to AHRQ (2011), risk assessment should be conducted on all individuals who are:

▶ Immobile

▶ Protein-calorie malnourished

▶ Incontinent

▶ Frail

▶ Disabled

▶ Nutritionally compromised

▶ Mentally compromised

At-risk individuals should be reassessed frequently. According to AHRQ (2011), the Norton and Braden risk assessment tools have undergone the most evaluation, and they are the risk assessment tools suggested by this organization.

The Hartford Institute of Geriatric Nursing recommends use of the Braden scale, which is highly reliable. This scale assesses risk in six areas (sensory perception, skin moisture, activity, mobility, nutrition, and friction/shear). An item score is then assigned ranging from one (highly impaired) to three/four (no impairment). Scores of 15 to 18 indicate at risk, 13 to 14 indicate moderate risk, 10 to 12 indicate high risk, and ≤ 9 indicate very high risk. The recommended intervals for use include acute care every 24–48 hours; critical care every 24 hours; home care every RN visit; institutional long-term care weekly, first 4 weeks after admission; and then monthly to quarterly (www.bradenscale.com; Hartford Institute of Geriatric Nursing, 2012).

Written policies and procedures should be in place to guide and encourage the healthcare team to act independently in prevention. Every at-risk patient should have a daily skin assessment. The soiled skin of patients who are incontinent should be cleaned and dried promptly. Moisturizers, such as emollients or lotions, should be used to prevent skin dryness and cracking. The AHRQ (2012) states that the skin over bony areas *should not* be massaged, as that action may worsen damage. Turning patients every 2 hours (or more frequently) is mandatory. Patients should be turned at a 30° oblique angle; this method helps decrease pressure over the trochanter and lateral malleolus. A pillow should be put under the calves to keep the heels and feet off the bed and relieve pressure on the heels.

A patient who is considered at risk should have a support surface placed on the bed and chair. These devices redistribute weight over a larger area and reduce tissue interface pressure. The Center for Medicare & Medicaid Services has divided support surfaces into three categories for reimbursement purposes:

▶ Group 1 devices are static; they do not require electricity. Static devices include air, foam (convoluted and solid), gel, and water overlays or mattresses. These devices are ideal when a patient is at **low risk** for pressure ulcer development.

▶ Group 2 devices are powered by electricity or a pump and are considered dynamic in nature. These devices include alternating and low-air-loss mattresses. These mattresses are good for patients who are at **moderate to high risk** for pressure ulcers or have full-thickness pressure ulcers.

▶ Group 3 devices, also dynamic, are air-fluidized beds. These beds are electric and contain silicone-coated beads. When air is pumped through the bed, the beads become liquid. These beds are used for patients at **very high risk** for pressure ulcers (Lyder & Ayello, 2011).

Other interventions to prevent ulcer formation include:

▶ *Avoid shear and friction.*

▶ *Monitor nutritional status:* Assess caloric intake, weight, serum albumin and pre-albumin, cholesterol, and total lymphocyte count (TLC).

▶ *Ensure adequate hydration:* Air-fluidized and low-air-loss beds increase insensible water loss, so patients should attempt to drink 2,000–2,500 cc of fluid per day unless contraindicated (e.g., HF, renal insufficiency).

Monitoring of nutritional parameters is an important task for gerontological nurses. Patients should be weighed monthly, as weight changes slowly in most individuals. Interventions should be taken immediately for patients who lose 5%–10% of their ideal body weight (IBW). If a patient loses one-third of the IBW, the healthcare team should view this as an ominous sign.

Serum albumin is another important marker in nutritional adequacy. Albumin values of < 3.5 g/dL are known to be associated with protein calorie malnutrition and increased morbidity and mortality. Pre-albumin is another nutritional indicator with a short half-life of 2 to 3 days. Pre-albumin levels can provide important information regarding the older patient's recent nutrional status, whereas serum albumin is a more stable marker. Additional monitoring parameters include total lymphocyte count and serum total cholesterol. Without adequate nutrition, patients' wounds will not heal. In addition, patients are at high risk for developing new wounds in spite of adequate prevention strategies. Consultation with a dietitian is needed for malnourished patients, and high-protein nutritional supplements can be used to promote healing.

Knowing the physiology of wound healing is important for nurses to determine the best way to heal an ulcer. Wound healing consists of three major stages: inflammation, proliferation, and maturation. The *inflammatory stage* begins immediately and lasts 4 to 5 days. During that time, the wound is red, warm, and painful. The inflammation stabilizes the wound through platelet activity that stops bleeding. The immune system is heavily involved, sending neutrophils, macrophages, and monocytes to the site to control bacteria and clean up debris. This stage often is impaired in older adults. Medications that older patients are required to take, such as steroids; nutritional deficiencies; and decreased immune response seen with normal aging markedly interfere with the speed of this stage (AHRQ, 2012).

The *proliferative stage* (or *granulation stage)* begins within 24 hours of injury and can last up to 3 weeks. During this time, three important processes occur: epithelialization, neovascularization (or granulation), and collagen synthesis. *Epithelialization* seals the wound and protects it from fluid loss; this process is hastened by a moist wound bed. During *neovascularization,* new capillaries are formed that feed the new tissues; these capillaries give the wound bed a beefy red appearance, and it bleeds easily. *Collagen production* gives the healing wound a new matrix for support. This first phase is dependent on oxygen, iron, vitamin C, zinc, and magnesium for healthy progression. Other factors that affect this stage of wound healing are an effective inflammatory reaction and a moist wound environment.

That being said, it should be assumed that individuals who cannot mount an adequate immune response (e.g., frail older adults, those taking steroids) and those who have wound beds that are dry or macerated may not have normal wound proliferation.

The *maturation stage,* sometimes referred to as *differentiation* or *remodeling*, begins about 3 weeks after the injury and may take years to complete. During this time, tensile strength is created through collagen deposition; the wound bed becomes thickened and more compact. At completion, the tensile strength of the area is only 80% of what it was before injury.

After wound healing has begun, healthcare providers should facilitate this process by staging and specific interventions to the wound itself. Staging of pressure ulcers requires assessment and documentation of the wound bed and surrounding bony prominences. Aspects to ascertain include: How deep is the lesion? Are the underlying structures involved? Is there exudate or infection in the wound bed? According to AHRQ (2012), wounds cannot be staged when they are covered with eschar. For the most part (exceptions are discussed below), eschar should be removed, then the wound should be staged. Table 19–4 reviews the different stages of pressure ulcers, based on AHRQ (2012) guidelines.

TABLE 19–4.
PRESSURE ULCER STAGING

	DESCRIPTION	TYPE OF LESION
Stage I	Nonblanchable hyperemia	None
Stage II	Extension through the epidermis	Abrasion Blister Shallow crater
Stage III	Full-thickness wound involving subcutaneous tissue	Deep crater with or without undermining
Stage IV	Full-thickness wound with extension into muscle, bone, or supporting structures	Deep wound usually involves undermining and sinus tracts
Unstageable	Eschar or slough overlying the wound	Base is covered in slough (yellow, tan, gray, green, or brown) and/or eschar (tan, brown, or black) renders the wound unstageable
Suspected deep tissue injury and unstageable		Purple or maroon discolored intact skin or blood-filled blister Surrounding skin is painful, firm, mushy, boggy, warmer, or cooler compared to adjacent tissue

Adapted from *Treatment of Pressure ulcers* (CPG No. 15), by the Agency for Healthcare Research and Quality, 2012.

After the wound is staged, the ulcer must be managed to facilitate healing. Basic principles of pressure ulcer management include:

▶ Eliminate or minimize pressure, friction, and shearing

▶ Monitor and optimize nutrition

▶ Create and maintain a clean, moist wound bed

▶ Ensure adequate circulation and oxygenation

Assuming a moist healing environment, the wound must be gently cleansed of necrotic tissue and infection, being careful not to disrupt the granulation tissue where healing may be starting to occur. Topical therapies (other than normal saline or those produced specifically for cleansing) should be used only in wound beds that are infected, because they kill healthy granulation tissues.

324 GERONTOLOGICAL NURSING REVIEW AND RESOURCE MANUAL, 3RD EDITION

Antiseptic solutions should be discontinued when the exudates or signs of infection have abated. Common antiseptic solutions that may be used in wounds include povidone–iodine (Betadine), acetic acid, hydrogen peroxide, or sodium hypochlorite (Dakin's, Clorpactin).

These agents are all cytotoxic and destroy healthy fibroblasts. Betadine can cause iodine toxicity if used undiluted for long periods of time (Friedman, 2006). When using the aforementioned solutions, Friedman (2006) provides some helpful information to keep in mind, which is summarized in Table 19–5.

TABLE 19-5.
CONSIDERATIONS FOR USE WITH WOUND ANTISEPTICS

SOLUTION	INDICATIONS FOR USE	NURSING CONSIDERATIONS
Povidone–iodine	Can be used short term if diluted; limit to 3–5 days	Never use on healthy, granulating tissues
Acetic acid	Can be used on wounds infected with *Pseudomonas aurigenosa*	▶ Suitable for use for wounds with a malodorous, green drainage ▶ Culture positive for Pseudomonas is preferred indication for use
Hydrogen peroxide	Provides débridement by effervescent action	Do not use in a sinus tract or deep crater
Sodium hypochlorite	▶ Can be used for fungal-type pathogens ▶ Ideally, solution should be diluted, as it is essentially bleach (with only a mild dilution factor)	Can affect clotting abilities and burn intact skin

Adapted from "Integumentary Function," by S. Friedman, 2006, in S. E. Meiner & A. G. Lueckenotte (Eds.), *Gerontological Nursing* (pp. 693–729), St. Louis, MO: Mosby/Elsevier.

Gerontological nurses should examine a wound and note the following:

▶ Color

▶ Presence of discharge, bleeding, or odor

▶ Degree of undermining or sinus tract formation

▶ Any necrotic tissue

▶ Any pain or tenderness

▶ Any erythema surrounding the wound edges

The wound bed should be beefy red, which indicates healthy granulation.

All wounds should be reassessed on an ongoing basis. All new wounds should be described using the aforementioned criteria. Other important information that should be documented includes:

▶ Location

▶ Dimensions (e.g., length, width, depth)

▶ Wound stage

Ideally, a wound will progress through the normal stages of healing. However, exudates and necrotic tissue can interfere with this process. *Débridement* involves removing necrotic material. In addition, dry, hard eschar should be removed. Both entities slow the migration of epithelial cells and delay the healing process. The exception to this recommendation is eschar on the heels. Eschar in this location should be left in place as long as it is dry, because it provides a protective shield for the heel. If it becomes soft or mushy, it should be removed, because that suggests that fluid (or pus) has accumulated beneath the eschar.

The modes of débridement are mechanical, autolytic, chemical, and surgical. Table 19–6, based on Friedman's (2006) work, summarizes these different types.

TABLE 19–6.
TYPES OF DÉBRIDEMENT

TYPE	DESCRIPTION	INDICATIONS	NURSING CONSIDERATIONS
Mechanical	▶ Method of removing slimy or stringy exudates that cannot be removed by other mechanisms ▶ Usually carried out by wet-to-dry dressings or whirlpool	▶ Shallow or deep smaller wounds that are difficult to access with other types of dressings (or too small to justify surgical intervention) ▶ Whirlpool or handheld irrigation devices (e.g., Water-Pik) can be used once or twice a day	Requires much nursing time and can be uncomfortable for patients
Autolytic	▶ Uses the body's own enzymes to provide débridement and cleansing ▶ Hydrocolloid or hydrogel dressings are used to soften and help remove exudate	Removes stringy slough when < 50% of the wound bed is covered and there are no signs of infection	▶ Cannot be used with infected wounds ▶ Causes a larger-appearing wound as debris is being removed ▶ Creates a brownish-yellow fluid that may have the appearance of pus (dead cells and neutrophils constitute the fluid)
Chemical	Use of chemicals to remove necrotic areas or tender yellow slough that is difficult to remove surgically	Small wounds	▶ Time-consuming and expensive ▶ Can be used at home and in long-term-care facilities ▶ With the exception of collagenase, the product cannot be used on healthy tissues

CONTINUED ▶

◄ **TABLE 19-6 CONTINUED**

TYPE	DESCRIPTION	INDICATIONS	NURSING CONSIDERATIONS
Surgical	Surgical removal of necrotic tissue quickly; done at the bedside with scalpel and scissors or in the operating room	► Dry, rubbery eschar ► Wound is infected and needs prompt removal of nonviable tissues	► Stop when bleeding (have reached healthy tissue) occurs ► Aseptic technique required to prevent "auto-infecting" the wound bed

Adapted from "Integumentary Function," by S. Friedman, 2006, in S. E. Meiner & A. G. Lueckenotte (Eds.), *Gerontological Nursing* (pp. 693–729), St. Louis, MO: Mosby/Elsevier.

Once proper débridement has occurred, the nurse must ensure that the wound has a nourishing environment to heal in. Maintaining a moist wound environment is the rule; if satisfactory wound healing is not seen in 2 to 4 weeks, the nurse must reevaluate the dressing selection.

Some general guidelines to remember with evaluating and treating pressure ulcers include:

► Gently irrigate all wounds with 1–2 ounces of normal saline at each dressing change

► Evaluate the wound border for *Candidiasis* with each dressing change

Superficial *Candidiasis* appears as small areas of erythema that can itch. Fungal infections of the skin grow in warm moist environments, so nurses must have a high index of suspicion for these pathogens with each dressing change.

Wound care dressing products include:

► Gauze products

► Nonadherent products

► Foam dressings

► Transparent films

► Hydrocolloids

► Hydrogels

► Alginates

Because nursing judgment determines what product should be used on each particular wound, gerontological nurses should be well informed about the attributes of each category of products. Based on Friedman's (2006) work, Table 19–7 depicts general information and indications for each category of wound care products.

TABLE 19-7.
WOUND CARE PRODUCTS

CATEGORY	MECHANISM OF ACTION	INDICATIONS	NURSING CONSIDERATIONS
Gauze dressings	Damp gauze is placed into the wound bed and allowed to dry to a modest degree; it is removed, taking with it exudate and necrotic materials	▶ Débriding and cleaning wound bed ▶ If wound has tunneling or undermining, the cavity can be loosely packed with moist gauze to maintain a moist environment and prevent walling off of the cavity	▶ Gauze should not be allowed to dry completely because it will remove normal healthy granulation tissues when removed ▶ Gauze comes impregnated with different products—povidone–iodine, Vaseline, and hypertonic saline—that can be used in selected scenarios
Nonadherent dressings	Protects the wound bed by leaving the epithelial cells undisturbed	Used for skin tears, skin grafts, or other wounds that require minimum intervention	Topical antibiotics can be used beneath these dressings, which are changed once or twice a day
Foam dressings	Absorbent dressings that protect ulcer and minimize maceration	Useful for wounds with excess drainage or exudates	▶ Can be used under films or other primary dressings ▶ Topicals can be applied beneath the foam
Transparent films	▶ Facilitates autolysis ▶ Dressings are semipermeable to allow air exchange ▶ Opsite or Tegaderm	▶ Used on superficial wounds ▶ Can be used to secure other dressings and to protect vulnerable areas from friction	▶ Usually left on for 3–7 days ▶ Can cause fluid build-up beneath dressing, leading to leakage and maceration of healthy tissues (nonadherent or alginate product can be placed beneath film can prevent)
Hydrocolloids	▶ Sticky, nonpermeable wafers that contain hydrocolloid material that melts and combines with natural body fluids to keep the wound bed moist ▶ Nonpermeable dressing is a barrier that creates a hypoxic wound bed that stimulates granulation (as long as peripheral circulation is adequate) ▶ DuoDerm	Can be used on Stage II and III wounds	▶ Can create a foul, sour odor, which is normal ▶ Usually left on for 3–7 days ▶ Should not be used if Candidiasis is present, infection or suspected infection is present, or the wound has purulent discharge

CONTINUED ▶

◀ TABLE 19-7 CONTINUED

CATEGORY	MECHANISM OF ACTION	INDICATIONS	NURSING CONSIDERATIONS
Hydrogels	Consists primarily of water; helps maintain a moist wound bed and facilitates healing	Can be used on superficial or deep wounds, as the product can be obtained in sheet or gel that can be spread into deep cavities	▶ Can be left in place for 1–7 days ▶ Should not be used on infected wounds ▶ Requires a cover dressing: gauze, foam, or transparent film (based on health of surrounding tissue and amount of exudate)
Alginates	Made of seaweed; products soak up drainage	Used to manage wounds with exudate	▶ Can use on infected wounds ▶ Helpful around drainage tubes and in wounds that are macerating healthy surrounding tissues

Adapted from "Integumentary Function," by S. Friedman, 2006, in S. E. Meiner & A. G. Lueckenotte (Eds.), *Gerontological Nursing* (pp. 693–729), St. Louis, MO: Mosby/Elsevier.

Pressure ulcers are associated with increased mortality. Complications include pain, cellulitis, osteomyelitis, systemic sepsis, and prolongation of hospital or nursing home length of stay. Electrical stimulation, vacuum drains, surgical débridement, and possible skin grafting should be considered for large or nonhealing wounds (McPhee & Papadakis, 2011).

REFERENCES

Agency for Health Care Policy and Research. (2011). *Comprehensive hospital-based program significantly reduces pressure ulcer incidence and associated costs.* Retrieved from http://www.innovations.ahrq.gov/content.aspx?id=1851

Food and Drug Administration. (2012). *Zostavax (herpes zoster vaccine) questions and answers.* Retrieved from http://www.fda.gov/BiologicsBloodVaccines/Vaccines/QuestionsaboutVaccines/UCM070418

Friedman, S. (2006). Integumentary function. In S. E. Meiner & A. G. Lueckenotte (Eds.), *Gerontological nursing* (pp. 693–729). St. Louis, MO: Mosby/Elsevier.

Hartford Institute for Geriatric Nursing. (2012). *Predicting pressure ulcer risk. Try this: Best practices in nursing care for older adults.* Retrieved from http://consultgerirn.org/uploads/File/trythis/try_this_5.pdf

Huether, S., & McCance, K. (2012). *Understanding pathophysiology* (5th ed.). St. Louis, MO: Mosby.

Lyder, C., & Ayello, E. (2008). *Pressure ulcers: A patient safety issue. Patient safety and quality: An evidence-based handbook for nurses. Agency for Healthcare Policy and Research.* Retrieved from http://www.ahrq.gov/qual/nurseshdbk/docs/lyderc_pupsi.pdf

McPhee, S., & Papadakis, M. (2011). *Current medical diagnosis and treatment* (50th ed.). New York: McGraw Hill Medical.

MedicineNet.com. (2012). *Parkinson's disease.* Retrieved from http://www.medicinenet.com/parkinsons_disease/article.htm

Meiner, S. E. (2001). Gastrointestinal problems. In A. S. Luggen & S. E. Meiner (Eds.), *NGNA Core curriculum for gerontological nursing* (pp. 73–161) St. Louis, MO: Mosby.

Nurse practitioners' prescribing reference. (2012). New York: Haymarket Media Publication.

Reuben, D., Herr, K., Pacala, J., Pollock, B., Potter, J., & Semla, T. (2011). *Geriatrics at your fingertips* (13th ed.). New York: American Geriatrics Society.

ADDITIONAL RESOURCES

Chronic and Disabling Conditions: www.agingsociety.org/

Healthy People 2020: www.healthypeople.gov/2020/

SLEEP DISORDERS AND SENSORY DISORDERS

Sleep is an important biological process necessary for the maintenance of bodily functions. Insomnia, frequent nighttime awakenings, early morning awakening, sleep apnea, restless leg syndrome, and periodic limb movement disorder are all symptoms of sleep disorders. Sleep complaints in older adults are common. Older adults also experience secondary problems that disrupt sleep, such as nocturia, depression, or chronic pain. Sleep disruption has been shown to affect cognitive function and lead to poor health status, low quality of life, and increased mortality (Crowley, 2011).

BOX 20-1.
RISK FACTORS FOR SLEEP DISORDERS IN OLDER ADULTS

- ► Chronic pain
- ► Heart failure (nocturnal dyspnea)
- ► Chronic obstructive pulmonary disease (nocturnal dyspnea)
- ► Gastroesophageal reflux disease
- ► Urinary problems (e.g., benign prostatic hyperplasia, incontinence)
- ► Depression and anxiety
- ► Drug or alcohol addiction
- ► Poor sleep habits (daytime naps)
- ► Medications or substances (bronchodilators, beta-blockers, caffeine, nicotine, antidepressants, corticosteroids)

Normal adult sleep occurs in two phases: REM (rapid eye movement) and non-REM sleep. *REM sleep* is characterized by muscle atonia and rapid eye movements. *Non-REM sleep* is divided into four stages, with Stages 1 and 2 being light sleep and Stages 3 and 4 being deep sleep. Normal sleep goes through Stages 1–4, then briefly back to 2, and finally to REM. This pattern occurs about every 90 minutes and repeats several times during a sleep period (Crowley, 2011).

Older adults experience a decrease in deep sleep (Stage 4 and REM). Consequently, they are more easily awakened. In addition, they take longer to fall asleep and "perceive" that their sleep is poor, because they spend more time in bed but less of that time sleeping. They also tend to wake earlier in the morning and, if bedtimes are earlier, they may awaken in the middle of the night. This occurrence is called *circadian advancement*.

Insomnia

Sleep patterns can give clues to possible causes of insomnia. For example, difficulty falling asleep (sleep latency) may be due to anxiety or bereavement, while the usual disturbance of patients with clinical depression is early morning awakening. Often, older adults will reach for over-the-counter (OTC) sleep medications to help them sleep better. Most of these remedies contain diphenhydramine as the active ingredient, which is an antihistamine, better known as Benadryl. Diphenhydramine is heavily sedating in most older adults and can lead to an increased risk of falls or cognitive impairment.

Older adults may turn to alcohol to improve sleep; however, alcohol actually causes more sleep fragmentation. Combining alcohol and hypnotic medications not only can be particularly dangerous, but also worsens sleep.

Obstructive Sleep Apnea

Obstructive sleep apnea (OSA) affects 18 million people in the United States and another 5.4 million are thought to be undiagnosed (Sleep Apnea Disorder, 2011). OSA is characterized by upper-airway collapse, resulting in decreased ventilation despite continued effort to breathe. Risk factors for OSA include:

▶ Obesity

▶ Alcohol

▶ Sedatives

▶ Sleeping supine

The condition often is suspected when one or more of the following symptoms are present:

▶ Daytime somnolence or fatigue

▶ Loud snoring (reported by bed partners)

▶ Morning headaches

▶ Poor attention, memory, or both

▶ Personality changes

However, the consequences of OSA are far worse than the symptoms. Left untreated, nocturnal hypoxemia can lead to cardiac complications such as arrhythmias, hypertension (HTN), heart failure (HF), and even sudden cardiac death. In addition, patients may fall asleep at undesirable times, such as when driving, which can lead to fatal accidents.

Diagnosis is made by a polysomnogram (PSG) or overnight sleep study. The most effective treatment is nocturnal continuous positive airway pressure; however, managing such a device is difficult for some older adults. In these cases, they often decline therapy. "Position therapy" for sleeping is effective for some patients. The most cost-effective way to ensure that someone does not sleep on his or her back is to sew tennis balls into the back of a sleep shirt or nightgown.

Sleep-Related Movement Disorders

Periodic leg movements of sleep (PLMS) and *restless leg syndrome* (RLS) are sleep-related movement disorders. RLS is often diagnosed by history, when patients experience an uncontrollable desire to move their legs while at rest (in bed before falling asleep). Some sort of paresthesia usually accompanies the movement, such as aching, itching, or a sense of "bugs crawling on me." Suspicion of PLMS often requires a bed partner to report the "kicking" that occurs. Patients will experience symptoms similar to those of OSA, such as daytime somnolence and poor concentration, but will think that they are "sleeping fine." PLMS is usually diagnosed by overnight PSG (Reuben et al., 2011). Medications that may be prescribed to treat these disorders are listed in Box 20–2.

Nurses play a key role in educating older adults about age-related sleep changes and sleep hygiene measures that can improve sleep (see Box 20–3). For most older adults, behavioral therapy should be the initial treatment. If a sleeping medication is prescribed, the lowest effective dose should be used; the older person should be informed that fall risk increases with all sleeping medications; these agents should not be prescribed for more than 3 to 4 weeks; and the dosage should be tapered down to prevent rebound insomnia and wean the patient off the medication gently (Reuben et al., 2011). Many "sleeping myths" must be addressed, such as that poor sleep at night requires daytime naps, or that getting in bed earlier facilitates or improves sleep.

> **BOX 20–2.**
> **TREATMENTS FOR SLEEP-RELATED MOVEMENT DISORDERS**
>
> ▸ Exercise
> ▸ Warm or hot bath
> ▸ Caffeine avoidance
> ▸ Alcohol avoidance
> ▸ Analgesic at bedtime (e.g., Tylenol)
> ▸ Sinemet
> ▸ Lyrica
> ▸ Mirapex
> ▸ Clonazepam

> **BOX 20-3.**
> **RULES FOR SLEEP HYGIENE**
> ► Establish a consistent time for going to sleep and waking.
> ► Avoid daytime naps, or limit naps to early afternoon and less than 1 hour.
> ► Exercise daily, but early in the day.
> ► Increase bright-light exposure during the evening (especially 7–10 p.m.).
> ► Avoid food or fluids before bedtime.
> ► Avoid caffeine, nicotine, or alcohol in the evening.
> ► Develop a bedtime routine (including a hot bath).
> ► Don't read, watch TV, or eat in bed.
> ► Don't get in bed until sleepy and not before 10:30 p.m.
> ► If unable to fall asleep within 20 minutes, get up and perform some activity (e.g., writing, reading, cleaning).
> ► Once sleepy, return to bed.
> ► Minimize light and noise in the bedroom.

Adapted from *Gerontological Nursing* (2nd ed.), by P. Tabloski, 2010, Upper Saddle River, New Jersey: Pearson Prentice Hall.

Sensory Disorders

Common sensory disorders in older adults include hearing and vision disorders.

Hearing Disorders

Hearing loss affects about one-third of adults age 65 or older and half of those over age 85 (McPhee & Papadakis, 2011). Hearing loss can lead to a significant decrease in functional ability and has been associated with frustration and embarrassment, leading to social isolation and depression. Hearing loss is often underrecognized by older adults, who may deny that they have a problem or blame others for "mumbling." Others may recognize the decline in hearing but attribute it to "normal aging" and fail to report it to healthcare providers.

Types of hearing loss include:

► *Conductive:* Impaired transmission of sound through the auditory canal, tympanic membrane (TM), or middle ear; causes include ear wax and TM perforation

► *Sensorineural:* Caused by dysfunction of the inner ear, eighth cranial nerve, brain stem, or cortical auditory pathways; causes include age, previous noise exposure, and medications (e.g., aminoglycoside antibiotics, aspirin, loop diuretics, some anti-neoplastic drugs)

► *Presbycusis:* The most common form of hearing loss in older adults; characterized by bilateral, symmetric loss of high-frequency tones. Several risk factors can accelerate this loss, including history of frequent middle-ear infections, previous noise exposure, heredity, and atherosclerosis. Presbycusis is sensorineural loss that occurs as result of the following changes:

  ► Atrophy of sensory cells and calcification of membranes in the inner ear

  ► Degeneration of eighth cranial nerve

  ► Degeneration of cells in auditory cortex

Functional changes in hearing involve loss of ability to hear pure tones and inability to understand speech in the presence of background noise (e.g., loss of "cocktail conversation").

Tinnitus, or noise (ringing) in the ear, is commonly reported by older adults. Tinnitus often is a symptom of sensorineural hearing loss and can be classified as subjective or objective.

▶ *Subjective tinnitus:* Audible only to the patient; characterized by buzzing, ringing, or humming

▶ *Objective tinnitus:* Audible to patient and examiner; most commonly referred to as vascular noise from a heart murmur or carotid bruit

Sometimes tinnitus is a symptom of another condition, such as Ménière's disease or a tumor.

Tinnitus can be annoying and difficult to treat. Sounds often are more noticeable at night and can be masked by various forms of ambient "white" noise (e.g., loud ticking clock, fan, soft music).

Physical examinations for hearing loss should always begin with an otoscopic exam of the ear, which may reveal cerumen impactions, a very common cause of conductive hearing loss in older adults. Visualization of the TM may reveal perforation or evidence of a middle-ear infection (otitis media). Pure-tone audiometry can be checked with a handheld device; however, audiologic evaluation in a soundproof room is considered the gold standard for assessing hearing loss.

One simple test is the "whisper" test, during which the examiner stands 1 to 2 feet from the patient on one side and whispers one- or two-syllable words, then has the patient repeat those words.

The Rinne and Weber tests (Reuben et al., 2011) are helpful for distinguishing conductive from sensorineural hearing loss. The Weber test involves striking a tuning fork and placing it in the middle of the patient's forehead. Sound will lateralize to the ear with a conductive loss if there is no sensorineural loss. If sensorineural loss is present, sound will lateralize to the better ear. The Rinne test involves striking a tuning fork and placing it on the mastoid bone. The patient indicates when he or she can no longer hear the sound, and that time is noted. The tuning fork is then held in front of the ear, and again the patient indicates when it can no longer be heard. Under normal circumstances, the air to bone ratio will be 2:1. If sensorineural loss is present, the ratio will be < 2:1.

To improve communication with older adults, the following steps are recommended:

▶ Face patients directly when speaking.

▶ Use normal volume and tone, and enunciate clearly without exaggerated lip movement.

▶ Don't cover the mouth with the hand.

▶ If asked to repeat something, rephrase the question or instruction.

▶ Ensure that hearing aids are in place and batteries are working.

▶ Encourage eye glasses when needed.

Older adults with evidence of hearing loss should be referred to an audiologist for evaluation. Hearing aids can be helpful for some patients, but they only amplify sounds, so they may not help patients who have problems with speech discrimination. Cochlear implants are useful in deaf children and younger adults, but not a realistic option for some older adults with advanced hearing loss because these devices require a long period of adjustment and training before the benefit is attained (Friedland et al., 2010). Pocket amplifiers, which can be useful for communicating one-on-one, are inexpensive headphone devices that amplify sound and are available at most electronics stores. Various assistive devices, such as telephone amplifiers and visual alarms for household use (e.g., door bell, smoke alarm, alarm clock), are available through hearing rehabilitation programs.

Vision Disorders

Vision disorders are the most common sensory problem in older adults, and blindness is the most feared disability. Visual acuity of less than 20/40 is defined as *vision impairment*, although visual acuity testing is not the best predictor of impairment because it does not simulate environmental context (e.g., low light, glare). *Blindness* is defined as visual acuity of 20/200 or worse in the "good" eye.

Like hearing impairment, vision loss leads to decreased functional ability and reduced quality of life, but the effect is more severe. Loss of vision has been associated with the following problems:

- ▶ Depression
- ▶ Inability to perform activities of daily living
- ▶ Inability to drive
- ▶ Falls
- ▶ Medication errors
- ▶ Increased risk of injury

Presbyopia, the age-associated vision loss that starts in the fourth decade, occurs as a result of increased lens density and loss of lens elasticity. Other effects include higher light requirements, decreased contrast sensitivity, and increased susceptibility to glare.

Cataracts are the most common ocular disease of aging and result from the cumulative effect of UVB light exposure plus other risk factors (Box 20–4). Cataracts cause progressive visual blurring. The best prevention involves protecting the eyes from sunlight and modifying risk factors. When impaired vision has a negative impact on function, the cataract should be surgically removed.

> **BOX 20-4.**
> **RISK FACTORS FOR CATARACTS**
> ▸ Smoking
> ▸ Age
> ▸ Heavy alcohol consumption
> ▸ Low educational level
> ▸ Diabetes
> ▸ Sun exposure
> ▸ Corticosteroids

Adapted from *Cataracts: Risk Factors* by the Mayo Clinic, 2010, retrieved from http://www.mayoclinic.com/health/cataracts/ds00050/dsection=risk-factors.

Primary open-angle glaucoma (POAG) is the second-most-common cause of blindness in the United States and the leading cause of blindness in African Americans (American Academy of Ophthalmology, 2010). Glaucoma causes progressive loss of peripheral vision due to increased intraocular pressure that produces a gradual optic neuropathy. Risk factors include:

▸ Family history

▸ Race (Black)

▸ Enlarged optic cup

▸ Diabetes

▸ Cardiac vascular disease (CVD)

There are two types of glaucoma: *open-angle* and *closed-angle glaucoma* (CAG). POAG develops slowly and is generally asymptomatic. CAG, on the other hand, is caused by a sudden increase in pressure due to blockage of vitreous outflow, which is caused by a foreign body or pupil dilation from medications.

POAG can be treated with topical medications, surgery, or lasers. Medications include beta-blockers, prostaglandin analogs, carbonic anhydrase inhibitors, and alpha²-agonists. Note that medications given in the eye may be absorbed systemically and, thus, cause side effects.

Age-related macular degeneration (AMD) is the leading cause of blindness in older adults in the developed world. The condition occurs in the fovea of the macula and results in central vision loss. AMD affects Whites more than other racial groups. Risk factors are the same as those for CAD. Other possible risk factors still under study are phototoxicity, inflammation, and diet.

There are two types of occurs over a long period of time. *Wet MD* is caused by growth of new blood vessels beneath the macula that often break and leak blood and fluid, causing a more abrupt loss of vision. *Dry MD* accounts for 90% of cases and wet MD for only 10%. There are no medical treatments for either type; however, wet MD can be treated with laser photocoagulation to reduce vision loss (Reuben et al., 2011). For patients with wet MD, anti-VEGF (Macugen) injections into the globe may slow vision loss (Macular Degeneration Research, 2012).

REFERENCES

American Academy of Ophthalmology. (2010). *Primary open angle glaucoma PPP. Preferred Practice Pattern Guidelines.* Retrieved from http://one.aao.org/CE/PracticeGuidelines/PPP_Content.aspx?cid=93019a87-4649-4130-8f94-b6a9b19144d2

Crowley, K. (2011). Sleep and sleep disorders in older adults. *Neuropsychological Review,* 21(1), 41–53.

Friedland, D., Runge-Samuelson, C., Baig, H., & Jenson, J. (2010). Case control analysis of cochlear implant performance in elderly patients. *Archives of Otolaryngology Head and Neck Surgery, 136*(5), 432–438.

Huether, S., & McCance, K. (2012). *Understanding pathophysiology* (5th ed.). St. Louis, MO: Mosby.

McPhee, S., & Papadakis, M. (2011). *Current medical diagnosis and treatment* (50th ed.). New York: McGraw Hill Medical.

Macular Degeneration Research. (2012). *Treatments for macular degeneration.* Retrieved from http://www.ahaf.org/macular/treatment/common/

Mayo Clinic. (2010). *Cataracts: Risk factors.* Retrieved from http://www.mayoclinic.com/health/cataracts/ds00050/dsection=risk-factors

Nurse practitioners' prescribing reference. (2012). New York: Haymarket Media Publication.

Reuben, D., Herr, K., Pacala, J., Pollock, B., Potter, J., & Semla, T. (2011). *Geriatrics at your fingertips* (13th ed.). New York: American Geriatrics Society.

Sleep Apnea Disorder. (2011). *Sleep apnea on quantum rise among the Americans.* Retrieved from http://sleepapneadisorder.info/2011/03/15/sleep-apnea-on-quantum-rise-among-the-americans/

Tabloski, P. (2010). *Gerontological nursing* (2nd ed.). Upper Saddle River, NJ: Pearson Prentice Hall.

ADDITIONAL RESOURCES

Chronic and Disabling Conditions: www.agingsociety.org/

Diabetes and the Older Adult: http://ohioline.osu.edu/ss-fact/0166.html

Healthy People 2020: www.healthypeople.gov/2020/

Hearing Disorders and Deafness – Hearing Disorders and Deafness: http://health.nih.gov/topic/HearingDisordersDeafness/

National Eye Institute – National Institutes of Health: http://www.nei.nih.gov/

Sleep Hygiene: www.sleepfoundation.org/

APPENDIX A

REVIEW QUESTIONS

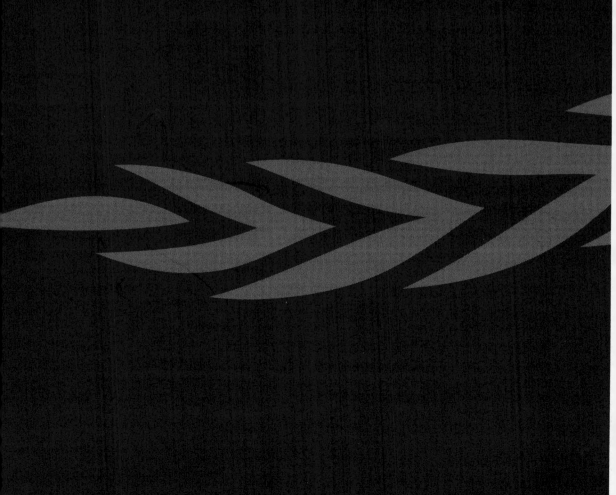

1. When an older patient is hospitalized, Medicare reimburses for this inpatient care by which of the following mechanisms?

    a. Medicare B

    b. Medicare A

    c. Medicare D

    d. Medigap

2. Gerontological nurses are expected to evaluate research to implement evidence-based practice. Which of the following studies provides the strongest evidence to change practice?

    a. Randomized control clinical trial

    b. Qualitative phenomenological study

    c. In-depth case study

    d. Cohort study

3. The landmark Institute of Medicine (IOM) report entitled *The Future of Nursing* advances which of the following positions?

    a. Nursing faculty will be required to pursue postdoctoral training.

    b. Nursing curriculum will require advanced aging content.

    c. Physicians will no longer be allowed to direct care in long-term-care facilities.

    d. Nurses should practice to the full extent of their education and training.

4. The biggest risk factor for developing a cognitive impairment is

    a. socioeconomic status.

    b. poor nutrition.

    c. age.

    d. female gender.

5. A 76-year-old woman presents at an ambulatory clinic. About 2 weeks ago, she had difficulty finding words, felt weak, and noticed her right hand felt numb for several hours. Although she has recovered most of her function, she continues to have difficulty with her short-term memory. The most likely cause of these symptoms is:

    a. Alzheimer's disease.

    b. organic delusional syndrome.

    c. vascular dementia.

    d. acute depressive syndrome.

6. An 85-year-old woman with advanced cancer asks the nurse, "What is wrong with me? My doctor won't tell me anything. The chemotherapy is making me sick and if I knew it wasn't helping, I would stop taking it." The nurse decides to tell the patient the truth. Which ethical principle is the nurse upholding?

    a. Fidelity

    b. Autonomy

    c. Justice

    d. Nonmaleficence

7. Higher RN staffing levels in long-term-care settings are known to be associated with which of the following factors?

    a. Lower costs to the facility

    b. Higher fall rates

    c. Lower rates of decubitus ulcers

    d. More medication use

8. The process of gerontological nursing certification by the American Nurses Credentialing Center is best described as a(n)

    a. formal process to validate clinical competence in a specialty area of practice.

    b. formal process to obtain a nursing license.

    c. informal process necessary for those considering graduate study.

    d. requirement only for those working in long-term care.

9. Mrs. Jones is a 78-year-old female with a history of severe degenerative arthritis of her lower back. She suffers from chronic pain much of time, rated between 4 and 6 on a 1–10 scale. She describes the pain as burning and tingling. Over the past few months, she has been on a variety of analgesics without much effect on her pain. Her current regimen includes tramadol 50 mg twice daily and gabapentin 300 mg at bedtime. She states that she sleeps well and that, for the most part, this regimen works better than previous ones that included hydrocodone. This scenario describes which of the following categories of pain?

    a. Nociceptive

    b. Neuropathic

    c. Visceral

    d. Unspecified

10. An 80-year-old man reports to his nurse that he is having trouble initiating the flow of urine, has to void every hour or so, and never feels his bladder is empty. The nurse realizes that these symptoms are most probably the result of which of the following conditions?

    a. Prostate cancer

    b. Neurological changes of aging

    c. Anemia

    d. Benign prostatic hypertrophy

11. Which virus is spread by the fecal-oral route, is usually transmitted by contaminated food or water, and has no chronic form?

    a. Hepatitis A

    b. Hepatitis B

    c. Hepatitis C

    d. Hepatitis D

12. A 70-year-old man is admitted to the hospital following a visit to his physician's office. He says that he is recovering from the flu and feels very weak. Initial nursing assessment reveals that his BP is 90/60, temperature is 98° F, pulse is 108/min, and respirations are 20/min. His skin and mucous membranes are dry. He is 5 ft 9 in and weighs 160 lb. He states that he takes "a little white pill" for his heart and another pill for "passing water." His wife reports that his memory is pretty good, but he has fallen 3 times in the last 2 days. He has taken his medication, but has had no desire to eat or drink. Based on the data given, what is the most serious problem to be addressed in the nursing care plan?

    a. Malnutrition

    b. Dementia

    c. Anxiety

    d. Dehydration

13. Who of the following patients is most prone to developing hyperkalemia?

    a. A 65-year-old woman with a fractured humerus

    b. A 78-year-old man with a decreased creatinine clearance who takes ibuprofen daily for joint pain

    c. An 85-year-old man with no health problems who eats a banana every day

    d. An 88-year-old woman who takes amlodipine 5 mg daily for her high blood pressure

14. Which of the following health promotion activities is labeled correctly?

    a. Influenza vaccine: primary prevention

    b. Blood pressure screening: primary prevention

    c. Diabetic education: secondary prevention

    d. Mammography: tertiary prevention

15. Retirement at the age of 65 reflects the thinking in which of the following theories of aging?

    a. Orem's self-care theory

    b. Activity theory

    c. Disengagement theory

    d. Free radical theory

16. Which of the following older persons should receive the zoster vaccine?

    a. A 70-year-old man who has had Herpes zoster

    b. An 80-year-old woman who has not had Herpes zoster

    c. A healthy 65-year-old man

    d. All of the above

17. The general recommendation regarding screening for prostate cancer by prostate-specific antigen (PSA) is that screening may be appropriate in patients 75 years of age and older with at least a ___ -year life expectancy.

    a. 10

    b. 5

    c. 2

    d. 1

18. Ms. Jones is a 75-year-old woman with several risk factors for cardiovascular disease. Which of her risk factors can be modified to reduce her risk of a cardiovascular event?

    a. Advancing age

    b. Postmenopausal status

    c. High blood pressure

    d. Family history

19. The gerontological nurse knows that acute conditions often present with atypical signs and symptoms in older adults. Which of the following might be an example of an *atypical* presentation of pneumonia?

    a. Fall
    b. Cough
    c. Fever
    d. Chest pain

20. The older adult with Parkinson's disease is often plagued with some sort of gait disturbance. If the patient has a tendency to fall backward when he or she walks, the person is said to have which of the following?

    a. Festination
    b. Propulsive gait
    c. Retropulsion
    d. Akinetic gait

21. Mrs. Blair comes into the clinic complaining of a skin rash on her forearms. She states that the areas of concern have been there for many years, and they seem to be getting worse. The patient is an 82-year-old female who appears younger than her stated age. She is well groomed. On and about her forearms and anterior thorax, she has several 3–4-mm brownish-black lesions that have a "stuck-on" appearance. The lesions have a greasy, brown appearance, and the patient tells you that she can sometimes rub them off with a towel after her bath. She wants to make sure they are not skin cancers. Given this information, the gerontological nurse recognizes Mrs. Blair's lesions as

    a. cherry angiomas.
    b. seborrheic keratosis.
    c. psoriasis.
    d. eczema.

22. Overdoses of acetaminophen have been linked to

    a. weight loss.
    b. falls.
    c. liver failure.
    d. constipation.

23. Which of the following is the best definition of the advance directive known as a "living will"?

    a. A statement of a person's wishes for how he or she would like to die and be treated at the end of life

    b. Naming another to make decisions in case the patient cannot make his or her own decisions

    c. Seeking advice from a judge in a court of law

    d. Asking the next of kin to make decisions consistent with the older person's values and beliefs

24. Which of the following behaviors in a grieving older widow may indicate the need for a mental health referral and counseling?

    a. Feelings of sadness 3 months after a loved one dies

    b. Feelings of sadness 3 months after the loss of a pet

    c. Failure to eat properly and refusal take medications to control hypertension and other signs of self-neglect

    d. Family reports that the grieving older person often talks about her dead husband

25. An older Arabic woman has requested that all her care be provided by female caregivers, according to her religious beliefs. The nurse should respond:

    a. "That is impossible. We have many fine male attendants and nurses on this floor."

    b. "I'll speak to the head nurse about this. No one has ever requested this before."

    c. "Did one of the male nurses or attendants offend you? Why have you made such a request?"

    d. "Yes, I understand your request and will make every attempt to accommodate your wishes. I'll make a notation on your nursing care plan."

26. One day after surgical repair of a hip fracture, an 89-year-old man becomes agitated and exhibits signs of visual hallucinations. The most likely cause of the symptoms is

    a. hypotension.

    b. delirium.

    c. Alzheimer's disease.

    d. Lewy body disease.

27. Which of the following is the best marker of adequate renal function in the older person?

    a. Voiding frequency in the daytime

    b. Voiding frequency at night

    c. Calculated creatinine clearance

    d. BUN (blood urea nitrogen) levels

28. A hospice patient on large doses of opioid medication has not had a bowel movement for 3 days and is complaining of abdominal discomfort. Which of the following is the most appropriate intervention?

   a. Increase fluids

   b. Administer a bulking agent such as Metamucil

   c. Decrease the dose of opioid medication to stimulate bowel function

   d. Administer a bowel stimulant

29. The gerontological nursing expert knows that acute conditions often present with atypical signs and symptoms in older adults. Which of the following might be an example of an *atypical* presentation of a urinary tract infection?

   a. Confusion and falls

   b. Blood in the urine

   c. Fever

   d. Painful voiding

30. Adult learning theory suggests which of the following?

   a. Teach the older person in simple terms, as you would teach a child.

   b. Provide information relevant to the older adult because he or she is a self-directed learner.

   c. Use your own unique style as a teacher, because it is more natural.

   d. Provide constant praise and encouragement to ensure the older person knows you are pleased.

31. A 78-year-old man is cognitively intact but suffers from severe degenerative joint disease. He recently has suffered urinary incontinence on occasion when he cannot get to the bathroom. The nurse notes that he has to be helped out of his chair or bed to get to his walker. This presentation of incontinence is called

   a. stress incontinence.

   b. functional incontinence.

   c. overflow incontinence.

   d. urge incontinence.

32. Respiratory acidosis would most likely occur in an older patient with

   a. renal failure.

   b. systemic infection.

   c. emphysema.

   d. anxiety.

33. An 89-year-old woman with chronic urinary tract infections has recently begun to have foul-smelling diarrhea. Last week, she completed a 10-day treatment of her UTI with levaquin. The nurse should

    a. administer Imodium and try to stop the diarrhea.

    b. make sure to urge additional fluid intake.

    c. notify the patient's healthcare provider to report the condition, and obtain a stool specimen for analysis while waiting for the callback.

    d. do nothing, because the diarrhea will probably resolve on its own.

34. Which electrolyte is a byproduct of purine metabolism, in which elevated levels are seen in patients with renal disease and gout?

    a. Folic acid

    b. Alkaline phosphatase

    c. Uric acid

    d. Amylase

35. An 85-year-old patient is dying of cancer. He is being cared for in his home. The visiting nurse notes his pain is increasing, despite the fact that he has been on a stable dose of opioids for the last several weeks. Which of the following actions is the most appropriate to recommend to the physician?

    a. Provide a short-acting opioid p.r.n. to be given when the patient states the pain is the worst

    b. Start an IV morphine drip

    c. Instruct the family to give subcutaneous morphine

    d. Increase the dose of the long-acting opioid to control the basal pain level with short-term p.r.n. medication for breakthrough pain as needed

36. An 80-year-old woman has been bed-bound for a week following a hip fracture and pneumonia. She takes a thiazide diuretic for control of her hypertension. You notice that the patient is more confused than at baseline and is unable to turn in bed. On assessment, you note that she has decreased deep tendon reflexes. This patient is most likely suffering from:

    a. hyperkalemia.

    b. hypernatremia.

    c. hypocalcemia.

    d. dehydration

37. Which of the following best describes "substituted judgment"?

   a. A guardian is appointed by the court system to make a decision that the patient would make if he or she were able to do so.

   b. The patient has chosen another person to make decisions if he or she is unable to do so and informs that person of the kind of care preferred.

   c. A person makes a decision to benefit another without any knowledge of the patient's stated preferences.

   d. A person designates in writing the kind of treatment that he or she does or does not want.

38. A nurse advocate can be best described as one who

   a. develops clinical pathways and implements evidence-based practice.

   b. collaborates with others to carry out nursing research.

   c. advances the rights of older people and speaks out against negative stereotypes of aging.

   d. organizes programs of instruction to teach students.

39. Which of the following signs and symptoms is most consistent with the diagnosis of deep vein thrombosis in a lower extremity?

   a. Bilateral ankle edema

   b. Unilateral ankle edema

   c. New onset urinary incontinence

   d. Elevated blood pressure

40. An 85-year-old woman was admitted to a long-term-care facility 2 days ago for recovery from an open reduction and internal fixation (ORIF), following a repair of a broken hip; she also has a diagnosis of late-stage Alzheimer's disease. Although verbal, she has not complained of pain since admission and has not received any pain medication. The best course of action for the nurse to carry out is

   a. observe the patient's oral and fluid intake, noting any deficiencies.

   b. assume the patient is in pain and administer the ordered pain medication, noting functional improvement (if any).

   c. praise the patient for her ability to tolerate pain.

   d. question the patient carefully about her level of pain using a validated pain scale.

APPENDIX B

ANSWERS TO THE REVIEW QUESTIONS

1. **Correct Answer: B.** Medicare A reimburses for hospital care. Medicare B reimburses for medical care and some durable equipment. Medicare D is the prescription drug benefit. Medigap is a term for private insurance that may be purchased to cover out-of-pocket expenses and deductibles.

2. **Correct Answer: A.** A randomized clinical trial is considered the "gold standard" and the highest level of research evidence. The randomized design eliminates selection bias, and the control and experimental groups provide evidence that any differences in outcomes at the end of the study are due to the study intervention and not chance. A phenomenologic qualitative study and a case study enable understanding of one person's "lived experience," which may or may not be typical of others. Outcomes from a cohort study may reflect differences in age groups found as a result of historical events and not necessarily changes as a result of research interventions.

3. **Correct Answer: D.** The IOM report advances that nurses should practice to the full extent of their training, nurses should be full partners with other professionals when redesigning the healthcare system, nurses should achieve higher levels of education and have opportunities for seamless academic progression, and nurses should participate in effective workforce planning and policy-making with a better data collection and information infrastructure.

4. **Correct Answer: C.** Cognitive impairments become more common with advanced age across all categories of older people.

5. **Correct Answer: C.** Vascular dementia is associated with sudden acute events, such as transient ischemic attacks or small strokes. Clinically, older patients suffering from vascular events will have sudden-onset presentation of their symptoms rather than slow, insidious onset.

6. **Correct Answer: B.** By telling the patient the truth about the cancer diagnosis, the nurse is supporting autonomy by providing information that supports self-determination. Justice involves treating patients fairly, nonmaleficence involves doing no harm, and fidelity involves faithful performance of duties and obligation to meet the needs of patients.

7. **Correct Answer: C.** Based on a study published by AARP, long-term-care facilities with higher RN staffing levels have higher quality indicators, including lower rates of decubitus ulcers, indwelling catheter use, and patient mortality.

8. **Correct Answer: A.** Certification is a voluntary process that occurs when a nurse passes an examination developed by experts in the field, assuring the public and other healthcare professionals that the nurse possesses knowledge of specialty content in a given area.

9. **Correct Answer: B.** Mrs. Jones is typical of the older client with chronic nonmalignant pain from inflammation of one or several spinal nerves. Her pain medication regimen includes an anticonvulsant and a nonopiate analgesic.

10. **Correct Answer: D.** Although the urinary symptoms listed could possibly suggest prostate cancer, benign prostatic hypertrophy is very commonly seen in older men and is more likely to be the cause. Anemia and urologic changes are unlikely to contribute to the symptoms listed in this question.

11. **Correct Answer: A.** Hepatitis A is a common viral hepatitis that has no chronic state. The other options are viral hepatitides that have chronic states and are transmitted by blood and body fluids.

12. **Correct Answer: D.** The patient's imminent problem is dehydration, probably from taking a diuretic for several days without adequate fluid intake. He could have any of the other problems listed, but these would be less critical.

13. **Correct Answer: B.** Any patient with a degree of renal failure is at risk for elevated potassium; use of NSAIDs, such as ibuprofen, greatly increases this risk. Bone fracture can predispose a person to high calcium.

14. **Correct Answer: A.** All vaccinations are classified as primary prevention. Screening activities such as blood pressure and mammography are secondary, and diabetic education is tertiary.

15. **Correct Answer: C.** Retirement is consistent with disengagement theory, which advances that as people get older, they become more self-centered and it is advantageous for them to withdraw from society. Disengagement theory is the opposite of activity theory, which says that to be healthy in old age, it is better to stay active and engaged in society.

16. **Correct Answer: D.** The zoster vaccine is recommended for all people over the age of 50, regardless of their history of disease.

17. **Correct Answer: A.** Because of the slow progression of prostate cancer, men with less than a 10-year life expectancy are likely to die of something else before their prostate cancer (if detected) is fatal.

18. **Correct Answer: C.** The risk factors for cardiovascular disease that can be modified are tobacco use, hypertension, obesity, physical inactivity, and high cholesterol.

19. **Correct Answer: A.** Falls in older adults may herald a number of acute problems, such as pneumonia, stroke, or myocardial infarction. Cough, fever, and chest pain are common and typical symptoms of pneumonia that may be seen in patients of any age.

20. **Correct Answer: C.** When the patient walks and tends to fall backward, the term is retropulsion.

21. **Correct Answer: B.** The description is of seborrheic keratosis, which are benign, "stuck on"–appearing lesions, commonly seen in older individuals.

22. **Correct Answer: C.** Doses of acetaminophen over 4 grams per day have been associated with liver failure in older people.

23. **Correct Answer: A.** A living will simply provides a written statement of how an older person wishes to receive medical care and treatment at the end of life.

24. **Correct Answer: C.** Older people who neglect their self-care and fail to eat properly may be suffering from pathologic grief and profound depression. These signs and symptoms may require further evaluation and treatment from a mental health professional.

25. **Correct Answer: D.** Cultural sensitivity dictates that a patient's request for privacy should be honored if possible.

26. **Correct Answer: B.** Delirium, or acute onset cognitive disturbance, can be triggered by pain, dehydration, administration of general anesthesia, or a combination of these, and is a common postoperative problem.

27. **Correct Answer: C.** Calculated creatinine clearance accounts for age and body size, which affect creatinine production, making it the most important assessment for adequate renal function. Urinary frequency is not related to kidney function or adequacy. Serum creatinine may be within "normal limits" in older people of small stature with severely diminished renal function.

28. **Correct Answer: D.** Constipation is a common side effect of opioid medications. A stimulant usually is needed to avoid constipation and fecal impaction. Fluids and bulking agents may not be effective and may cause further discomfort in the dying patient.

29. **Correct Answer: A.** Confusion and falls in older adults may herald a number of acute problems, such as urinary tract infection. Blood in the urine, fever, and painful voiding are common and typical symptoms of urinary tract infection that may be seen in patients of any age.

30. **Correct Answer: B.** Adult learning theory says that older adults do not learn like children. It says that teachers are most effective when they teach using the learner's preferred style. Choice B is the correct answer because this theory suggests that older persons are self-directed learners interested in information that will benefit them.

31. **Correct Answer: B.** This patient suffers from functional incontinence because his mobility deficits make him reliant on others to help him up from the chair or bed. Stress incontinence is characterized by loss of small amounts of urine when coughing, or sneezing; overflow is characterized by dribbling from an overfilled bladder; urge is characterized by inability to stop the flow of urine once the urge to void is felt.

32. **Correct Answer: C.** Emphysema or chronic obstructive pulmonary disease (COPD) may lead to respiratory acidosis from chronic air trapping and incomplete exhalation of carbon dioxide. Infection and renal failure cause metabolic acidosis; anxiety leads to respiratory alkalosis.

33. **Correct Answer: C.** Based on the case, it is probable that the patient has c-difficile or pseudo-membranous colitis and the patient's healthcare provider should be notified.

34. **Correct Answer: C.** Uric acid levels are elevated in patients with gout. Folic acid is a water-soluble B vitamin; alkaline phosphatase is an enzyme related to bone metabolism; amalyase is an enzyme that breaks down starch into sugar.

35. **Correct Answer: D.** The combination of a long-acting opioid to control baseline pain and a short-acting medication for breakthrough pain will provide optimal pain control in the older adult with end-stage cancer pain. If the p.r.n. is frequently administered (more than twice/day), the baseline dose of the long-acting opioid medication should be increased.

36. **Correct Answer: D.** Thiazide diuretics may be associated with any or all of the following electrolyte imbalances: low potassium (hypokalemia), low sodium (hyponatremia), or high calcium (hypercalcemia). Signs of muscle weakness and decreased deep tendon reflexes are found with dehydration.

37. **Correct Answer: C.** Answer A describes guardianship. The other choices describe a durable power of attorney for health care and a living will. Answer C is correct, because the person making decisions for another without benefit of knowing their preferences will be required to substitute his or her judgement.

38. **Correct Answer: C.** Nurse advocates serve important roles by educating the public and those in the healthcare system about issues relating to the care of older people, including normal changes of aging, false stereotypes, evidence-based practice principles, and policy improvements to ensure safe and effective nursing care.

39. **Correct Answer: B.** Answer A is suggestive of dependency edema often seen in heart failure; Answers C and D are nonspecific symptoms that may be associated with many acute and chronic conditions. Answer B, unilateral ankle edema, is most often seen with the diagnosis of DVT.

40. **Correct Answer: B.** Because older patients with advanced Alzheimer's may not be able to verbalize their pain and the nurse is aware that surgical procedures such as the one experienced by this patient (ORIF) are usually painful, the nurse should administer pain medication and carefully observe the patient's response.

INDEX

INDEX

Page numbers followed by *f* indicate figures; *t* tables; and *b* boxes.

E

O

ABOUT THE AUTHOR

Patricia A. Tabloski, PhD, GNP-BC, FAAN, FGSA, possesses three degrees in nursing. She received her BSN from Purdue University, her MSN from Seton Hall University, and her PhD from the University of Rochester. As a gerontological nurse and nurse practitioner, Dr. Tabloski has provided primary care to older patients in a variety of settings, including acute care facilities, geriatric outpatient clinics, long-term-care facilities, and hospice programs. She has taught graduate and undergraduate students about gerontology since 1981, and presently is an Associate Professor at the William F. Connell School of Nursing at Boston College. In 2002, Dr. Tabloski was honored as a Fellow in the Gerontological Society of America and in 2010 was honored as a Fellow in the American Academy of Nursing. She has numerous publications and presentations relating to gerontological nursing and has lectured internationally in Hungary, China, Switzerland, and the United Kingdom.

Dr. Tabloski has chaired the Test Development Committee for the Gerontological Nurse Practitioner examination by the American Nurses Credentialing Center and is a member of the American Nurses Association, the Gerontological Society of America, the American Geriatrics Society, the National Organization of Nurse Practitioner Faculties, Sigma Theta Tau, and the Eastern Nursing Research Society. Dr. Tabloski is a federally funded researcher and conducts clinically based outcome studies related to non-pharmacological interventions designed to improve sleep and ease agitation in older persons in community and institutional settings. Additionally, Dr. Tabloski has received federal funding to establish an Advanced Practice Nursing Program in Palliative Care.

21010325R00209

Made in the USA
Charleston, SC
04 August 2013